Professional
Nursing

Professional
Nursing
Concepts And Challenges

SECOND EDITION

Kay Kittrell Chitty, Ed.D., R.N., C.S.

Adjunct Associate Professor, School of Nursing
University of Tennessee at Chattanooga
Chattanooga, Tennessee

W.B. SAUNDERS COMPANY
A Division of Harcourt Brace & Company

Philadelphia London Toronto Montreal Sydney Tokyo

W.B. SAUNDERS COMPANY
A Division of Harcourt Brace & Company
The Curtis Center
Independence Square West
Philadelphia, Pennsylvania 19106

Library of Congress Cataloging-in-Publication Data

Professional nursing : concepts and challenges / [edited by] Kay
   Kittrell Chitty.   2nd ed.
      p. cm.
   Includes bibliographical references and index.
   ISBN 0-7216-6882-8
     1. Nursing—Vocational guidance.   2. Nursing—Social aspects.
  I. Chitty, Kay Kittrell.
   [DNLM: 1.   Nursing.   WY 16 P9644 1977]
  RT82.P755   1997
  610.73'069—dc2U
  DNLM/DLC   96-20037

ISBN   0–7216–6882–8

PROFESSIONAL NURSING: Concepts and Challenges

Printed in United States of America

Last digit is the print number: 9 8 7 6 5 4 3 2 1

The second edition of this book is dedicated to my parents,
who taught me to persevere,
and to my husband,
who makes it possible for me to do so.

CONTRIBUTORS

Virginia Trotter Betts, M.S.N., J.D., R.N.
Professor of Nursing,
Chairholder, National Health Care Chair
    of Excellence
Middle Tennessee State University,
Murfreesboro, Tennessee
and
President
Health Futures, Inc.
Nashville, Tennessee

Carol T. Bush, Ph.D., R.N.
Executive Director
Dekalb Region 6
Division of Mental Health, Mental
    Retardation, and Substance Abuse
Georgia Department of Human Resources
Atlanta, Georgia

Cathy Campbell, M.N., R.N.
Assistant Professor
Nell Hodgson Woodruff School of Nursing
Emory University
Atlanta, Georgia

Pamela S. Chally, Ph.D., R.N.
Associate Dean, Associate Professor
University of North Florida
Jacksonville, Florida

Catherine J. Futch, M.N., R.N., C.N.A.A., C.H.E.
Affiliate Faculty
Nell Hodgson Woodruff School of Nursing

Emory University
and
School of Nursing
College of Health Sciences
Georgia State University
and
Regional Clinical Services Coordinator
Kaiser Permanente,
Atlanta, Georgia

Pamela J. Holder, D.S.N., R.N.
Director, School of Nursing
University of Tennessee at Chattanooga,
Chattanooga, Tennessee

Jennifer E. Jenkins, M.B.A., R.N., C.N.A.A.
Vice President
Healthcare Concepts, Inc.
Memphis, Tennessee

Judith K. Leavitt, B.S.N., M.Ed., F.A.A.N.
Director, Generations United
and
Former Chair
American Nurses Association Political
    Action Committee
Washington, District of Columbia

Frances A. Maurer, M.S., R.N.
Instructor, Community Health
University of Maryland at Baltimore
Baltimore, Maryland

Carolyn Maynard, Ph.D., R.N.
Assistant Professor
Department of Family and Community
   Nursing
University of North Carolina at Charlotte
Charlotte, North Carolina

Elaine F. Nichols, Ed.D., R.N.
Associate Dean, Undergraduate Program
College of Nursing
The University of Akron
Akron, Ohio

Barbara R. Norwood, M.S.N., R.H.
Assistant Professor
School of Nursing
University of Tennessee at Chattanooga
and
Staff Nurse
Memorial Hospital
Chattanooga, Tennessee

Cheryl A. Peterson, M.S.N., R.N.
Associate Director
Federal Government Relations
American Nurses Association
Washington, District of Columbia

**Robert V. Piemonte, Ed.D., R.N.,
   C.A.E., F.A.A.N.**
Adjunct Professor of Nursing
Teachers College
Columbia University
New York, New York

**Barbara K. Redman, Ph.D., R.N.,
   F.A.A.N.**
Dean and Professor
School of Nursing
University of Connecticut
Storrs, Connecticut

Frances I. Waddle, M.S.N., R.N.
Health Facilities Consultant
Oklahoma State Department of Health
Oklahoma City, Oklahoma

PREFACE

The success of the first edition of *Professional Nursing: Concepts and Challenges* was personally and professionally gratifying to all those involved in its production. According to users of that edition, a number of whom were surveyed in preparing this revision, they were highly satisfied with its content, organization, and "readability." Because of their enthusiastic endorsements, the revision has retained its compact size, its assumption that some readers have no prior nursing knowledge, numerous photographs, and interesting features and sidebars. Research Notes, Self-Assessments, and News Notes have been updated and their number increased. New to this edition are letters from nurses and nursing students that provide insights into a variety of nursing issues about which they have first-hand knowledge. Every effort has been made to include clinical examples, even though this book deals mainly with nonclinical concepts of the nursing profession.

This second edition retains the interactive, student-centered style that characterized the first edition. The focus continues to be on the dynamic process of *becoming* a professional nurse. The values and skills needed by students in this era of dramatic changes in health care delivery are emphasized, but learning about oneself remains vitally important. To that end, a wealth of self-awareness and self-development activities are included to help students to build their critical thinking skills and evaluate their own points of view.

Because a number of schools select this textbook for use in the "bridge" course for registered nurses in degree completion programs, content has been enriched to reflect their broader experiential and knowledge bases. We combined or streamlined some chapters to reflect the sophistication of the RN student while making every attempt to include enough basic information for the student who is unfamiliar with nursing. Chapters remain "freestanding" and may still be used in any order.

Users of the second edition will notice that multicultural content is increased and that the spiritual aspects of nursing are integrated throughout the book. Gender-oriented content focuses on the relationship between gender and the development of nursing. Coverage of perspectives of patients with chronic illnesses and disabilities, nursing theory, legal and ethical concerns, and collaboration among health care professionals is also expanded. And an exciting new Instructor's Manual, written by Helene Charron, M.S., R.N. contains in-class and out-of-class activities designed to enhance students' learning and to enrich classroom experiences. The Instructor's Manual also includes chapter outlines, chapter objectives, suggested readings, and a comprehensive test bank.

It is my hope that the students and faculty who use this new edition will find it even more stimulating, enjoyable, and enlightening than the first edition and that it will continue to contribute to the positive development of our profession.

Kay K. Chitty

ACKNOWLEDGEMENTS

The second edition of *Professional Nursing: Concepts and Challenges* has been a joint effort of many individuals, all of whom played instrumental roles in its successful completion. First, I should recognize the many students and faculty members who enthusiastically used the first edition and, when asked, made helpful recommendations for revisions. Next my appreciation goes to Ilze Rader of W.B. Saunders, whose thoughtful and perceptive suggestions during the conceptual development of this edition were extremely useful. Her understanding of nurses, the nursing profession, and human nature is as deep as it is broad.

My gratitude also goes to the contributors, all of whom have busy professional and personal lives but who believed so strongly in the value of this book to the nursing profession that they were willing to participate in the revision process. I also wish to thank those nurses who were interviewed or who wrote letters included in the book for sharing their experiences on and insights into a variety of nursing issues.

Kadie Vandenburgh, my research assistant, was tireless in her search for the latest information and unfailingly cheerful and supportive. Will McDonald, Jean Payne, Kelly Whalen, Charlene Robertson, and many others at Memorial Hospital, Chattanooga, Tennessee, generously contributed their time to provide the majority of the photographs for this edition. Charles Field's patience and humor was refreshing during the production phase of the revision.

Last, my deepest appreciation goes to my husband, Charlie, and to Maura Connor and Stephanie Klein, of W.B. Saunders, all of whom kept me going when neither the spirit nor the flesh was willing.

CONTENTS

Professional
Nursing
Concepts And Challenges

1

Catherine J. Futch

History of Nursing

O B J E C T I V E S

- Describe how the nursing profession evolved from ancient to modern times.
- Discuss the influence of religious orders on the development of nursing.
- Describe Florence Nightingale's influence on nursing practice and nursing education.
- Describe the early nursing schools in the United States.
- Identify key accomplishments of nursing leaders who shaped the profession in the United States.
- Trace the history of African-American nurses and African-American schools of nursing in the United States.
- Explain the relationships among societal change, military conflicts, and the development of nursing in the United States.

V O C A B U L A R Y

Clara Barton	Martha Franklin	Isabel Hampton Robb
Mary Ann Ball/"Mother Bickerdyke"	Frontier Nursing Service	Margaret Sanger
	Goldmark Report	Jessie Sleet Scales
Mary Breckinridge	Annie Goodrich	Spellman Seminary
Namahyoke Curtis	Henry Street Settlement	Susie Taylor
Deaconess Institute at Kaiserswerth	Hippocrates	Sojourner Truth
	holism	Harriet Tubman
Dorothea L. Dix	Lucille Petry Leone	Lillian Wald
Lavinia Dock	Mary Eliza Mahoney	
Francis Reed Elliott	Florence Nightingale	

The history of nursing spans the history of humankind. For as long as there has been life, there has been the need to provide care and comfort to those suffering from illness and injury. "From the dawn of civilization, evidence prevails to support the premise that nurturing has been essential to the preservation of life. Survival of the human race, therefore, is inextricably intertwined with the development of nursing" (Donahue, 1985, p. 2).

THE JOURNEY

In looking at the evolution of nursing as a profession, we see that cultural and societal changes have shaped the profession of nursing as we know it today. This chapter traces the development of nursing from ancient times to the present.

Nursing from Ancient Times to the Nineteenth Century

"Nursing has been called the oldest of the arts and the youngest of the professions" (Donahue, 1985, p. 2). The word *nurse* evolved from the Latin word *nutricius*, which means "nourishing" (Kalisch and Kalisch, 1986, p. 1). The roots of medicine and nursing are intertwined and found in mythology, ancient Eastern and Western cultures, religion, and reasoned thinking.

Although modern nursing and medicine are distinct professions, for most of the history of humankind, nursing was not well differentiated. "Nursing of the sick was never seen as a professional activity by people in the ancient world. Greek and Roman doctors, usually male, attended serious or complicated cases; midwives, always female, attended births and newborns; and female kin cared for the sick in the context of the family and without pay" (Kampen, 1988, p. 7).

ANCIENT CIVILIZATIONS

The ancient Egyptians created an advanced civilization. Their medical practices were impressive. Egyptian physicians are believed to have specialized in certain diseases (such as internal diseases, fractured bones, and wounds), and they wrote textbooks of medicine as it was practiced at that time. They also hired women, later known as midwives, to assist with childbirth. These women were the first recorded nurses.

The ancient Hebrews practiced preventive medicine as long ago as 1200 to 600 B.C. The Hebrews isolated people with contagious diseases and actively quarantined contaminated wells. Their religious laws forbidding the eating of pork supported the avoidance of food-borne diseases such as trichinosis, which was transmitted by consuming infected pork.

Eastern cultures also influenced early healing practices. As early as 800 B.C., Indian physicians performed amputations and sophisticated procedures such as plastic surgery. Traditional Chinese medicine taught that disease results from an imbalance of the two life forces, *yin* and *yang*. To control the flow of these forces and thus cure disease, Chinese physicians inserted fine needles into specific body parts. This practice, acupuncture, is still in use today.

GREECE AND THE ROMAN EMPIRE

Belief in Apollo, the Greek god of healing, and Asclepius, the Greek god of medicine, predominated in the Greek civilization, which reached its peak around 400 B.C. The Greeks prayed to Apollo and Asclepius for magical cures for their illnesses.

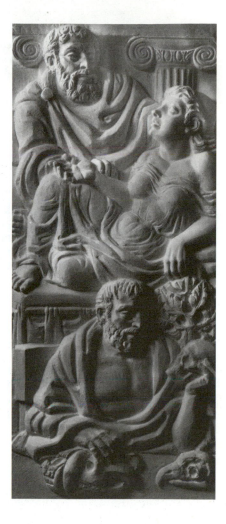

F I G U R E   1 – 1
First Relief Panel, West Virginia University Medical Sciences Building Pylons, depicting Hippocrates (father of medicine) administering to a seated woman and, below them, Aristotle, seated at a table examining a human skull. Artist: Milton Horn. (Reprinted with permission of the West Virginia and Regional History Collection, West Virginia University Libraries, Morgantown, West Virginia.)

Belief in gods and magical cures gave way to understanding through the work of early scientists such as the Greek physician **Hippocrates** (400 B.C.) (Fig. 1–1). Hippocrates believed that disease had natural, not magical, causes. His work marked the separation of medicine from religion for the first time in history.

After 300 B.C., the Roman Empire dominated the ancient world, conquering Egypt and Greece. Roman noblewomen, including the wives of emperors, cared for the sick. Early Roman physicians built on the groundwork of their Egyptian and Greek predecessors.

The Romans are best known for advances in the health of the public. They constructed an impressive network of aqueducts and sewers that provided Rome with both a continuous supply of fresh water and a waste disposal system, making a high level of sanitation possible.

Galen, a Greek physician living in Rome about 100 B.C., performed numerous experiments on animals to learn about anatomy and disease. Although

Galen's influence lasted hundreds of years, many of his animal experiments led to erroneous conclusions when applied to human beings. Although some of their information was later proved inaccurate, these early scientists began erasing the mystique surrounding the human body's processes and replacing it with knowledge.

THE MIDDLE AGES

Progress in Western civilization's quest for knowledge about disease and the human body slowed during the early part of the Middle Ages, known as the Dark Ages, which lasted from A.D. 400 to 900. In the Muslim empire of southwest and central Asia, however, advances continued.

Avicenna, an Arab physician, wrote a volume called the *Canon of Medicine* that outlined all the diseases and treatments known at that time. This book was used by physicians for hundreds of years. In western Europe, deep in the anti-intellectualism that characterized the Dark Ages, "scientific medicine survived . . . chiefly through the efforts of Jewish physicians who translated Greek and Arabic medical treatises into Latin and who circulated Greco-Arabic medical knowledge throughout Christendom" (Kalisch and Kalisch, 1986, p. 7).

Following the Dark Ages, interest in care of the sick was sparked by the effects of poverty, disease, the ravages of war, and a renewed quest for knowledge. There were massive epidemics of diseases such as leprosy and bubonic plague. From A.D. 500 to 1400, 25 percent of the population of Europe died in epidemics. Widespread disease stimulated the building of hospitals. The oldest known hospital was the Hôtel-Dieu (House of God), built in Lyons, France, in 542. Medical schools multiplied rapidly, and books were written describing smallpox, measles, and other infectious diseases.

Around 1060, Constantinus Africanus established a university at Salerno, Italy. This university was a dominant western European force in medical education until well into the twelfth century. It was particularly important to nursing because it provided women with the opportunity to study nursing and midwifery. The first known nursing publication was written by a twelfth-century midwife named Trotula. Her famous obstetrical treatise was entitled *Trotulae curandanum aegritudinum muliebrum* [Trotula on the cure of diseases of women].

RELIGION'S INFLUENCE

In 1099, the first separate military-nursing order was formed. Known as the Knights Hospitalers of St. John of Jerusalem, they "soon became famous and highly esteemed, providing thousands of pilgrims and crusaders in the Holy City with hospitality and care" (Kalisch and Kalisch, 1986, p. 9). This group is the first identifiable organization of nurses. Eventually, in addition to their commitment to the care of travelers, those who were ill, and those who were impoverished, they also became known as a powerful military order. Figure 1–2 depicts a scene from the Old Testament, from which nursing orders derived their mission of caring for the sick.

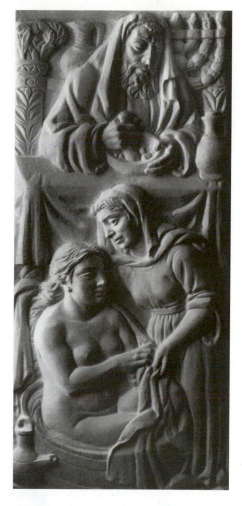

FIGURE 1-2
Second Relief Pylon, West Virginia University Medical Sciences Building Pylons, depicting the scriptural apothecary from Exodus (30:25). Scene includes a bearded, robed man seated at a table, using a mortar and pestle; the scene below depicts two female figures, one of whom is bathing, the other stands behind her with towel, representative of the rules of hygiene as set forth in the Old Testament. (Reprinted with permission of the West Virginia and Regional History Collection, West Virginia University Libraries, Morgantown, West Virginia.)

During the later Middle Ages, lasting from 900 to 1500, religious orders continued their interest in nursing. St. Benedict's Rule decreed that every monastery have a hospital, and although care for the ailing was at first directed mainly toward members of the order, workers on church-owned estates were eventually included. The masses, however, still had to depend on their womenfolk for treatment and care during illness (Kalisch and Kalisch, 1986, p. 11).

Nursing care during this period often was provided by monks and nuns who were members of Catholic nursing orders (Fig. 1–3). Care was segregated by sex, with women caring for women and men caring for men.

Many Catholic monasteries were closed after the rise of Protestantism during the Protestant Reformation of the fifteenth century, leaving only hospitals to

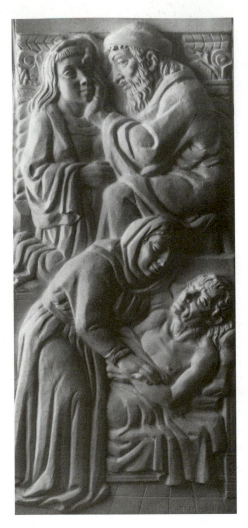

FIGURE 1-3
Fourth Relief Pylon, West Virginia University Medical Sciences Building Pylons, depicting Benevenutus Grassus conducting his studies on the structure of the eye; the lower scene shows a deaconess in a medieval hospital caring for a man in bed. (Reprinted with permission of the West Virginia and Regional History Collection, West Virginia University Libraries, Morgantown, West Virginia.)

care for the poor sick. The wealthy never used hospitals, preferring to be cared for at home. It is little wonder, as sanitation in hospitals was an unknown concept, and conditions were often desperate.

> In a typical hospital of the 1400s, the daily work of the nurses began at 5:00 A.M., when, after rising and washing, they went downstairs to church service. Then the sister nurses went about their work in areas such as the laundry, the wards, and the hall for admittance. When the patients were awake, each nurse would make the rounds with a basin in one hand and a towel in the other. Later, while beds were being made, the healthier patients were allowed to get up while the more seriously ill were moved to vacant beds. Each bed, a straw-filled mattress suspended on cords stretched from four corner posts, held at least two and in many cases three patients. . . . Sister nurses were forbidden to witness childbirths, to help

with gynecologic examinations, or even to diaper boy babies. Close contact with male patients, such as administering enemas, was also prohibited, as was the care of patients suffering from venereal diseases. Servants were employed to carry out these tasks (Kalisch and Kalisch, 1986, p. 17).

THE DARK PERIOD

In the sixteenth and seventeenth centuries, plague and pestilence again wrought havoc throughout the civilized world. The few medicines in existence were herbs or concoctions consisting of "urine, animal excreta, powdered earthworms, and the like" (Kalisch and Kalisch, 1986, p. 17). Such factors as an incomplete understanding of how the human body functioned, lack of basic hygiene, and no understanding of the role of yet-to-be-discovered microorganisms in illness resulted in millions of additional deaths from measles, leprosy, typhus, bubonic plague, and other infectious diseases.

The years from 1600 to 1850 have been described as the darkest period of nursing history. Hospitals were charitable institutions staffed by untrained women of the lower classes, many of ill repute. Nurses and physicians themselves often contracted and died of the same diseases they were treating in others.

By the middle of the eighteenth century, life expectancy was still short, infant mortality was still high, and crowded conditions in city slums continued to breed disease. Most nursing care was provided in the home, and those who were exposed to hospital care were often at great risk. The following description of a late-eighteenth-century European hospital illustrates the terrible conditions therein:

> In one bed of moderate width lay 4, 5, or 6 sick persons beside each other, the feet of one to the head of another. . . . In the same bed lay individuals infected with infectious diseases beside others only slightly unwell; on the same couch, body against body, a woman groaned in the pains of labor, a nursing infant writhed in convulsions, a typhus patient burned in the delirium of fever, a consumptive coughed his hollow cough, and a victim of some disease of the skin tore with furious nails (Kalisch and Kalisch, 1986, p. 24).

Medical education in the eighteenth century was better than it had been and more plentiful, but not enough was known about health and illness to make a difference (Fig. 1–4). Although scientists had suspected that "seeds" created disease, it was not until the late 1800s that Louis Pasteur and Robert Koch demonstrated that microorganisms caused disease. This was a turning point for health care worldwide.

Nursing in America from Colonization to Independence

As America was colonized, the same health care problems were encountered here that occurred throughout Europe. The first hospital built in the colonies was located in what later became known as New York. Its doors opened in 1658 (Selavan, 1984). Most patients suffering from contagious diseases, however, were placed in what were called "pest houses," such as those in Boston, New York,

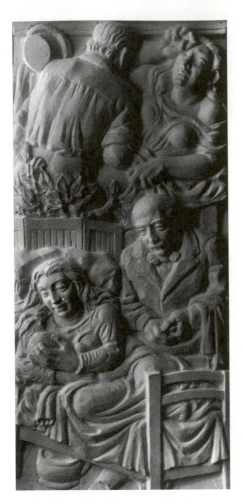

FIGURE 1–4
Fifth Relief Pylon, West Virginia University Medical Sciences Building Pylons, depicting Ephraim McDowell (1771–1830) removing an ovarian tumor; lower scene shows Ignaz Semmelweis (1818–1865), known for instituting sterilization methods in obstetrics. (Reprinted with permission of the West Virginia and Regional History Collection, West Virginia University Libraries, Morgantown, West Virginia.)

Philadelphia, and Charleston. By 1776, Virginia had two private hospitals as well as a hospital for the insane. Philadelphia had Pennsylvania Hospital, owing, in part, to the influence of Benjamin Franklin.

Early American physicians were prepared through courses of study in Europe and a variety of apprenticeships. Untrained and uneducated nurses provided "care" to those unfortunate enough to be hospitalized. Physicians were not required to have a license to practice medicine. There were fewer than 500 licensed physicians of 3500 practicing at the time of the Revolutionary War. Female members of each household continued to be the primary providers of nursing care.

Soldiers who fought in the American Revolution (1775–1783) were more apt to die from disease or the effects of their care than they were from the wounds of battle. "Purging, blistering, and bleeding" were the treatments of choice, and when wounds became infected, amputation was the only option. They also had to contend with pneumonia, dysentery, lack of adequate food, impure water, and unclean camps and hospitals (Selavan, 1984, p. 19).

Two major health care victories emerged from the American Revolution. The first was the routine innoculation of troops against smallpox, which greatly decreased the spread of smallpox in the nation. The second was the recognition, attributed to Gen. George Washington, that the United States Army needed clean hospitals and nurses to participate in supervising the care provided in them.

In spite of the absence of army hospitals during this period, the names of paid nurses did appear on military payrolls and pension lists, and "women who acted as nurses were entitled to the same rations as soldiers" (Selavan, 1984, p. 21). Military leaders had recognized the value of proper nursing care for soldiers in combat.

The Dawn of Modern Nursing: Florence Nightingale

From the late 1700s through 1853, the manner in which the sick were cared for in America remained essentially unchanged. In Europe, however, the dawn of nursing was under way. "The **Deaconess Institute at Kaiserswerth,** Germany, was established in 1836 by Pastor Theodor Fliedner" (Donahue, 1985, p. 234). By 1842, the work of Pastor Fliedner and his followers resulted in a large hospital and planned training program for the deaconesses, who believed that their duty lay in the care of the sick and the provision of social services (Donahue, 1985, p. 234).

> The program in nursing included a rotation in hospital clinical services (experience on wards for men, women, and children as well as those for communicable disease, convalescents, and sick deaconesses), instruction in visiting nursing, theoretical and bedside instruction in the care of the sick, instruction in religious doctrine and ethics, and enough pharmacy to pass the State examination for pharmacists. Their program of study took three years. An interesting principle was enforced in that the nurses were required to follow the physician's orders exactly, and the physician alone was responsible for the outcome (Donahue, 1985, p. 235).

Graduates of the Kaiserswerth program spread their influence throughout the world. By 1849, four of the deaconesses were in Pittsburgh, Pennsylvania, where they assumed responsibility for the Pittsburgh Infirmary, later known as Passavant Hospital.

YOUNG FLORENCE NIGHTINGALE

Meanwhile, in England, **Florence Nightingale** was coming of age (Fig. 1–5). Nightingale, born to an upper-class English family, was shaped by three major influences in her life. First, she was dissatisfied with what she viewed as the dull, routine lifestyle of the upper-class women of her day. She had an active mind and an interest in her surroundings beyond household and social events.

Second, she had received "a classical education equal to that of most men of her day" (Smith, 1984, p. 9). This education provided her with an understanding of the circumstances of the world in which she lived. This fueled her desire

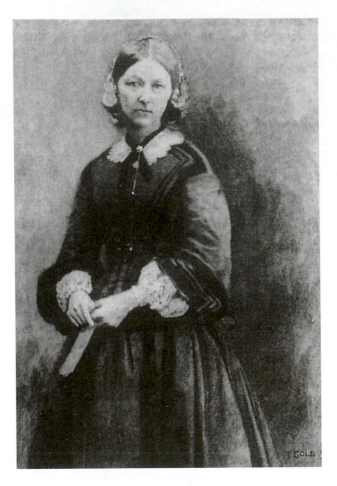

FIGURE 1–5
Florence Nightingale.

to secure the necessary financial and political influence to make a difference—
to create lasting changes in the provision of health care.

Third, she became aware of the inadequate care being provided in hospitals
as she accompanied her mother on visits to the ill. What Nightingale saw in those
hospitals intrigued her and made her want to become more involved. Refused
permission by her parents to attend nursing school, she spent three years studying parliamentary reports to become expert in issues relating to public health and
hospitals.

NIGHTINGALE AT KAISERSWERTH

In 1846, in spite of the concerns of parents and friends, Nightingale began to
visit and care for the sick both in her own family and in her community. In ad-

dition, she visited hospitals in England and throughout Europe. Out of her experiences came the recognition that nurses required knowledge, training, and discipline if they were to be effective. She discussed her beliefs with her friend Elizabeth Fry, herself an advocate for more humane treatment in prisons. Through her, Nightingale learned about the school at Kaiserswerth, and in 1850 she was admitted to their training program.

The three years of training she received were rigorous but helped her clarify what was lacking in the current training of English nurses. Upon her return to England, to the great consternation of her family and friends, Nightingale embarked on a career that would have lasting impact on nursing in England, in the United States, and throughout the world. In 1853, she was appointed superintendent of the Institution for the Care of the Sick Gentlewomen in London.

IN THE CRIMEA

Nightingale's work began in earnest during the Crimean War (1854–1856). She and a small band of untrained nurses went to the British hospital at Scutari in Turkey, where she wanted to make a difference in the care of British soldiers. What she found was a hospital "so crowded that patients lay on the floor, still in bloody uniforms. Bath equipment, sheets, cutlery, and laundry facilities were either non-existent or nearly so" (Smith, 1984, p. 10). With great compassion and in spite of the unwelcoming attitude of some military officers with whom she worked, she set about the task of organizing and cleaning the hospital and providing care to the wounded soldiers.

Through her efforts and the help of others she enlisted to assist with her causes, Nightingale introduced numerous improvements in the military hospital care of this period. Her efforts were largely responsible for dramatic reductions (42 percent to 2 percent) in the wartime death rate of British soldiers in this conflict.

AFTER THE WAR

Following Scutari, Nightingale almost single-handedly tried to change health care in England.

> [She] protested against the corridor system of hospitals and fought for pavilions (1850); printed her extensive octavo on the health of the Army (1858); issued the anonymous blue book on military sanitation in which she demonstrated the frightful but preventable mortality of the recent Crimean War (1859); showed the relationship of sanitary science to medical institutions (*Notes on Hospitals*, 1859); established the Army Medical School at Fort Pitt, Chatham, and chose its faculty (1860); and founded the first training school for nurses (St. Thomas's Hospital, London, 1860). Florence Nightingale epitomized her life work when she wrote in a private note: "I stand at the alter of the murdered men, and, while I live, I fight their causes" (Robinson, 1946, p. 129).

In addition to being a great war nurse, Nightingale also was the founder of modern nursing education. Through the publication of countless articles and pa-

pers, she shared her ideas about nursing and nursing education. Her most famous written document, *Notes on Nursing: What It Is and What It Is Not*, was
published in 1859. Miss Nightingale was the first to mention **holism** (treating the
whole patient) in nursing and the first to state clearly that a unique body of
knowledge was required of those wishing to practice professional nursing. These
ideas are as current today as they were nearly 150 years ago. Although Nightingale never set foot on American soil, her work served as a catalyst for the development of the foundations of American nursing, and her influence is felt even
today.

Nursing in America: The Civil War, 1861–1865

While Florence Nightingale was involved with the founding of her training school
for nurses at St. Thomas's Hospital, the United States was moving toward a civil war that would divide the nation and result in huge casualties and loss of life
for both sides. Neither North nor South was prepared to care for large numbers
of sick and injured soldiers, but as war became imminent, women once again mobilized an effort to care for those they loved. Black and white, rich and poor,
married and single women cared for sick and wounded soldiers in hospitals, provided clothing and food for soldiers, developed aid societies, and secretly shel-
tered fugitive black slaves. The care provided by women during America's Civil
War was profoundly influenced by what they had learned of the work of Nightingale in the Crimea.

Following an 1861 meeting that involved Dr. Elizabeth Blackwell of New York
and President Abraham Lincoln, Lincoln created the United States Sanitary
Commission. This commission was given responsibility for planning the care of
the war's wounded.

THE INFLUENCE OF DOROTHEA DIX

Dorothea L. Dix, a Boston schoolteacher who had devoted herself to the care of
the mentally ill, volunteered her services to the newly formed United States San-
itary·Commission. She was immediately appointed superintendent of Women
Nurses of the Army (Austin, 1984, p. 22).

Dix listed the following criteria for the selection of army nurses: "age, at least
30 and not over 50; good health and endurance; matronly demeanor, with experience and good character; plainly dressed, with no ornaments, and no hoops"
(Austin, 1984, p. 22). Dix's selection process was directed toward excluding those
women she judged too pretty, too popular, or too fun-loving to serve as effective
nurses. Many women who did not meet her stringent criteria, however, provided active and valuable service during the war. Soon 100 young women who met
the Dix qualifications went to Bellevue and New York Hospital for a month's
training by hospital staff physicians to prepare them to supervise care of the
wounded.

In the South, volunteers provided care in hospitals or in their own homes.
With the establishment of a medical department under Confederate Surgeon
General Samuel Preston Moore, "Richmond, Virginia, became a vast hospital

center for the South. . . . Some hospitals like the Chimborazo Hospital in Richmond were large, having several divisions with 'lady' nurses in charge" (Austin, 1984, p. 24).

Kate Cumming was actively involved in providing care to the Southern wounded. She was inspired by Nightingale, believing that "What one woman has done another could do also" (Parsons, 1984, p. 27). Cumming kept a diary of all her experiences as a hospital matron from April 1862 until the end of the war. Her work is recognized as the most comprehensive documentation of the work of Confederate hospital matrons in existence. She and the other military hospital matrons endured tremendous hardships hardly imaginable today. Cumming herself survived two hospital fires, whereas others contracted infectious diseases, such as typhoid fever, and died.

CONTRIBUTIONS OF AFRICAN-AMERICAN NURSES

Many African-American women, both free and slave, made contributions during the Civil War. Most famous are **Sojourner Truth** (Fig. 1–6), **Harriet Tubman,** and **Susie Taylor.**

> Born a slave in New York State and freed by the New York State Emancipation Act of 1827, Sojourner Truth (1797–1881) was not only a famous abolitionist and underground railroad agent, itinerant preacher and lecturer, women's rights worker, and humanitarian, but also a nurse during the Civil War and immediately thereafter (Carnegie, 1986, p. 6).

Having changed her name from "Isabella" to "Sojourner" after her emancipation in 1827, she spent her life as her name implied, traveling and telling about slavery wherever she went. After the war, she continued her work in the Washington, D.C. area as a nurse/counselor for the Freedmen's Relief Association.

FIGURE   1 – 6
Sojourner Truth: a nurse in the Civil War. (Courtesy of Joyce A. Elmore.)

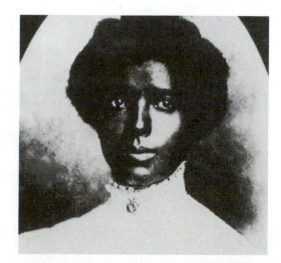

She helped find homes and jobs for freedmen and worked in Freedmen's Village, caring for the ill in the hospital. She gathered together a group of women to clean the Freedmen's Hospital because of her concern about the unhygienic conditions there.

Harriet Ross Tubman (1820–1913) was an abolitionist who was sometimes called "Conductor of the Underground Railroad." Tubman "made 19 secret trips below the Mason and Dixon line, leading more than 300 slaves to freedom. She served as a nurse in the Sea Islands off the coast of South Carolina, caring for the sick and wounded without regard to color" (Carnegie, 1986, p. 9). Tubman was later commended by Acting U.S. Assistant Surgeon General Henry K. Durrant for her "kindness and attention to the sick and suffering" (Carnegie, 1986, p. 9).

Susie King Taylor (1848–1912) was a young African-American girl who learned to read and write in secret at a time when these skills were forbidden to slaves. When Fort Pulaski, South Carolina, fell to Union troops, a Union officer assigned the 14-year-old Susie to teach African-American refugee children to read and write. Following her marriage, she was employed by Company E of the First South Carolina Volunteers as a laundress but continued her work as a teacher and nurse in her free time.

> At Beaufort, South Carolina, during the summer of 1863, Susie King Taylor met Clara Barton, later to be the great "moving spirit" in the founding of the American Red Cross. She frequently accompanied Miss Barton, who treated her very cordially, on rounds in the hospitals at the front (Carnegie, 1986, p. 11).

Working as a volunteer nurse, she served the Union for more than four years.

"THE LITTLE LADY IN BLACK SILK" AND "MOTHER BICKERDYKE"

Clara Barton (1821–1912) (Fig. 1–7), perhaps the best-known Civil War nurse, was called the "little lone lady in black silk" (Donahue, 1985, p. 294). She was, however, a little lady of iron will, preferring to act on her own and free from the direction of others.

> [Barton] . . . independently operated a large scale war relief operation in which she arranged for huge quantities of supplies to be furnished to the Army and the hospitals. . . . She nursed in Federal hospitals and with the armies on the battlefield and cared for the wounded of the Confederate Armies. Her impartiality was expressed in the nursing care she extended to both whites and blacks, Northerners and Southerners. . . . On more than one occasion, bullets made holes in her dresses and she became one of the most prominent figures among the lay nurses of the Civil War. Her work embodied the ideals now characteristic of the Red Cross and became the foundation of her later success in the development of the American Red Cross in 1881 (Donahue, 1985, p. 294).

A final Civil War–era woman known for her nursing skill was **Mary Ann Ball** (1817–1901). She answered the call for women to help in caring for the wound-

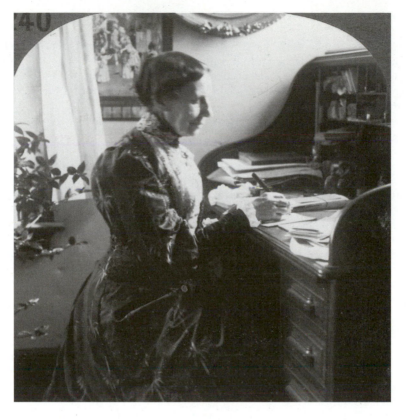

ed and dying. A widow with two small sons, she was affectionately called **"Mother Bickerdyke."**

> [She] . . . served under fire in nineteen battles from Fort Donelson in Tennessee to Savannah, Georgia. She organized diet kitchens, laundries, and an ambulance service. She supervised the nursing staff and distributed supplies. At night she often walked through the abandoned battlefields, afraid that someone who was still alive would be left uncared for. She became known as one of the greatest nurse heroines of the Civil War (Donahue, 1985, p. 302).

Throughout the Civil War, nurses and laywomen in both the Union and the Confederacy were empowered by their patriotism, caring, and Nightingale's Crimean example to do more than they dreamed they could do.

The Birth of a Profession: 1870–1900

With the final shots of the Civil War still ringing, the stage was set for the birth of organized nursing in the United States. Nightingale had broken the ground, and many who knew of her work recognized the wisdom of her efforts. Those who had served in the war and recognized the need for trained nurses were poised to lead the way.

The years following the Civil War saw a number of events merge to support the founding of training schools for nurses. In 1869, Dr. Samuel Gross recommended to the American Medical Association that large hospitals should begin the process of developing training schools for nurses. He proposed that the students in these schools would be taught by medical staff and resident physicians. Simultaneously, members of the United States Sanitary Commission who served during the war began to lobby for the creation of nursing schools. Support for their efforts gained momentum as supporters of social reform reported the results of their visits to existing hospitals.

Although intended to be helpful in the overall goal of establishing training schools for nurses, the recommendations of Gross and his colleagues were often in direct opposition to the teachings and recommendations of Nightingale, who believed nurses should be trained and supervised by other nurses. These conflicting viewpoints heralded the beginning of a long and heated conflict between medicine and nursing regarding the proper education and supervision of nurses.

During this postwar time, society was also changing. Immigration, industrialization, and urbanization were altering the face of the United States. More and more people were in need of care that could no longer be provided by family members because many families were separated by immigration and migration from farms to cities.

Women, out of both economic necessity and the wish to leave the confines of home, were entering the workplace. They sought jobs in factories and workshops and as teachers, clerks, seamstresses, and untrained nurses in hospitals and homes. Societal changes and the movement to provide formal training for nurses dovetailed at this point in history.

The movement to formalize nurses' training found an advocate in Sarah J. Hale, editor of *Godey's Lady's Book and Magazine* for more than 30 years. She published an editorial entitled "Lady Nurses" in the February 1871 issue:

> Much has been lately said of the benefits that would follow if the calling of the sick nurse were elevated to a profession which an educated lady might adopt without a sense of degradation, either of her own part or in the estimation of others. . . . There can be no doubt that the duties of sick nurse, to be properly performed, require an education and training little, if at all, inferior to those possessed by members of the medical profession. To leave these duties to untaught and ill-trained persons is as great a mistake as it was to allow the office of surgeon to be held by one whose proper calling was that of a mechanic of the humblest class. The manner in which a reform may be effected is easily pointed out. Every medical college should have a course of study and training especially adapted for ladies who desire to qualify themselves for the profession of nurse; and those who had gone through the course, and passed the requisite examination, should receive a degree and a diploma, which would at once establish their position in soci-

ety. The "graduate nurse" would in general estimation be as much above the ordinary nurse of the present day as the professional surgeon of our times is above the barber-surgeon of the last century (Donahue, 1985, p. 310).

FORMATION OF TRAINING SCHOOLS FOR NURSES

Training schools for nurses did evolve but not exactly in the manner Hale had envisioned. Following the 1872 opening of the New England Hospital for Women and Children training school for nurses with a class of five students, a number of other schools were established. These early schools were founded on the basic principles of the Nightingale schools. The first professional nurses were being trained in the United States (Fig. 1–8).

These early nurse training schools brought about slow and gradual change in the practice of nursing. The impact of professionally trained nurses was seen in the gradual creation of order and cleanliness out of the chaos and filth that had existed in hospitals up to this time. More about the growth of schools of nursing in the United States is found in Chapter 2.

TRAINING OF AFRICAN-AMERICAN NURSES

On August 1, 1879, **Mary Eliza Mahoney** (1845–1926) completed the 16-month course of training at the New England Hospital for Women and Children and became the first African-American "trained nurse" in the United States. At the time, only a few token admissions to training schools for nurses were granted to African-American or Jewish applicants. With segregation by law in the South and by choice in the North, it followed that African-American schools of nursing would have to be opened if African-American women were to enter the profession in large numbers.

In 1886, **Spellman Seminary** in Atlanta, Georgia, started the first nursing program for African-Americans. It was followed in 1891 by Dixie Hospital Training School in Hampton, Virginia, and in 1892 by Tuskegee Institute in Alabama. The Tuskegee program became the first baccalaureate program in a traditionally African-American institution in 1948 (Carnegie, 1986). These programs were largely responsible for the nursing education of generations of African-American nurses.

DEVELOPMENT OF NURSING ORGANIZATIONS

In 1893, **Isabel Hampton (Robb)** presented a paper at the International Congress of Charities, Correction, and Philanthropy at the Chicago World's Fair "protesting the lack of uniformity of instruction in training schools and the completely inadequate education being provided" (Christy, 1984, p. 38). Her presentation resulted in the formation of the American Society of Superintendents of Training Schools for Nurses (Fig. 1–9). This society changed its name in 1912 to the National League of Nursing Education (NLNE); in 1952, it was again re-

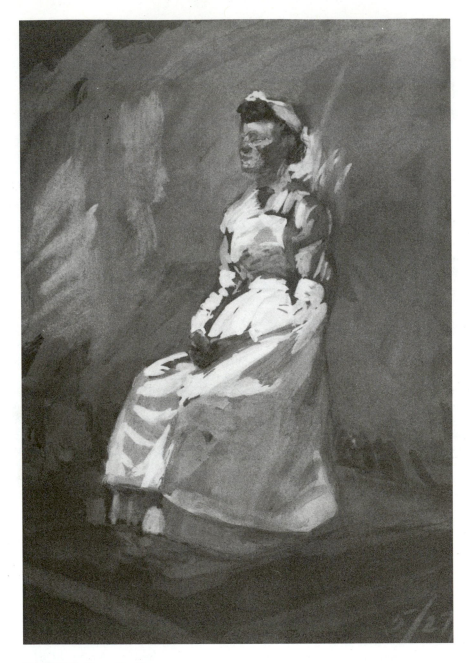

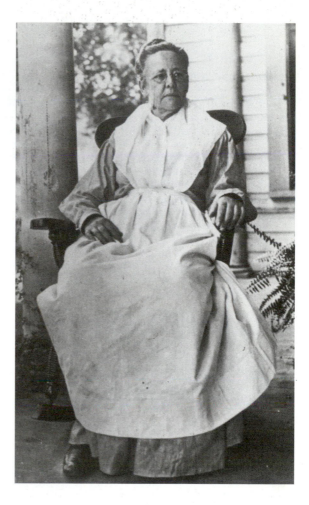

FIGURE 1–9
Annie Davis Baker, first head
nurse, Scott and White Hospital, Temple, Texas.
(Reprinted with permission
of Sarah Parisi, M.S.N.,
R.N., subject's great, great
granddaughter.)

organized and given its current name, the National League for Nursing (NLN)
(Christy, 1984).

In that same year, 1893, another nursing influential, **Lillian Wald,** underwent
a transformational experience that changed the direction of nursing profoundly. Her graphic description of this event in her life is reprinted in Box 1–1.

As a result of this experience, Wald and her colleague, Mary Brewster, moved
into a tenement on New York's Lower East Side. With the help of private philanthropists, they provided care to their neighbors and established the **Henry
Street Settlement** and public health nursing in the United States (Christy, 1984,
p. 38). Wald later formed the National Organization of Public Health Nurses
(1912), marking the beginning of specialization in nursing.

Isabel Hampton Robb recognized the need "to unite practitioners of nursing." She had already been instrumental in the formation of the National League
for Nursing Education. In 1896, she was again successful in her efforts, founding the Associated Alumnus of the United States and Canada, which in 1911 be-

BOX 1-1
Lillian Wald's Awakening

From the schoolroom where I had been giving a lesson in bed-making, a little girl led me one drizzling March morning. She had told me of her sick mother, and gathering from her incoherent account that a child had been born, I caught up the paraphernalia of the bed-making lesson and carried it with me.

The child led me over broken roadways . . . between tall, reeking houses . . . past odorous fish stands for the streets were a market-place, unregulated, unsupervised, unclean, past evil-smelling, uncovered garbage cans, and perhaps worst of all, where so many little children played. . . .

The child led me on through a tenement hallway, across a court where open and unscreened closets were promiscuously used by men and women, up into a rear tenement, by slimy steps whose accumulated dirt was augmented that day by the mud of the streets, and finally into the sickroom.

All the maladjustments of our social and economic relations seemed epitomized in this brief journey and what was found at the end of it. The family to which the child led me was neither criminal nor vicious . . . and although the sick woman lay on a wretched, unclean bed, soiled with a hemorrhage two days old, they were not degraded human beings. . . . It would have been some solace if by any conviction of the moral unworthiness of the family, I could have defended myself as part of a society which permitted such conditions to exist. . . . Miserable as their state was, they were not without ideals for the family life, and for society, of which they were so unloved and unlovely a part.

That morning's experience was a baptism of fire. Deserted were the laboratory and the academic work of the college. I never returned to them. . . . To my inexperience it seemed certain that conditions such as these were allowed because people did not *know*, and for me there was the challenge to know and tell. When early morning found me still awake, my naive conviction remained that, if people knew things,—and "things" meant everything implied in the condition of this family,—such horrors would cease to exist, and I rejoiced that I had training in the care of the sick that in itself would give me an organic relationship to the neighborhood in which this awakening had come.

(From *The House on Henry Street* by Lillian Wald. Copyright 1915, 1943 by Julia Wald Cordley. Henry Holt & Company, Inc., Publisher. Used by permission.)

came officially known as the American Nurses Association (ANA) (Christy, 1984, p. 38).

In October 1900, after years of dedicated work by Robb, Mary Adelaide Nutting, Lavinia Dock, and others, the first issue of the *American Journal of Nursing* was published (Christy, 1984, p. 39). Nurses now had both a professional organization and an official journal through which they could communicate with each other.

MILITARY NURSING ESTABLISHED

The Spanish-American War (1898) provided the first opportunity for trained nurses to be accepted in military hospitals. It also marked the first time a trained

African-American nurse, **Namahyoke Curtis,** was employed as a contract nurse by the War Department. Her efforts and the efforts of all graduate nurses involved in this war emphasized the importance and need for military nurses. This realization led to the formation of the Army Nurse Corps (1901) and the Navy Nurse Corps (1908).

Organized nursing in the United States had moved out of its infancy. By 1900, there were some 1200 trained nurses in addition to 109,000 untrained nurses practicing in homes, public health settings, hospitals, and the military (National League for Nursing, 1990). Although much was left to be accomplished, the trained nurse was destined to make a difference.

Nursing in the Twentieth Century—
In Step with a Changing Society

From its humble beginnings, nursing during the twentieth century grew into a respected profession, the development of which continued to parallel that of the United States.

1900–1920: SOCIAL AWAKENING, WORLD WAR I

The period from 1900 to 1920 was both a period of social awakening and a period of continued social injustices. The invention of the telephone, the airplane, and the automobile created more and faster avenues for communication and travel. Yet women still could not vote, and minorities were left to pave their own way in this changing society.

In 1900, **Jessie Sleet (Scales)** became the first African-American public health nurse. In 1908, the National Association of Colored Graduate Nurses (NACGN) was founded by **Martha Franklin.** Since some state nurses' associations still barred African-American nurses from membership, as late as 1916, they were prevented them from being eligible for membership in the ANA. Undaunted, **Francis Reed Elliott** became the first African-American nurse accepted by the American Red Cross Nursing Service in 1918.

Although minority groups in nursing were struggling, the profession as a whole continued to expand and establish new standards. In 1903, the first four state nursing licensure laws were passed in North Carolina, New Jersey, New York, and Virginia. These laws marked nursing's first successful efforts to become self-regulating and paved the way for licensing examinations nationwide. Progress during this era also included the 1912 establishment of the Town and Country Nursing Service by the American Red Cross and the opening of the first birth control clinic in the United States by **Margaret Sanger** in 1916. Sanger's clinic was the forerunner of Planned Parenthood.

In April 1917, the United States entered World War I, destined to become the bloodiest war of all time because of new weapons and military technology. The nation once again mobilized its resources. As young men were drafted into the armed services in large numbers, the Army Nurse Corps and Navy Nurse Corps made concentrated efforts to expand their forces. With too few nurses available to meet both civilian and military needs, controversy raged about how best to meet the critical nursing shortage. In spite of almost insurmountable pressure from all sides to create a quick solution, calmer heads prevailed, and the Army School of Nursing was formed in 1918. Designed to meet the military's increased need for nurses quickly but competently, the school was headed by **Annie Goodrich,** then president of the ANA and an assistant professor of nursing at Teachers College (Columbia University).

The war effort was severely hampered by the great influenza epidemic of 1918–1919. Physicians and nurses as well as troops and civilians were struck with influenza. "The death toll in the United States alone for the last four months of 1918 and the first six months of 1919 was 548,452—five times greater than the total World War I American military deaths" (Kalisch and Kalisch, 1986, p. 361). Health care resources were decimated by the epidemic. Because of the severity of the situation, 18 African-American nurses were ultimately accepted by the military, representing a breakthrough for this minority group. They were never actually able to participate in the war effort, however, because the war ended soon after their appointment.

The year 1919 marked the passage of the Nineteenth Amendment to the U.S. Constitution. That amendment extended voting privileges to women. Women's suffrage had been under active consideration for 40 years before it was approved, and nursing organizations had formally voted to support the amendment on a number of occasions before it was actually passed. **Lavinia Dock** (Fig. 1–10) was a well-known early twentieth-century nurse who was actively involved in women's rights issues and the suffragette movement. Dock, affectionately called "Little Dockie," was a small, red-haired woman whose appearance belied her leadership abilities. In 1925, looking back at the evolution of nursing and its involvement with societal issues, Dock and Isabel Stewart wrote:

> When we consider the whole movement of social progress, the breaking down of the spirit of hatred and prejudice, the promotion of kindlier and more humane relations between human beings, the organization of practical and effective measures for reducing human suffering and distress, it would be hard to find any group of workers who have contributed more to the sum total of social effort than have nurses (Donahue, 1985, pp. 13–14).

Trained nurses *had* been involved, even to the point of marching in public parades to support the causes they believed in, such as women's suffrage.

1920–1929: THE ROARING TWENTIES

The decade of the 1920s saw the beginning of unheard of freedom for women. Shortened hairstyles, rising hemlines, and the use of cosmetics were all part of the "flapper" era of the 1920s. Hospitals continued to expand, as did schools of nursing, yet they often did not employ their own graduates, preferring to staff the hospital with student nurses because student help was less expensive.

In 1923, the findings of a nursing report entitled *Nursing and Nursing Education in the United States* were published. Called the **Goldmark Report,** "this document emphasized the desirability of establishing university schools of nursing to train nurse leaders. It pointed out the fundamental faults in hospital train-

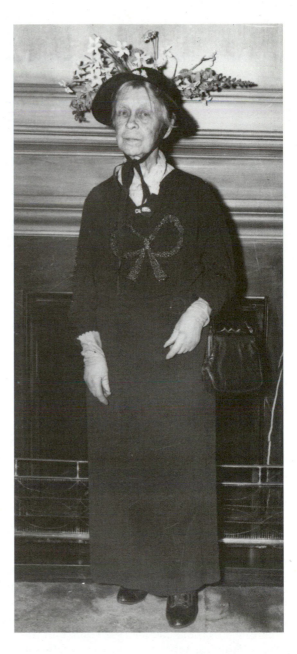

F I G U R E   1 – 1 0
Lavinia Dock. (Reproduced
with permission of the Special
Collections, Milbank Memorial
Library, Teachers College,
Columbia University.)

ing schools, and identified the primary obstacle to higher standards as the lack
of funds set apart specifically for nursing education" (Kalisch and Kalisch, 1986,
p. 374). Despite opposition by physicians, hospital-based training schools, and
some veteran nurses, collegiate nursing programs were under way.

During the 1920s, nursing was also progressing on another front—rural midwifery. Responding to the lack of maternity care for rural women, **Mary Breckin-ridge** founded the **Frontier Nursing Service** in 1925. Although untrained women had served as midwives for centuries, the Frontier Nursing Service provided "the first organized midwifery service in this country" (Donahue, 1985, p. 350).

1929–1937: THE DEPRESSION

By 1927, there were some 2286 schools of nursing in the United States, most of which were hospital based (Kalisch and Kalisch, 1986, p. 369). The prosperity of the United States was waning in these early days leading up to the Great Depression. The use of private-duty nurses declined as family resources diminished. There was insufficient funding for visiting nurse services. Soon there were too many trained nurses, and unemployment nationwide was on the rise. The stock market crash of 1929 marked the beginning of a long period of economic decline and further unemployment in the United States.

During the 1930s, the United States struggled to emerge from the economic depression that caused devastating hardships. Nursing unemployment hit an all-time high. Yet even in this time of economic depression, a number of medical advancements were achieved. As medical technology advanced and nurses demonstrated that they were well trained in the care of the sick, hospitals rapidly became the primary setting for health care. Health insurance plans evolved, Social Security was passed in 1935, and labor movements brought renewed attention to working conditions and child labor.

The labor movement forced hospitals and training schools to look more closely at the way in which they used student nurses. Training schools reduced the long duty schedules of student nurses, and hospitals actively recruited graduate nurses, which served to reduce nursing unemployment. The shift in employment of graduate nurses from homes to hospitals coincided with increasing hospital admissions and a decline in home-based care that was to last until the 1980s.

1937–1945: THE WAR YEARS

The decade of the 1940s found the United States emerging from a major economic depression, preparing for war, fighting the war, and recovering from it. It was also a time of prosperity and progress for nursing.

The 1941 Lanham Act supported the need for additional trained nurses by allocating funds for additions to dormitories, libraries, classrooms, and other physical facilities (Donahue, 1985, p. 413). Through the efforts of Frances Payne Bolton, federally funded support for nursing education came with the passage of the Appropriations Act for 1942 (Donahue, 1985, p. 412). It was followed by the Nurse Training Act of 1943, which was also sponsored by Bolton. Later, this act became known as the Bolton Act and resulted in the creation of the United States Cadet Nurse Corps. It was administered by the U.S. Public Health Service, Division of Nurse Education, led by **Lucille Petry (Leone)**. By the war's end, some 65,000 nurses had enlisted and graduated from the Cadet Nurse Corps (National League for Nursing, 1990), and nearly 69,000 nurses were serving in the Army and Navy Nurse Corps (Donahue, 1985, p. 415). In 1949, Petry, now known by her married name, Lucille Petry Leone, became the first woman appointed to the position of assistant surgeon general of the U.S. Public Health Service. At that time, this was the highest post ever held by a nurse.

World War II served as a catalyst for significant advances in medical science and in care given by nurses and physicians. Such advances as blood transfusions, early antibiotics, improved treatment for malaria, trauma care, rehabilitation, and other techniques were discovered out of the need to treat those ravaged by war. Science, medicine, and nursing were changing and expanding and becoming more proficient. Nurses, along with their physician colleagues and military corpsmen, were present on every battlefront—on the land, at sea, and in the air (Fig. 1–11). Some were wounded, some died, and some were captured and placed in prisoner-of-war camps. Once again, nurses played an instrumental role during wartime.

FIGURE   1–11

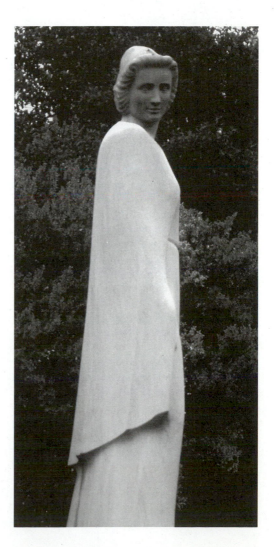

Nurse. A statue in Arlington Cemetery dedicated in 1971 "to commemorate devoted service to country and humanity by Army, Navy, and Air Force Nurses." (Reprinted with permission of the Smithsonian Institution, Washington, DC.)

The first Nurse Draft Bill was introduced late in the war, but the war's end made the bill unnecessary. Nurses who served in the war were officers and, when discharged following the war, had access to further education through the GI Bill of Rights. They entered undergraduate and graduate programs to earn advanced degrees in nursing. Many, however, chose to return to more traditional, non-working female roles following the war.

Discrimination against African-American nurses continued throughout the years surrounding the war. In 1940 in Mississippi, for example, there were three African-American public health nurses and 1 million African-American people. This disproportion was typical of the barriers African-Americans faced in entering all professional fields.

1945–1965: THE POSTWAR ERA AND TECHNOLOGICAL EXPLOSION

The postwar economic boom and the "baby boom" both served to stimulate the construction of hospitals. The nursing shortage once again became painfully acute in hospitals, and two new categories of workers emerged in response to the shortage. They were the nursing assistant (NA) and the licensed practical nurse (LPN). One-year practical nursing programs, begun during the war as an expedient way to supplement the numbers of registered nurses, became institutionalized with licensure of LPNs.

As with any labor shortage, working conditions in hospitals became increasingly difficult, with long hours, low pay, large work loads, and insufficient help. Many nurses were unhappy with both their working conditions and the quality of nursing care they were able to provide in these adverse conditions. In 1946, the ANA authorized its state units to form collective-bargaining units, and another conflict arose—to strike or not to strike. Heated debates throughout the United States defined the ethical dilemma of nursing professionals: the duty to care for patients and the personal duty to care for one's own welfare.

In the 20 years following World War II, the United States experienced an explosion of technology that profoundly affected health care. A vast store of medical knowledge and technical advances resulted from World War II, and within two decades, the United States was engaged in two more wars—Korea and Vietnam (Fig. 1–12). With each war, medical advances were made. As science and technology moved to the forefront of health care, the size, number, and distribution of hospitals rapidly expanded. Changes took place within nursing as well.

During the 1950s, a shorter educational route to becoming a nurse, the associate degree program, was added to the degree and diploma programs already in existence. The *Journal of Nursing Research* was founded in 1952 as the pace and quality of nursing research rapidly expanded. Military corpsmen entered nursing programs, and the number of male nurses increased. More nurses sought advanced degrees. State units of the ANA accepted African-American nurses for membership, as did the ANA itself. The National Association of Colored Graduate Nurses was dissolved in 1951 but was followed in 1972 by the formation of the National Black Nurses Association. Health insurance plans expanded during this era, creating a great demand for more health services. The Civil Rights Movement, which began in the early part of the 1960s, moved the United States into an era of social justice that broke down some barriers of inequality of the races

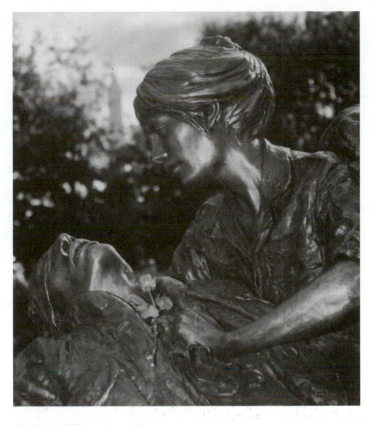

FIGURE 1–12
Vietnam Women's Memorial, dedicated November 11, 1993. (Reprinted with permission of the Smithsonian Institution, Washington, DC.)

and the sexes. Technological advances resulting from space exploration impacted medical science and nursing practice even further. Undreamed-of life-saving drugs and life-prolonging technologies were developed. Trauma care and care of premature infants saved thousands of lives that formerly would have been lost. To keep up with the new technologies, critical care nursing evolved as a specialty area of practice.

1965–1990: HEALTH CARE BOOM AND ESCALATING COSTS

The next 25 years saw unparalleled growth of hospitals and other health care agencies. As depicted in Figure 1–13, nurses increased their scope of practice and assumed roles and functions formerly restricted to physicians. Medical technology reached previously unheard-of heights with astounding new medical, surgi-

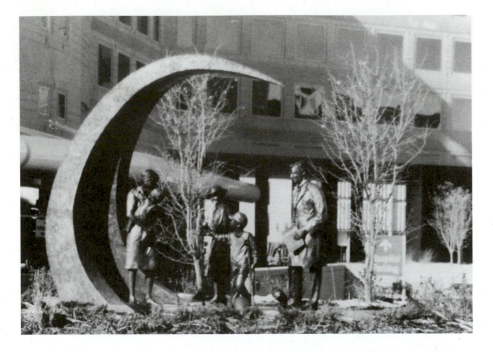

F I G U R E   1 – 1 3
Caring Hands. (Reprinted with permission of Phyllis C. Beattie, Sculptor.)

cal, and diagnostic techniques. Not unexpectedly, the costs of health care also rose steadily. Nursing's political agendas during this time centered around achieving parity with medicine and autonomy in practice (National League for Nursing, 1990).

Nursing specialization continued, and with it developed specialty-focused professional organizations. The nurse practitioner's role evolved to meet changing health care needs and eventually paved the way for increasingly collaborative relationships between nursing and medicine. It also created conflict, however, in some areas of the United States as physicians and nurses battled over the right to practice.

Lyndon B. Johnson's "Great Society" reforms reflected the prevailing social climate and demand for improved living conditions and access to health care. In 1965, Medicare and Medicaid were made law. Access to health care for the elderly, poor, and disabled in the United States seemed assured. Shortly thereafter, however, health care costs began to rise dramatically. In response, major legislative acts were passed to curtail these costs. Chapter 14 discusses this legislation in some detail.

Large numbers of nurses were employed outside hospitals: in business, industry, law, government, education, the military, and the community. Entrepreneurship prevailed as nurse-owned-and-operated businesses emerged. These new opportunities contributed to continued periodic nursing shortages, however.

By 1990, the face of both nursing and health care had changed. Hospitals cared predominantly for the acutely ill, as patients moved away from the hospital and back into community care settings and the home. Major health care issues centered around the uninsured, the elderly, the homeless, the disadvantaged, and the acquired immunodeficiency syndrome (AIDS) epidemic. As they had done throughout their history, nurses continued to reach out and provide care to the needy wherever they happened to be. Minority nurses continued to seek recognition for their accomplishments, and the nursing profession continued to grow and adapt to the rapidly changing health care needs of society (Fig. 1–14).

1990S: THE ERA OF COST CONTAINMENT— NURSING LEADS THE WAY

The decade of the 1990s has been characterized by public and private sector efforts toward cost containment and heightened efficiency and quality in health care. By 1992, the need for major health care reform was recognized by most thoughtful Americans and was widely debated in Congress and elsewhere.

Organized nursing assumed a major leadership role in the reform effort by submitting its *Agenda for Health Care Reform*. The plan for reform, discussed more fully in Chapter 4, was comprehensive and focused on restructuring the health care system in the United States, reducing costs, and improving accessibility to all in need of care. Nursing's *Agenda* received attention at the highest governmental levels and was widely recognized.

By 1996, although no major Federal legislation toward health care reform had been passed, the health care delivery system had nevertheless experienced rapid and dramatic changes. The focus of health care delivery was shifting from the treatment of illness to the prevention of illness. The primary site of care had moved from the hospital to the outpatient setting and the home. The role of advanced practice nurses had expanded as states recognized the cost savings to be realized by greater use of these nurses.

The vital role of nursing in the newly emerging health care system has been reaffirmed. Yet a number of challenges remain. A discussion of the challenges faced by the nursing profession in the future is covered in Chapter 22.

S U M M A R Y

The history of nursing is rich, filled with struggle, neglect, missed opportunities, vision, courage, and victory. A contemporary nursing leader, Margretta Styles, wrote "A Biblical Fable on Our Origins," from which the following is excerpted:

> In the beginning, God created nursing. He (or she) said, "I will take a solid, simple significant system of education and an adequate, applicable base of clinical research, and on these rocks will I build My greatest gift to mankind—nursing practice." On the seventh day He threw up his hands. And has left it up to us (Donahue, 1985, p. 434).

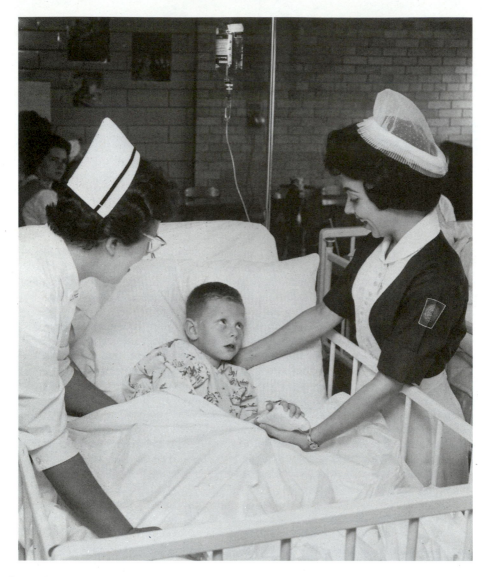

FIGURE 1-14

Nursing instructor, student nurse, and pediatric patient. (Reprinted with permission of the West Virginia and Regional History Collection, West Virginia University Libraries, Morgantown, West Virginia.)

And we have not done too badly! After years of apprenticeship learning and exploitation of students in the workplace, we now have a significant system of nursing education. After using research findings from other disciplines, we now have our own rapidly growing base of clinical research and a pool of nurses educated to pursue nursing research. After decades of basing our professional actions on theories from psychology, sociology, education, and medicine, we now are developing nursing theories on which to base our practices. We are a profession whose education and practice are founded on the basic sciences, reasoned thinking, and the questioning minds of researchers. We have strong, caring, committed practitioners, educators, and leaders who give nursing life, shape, and vitality. These words of Florence Nightingale are as appropriate today as when she wrote them:

> Nursing is an art; and if it is to be made an art, it requires as exclusive a devotion, as hard a preparation, as any painter's or sculptor's work; for what is the having to do with dead canvas or cold marble, compared with having to do with the living body—the temple of God's spirit? It is one of the Fine Arts; I had almost said, the finest of the Fine Arts (Donahue, 1985, p. 469).

Nurses, empowered by caring, commitment, and knowledge, will continue to have a significant impact on the continuing evolution of the practice and profession of nursing. They can be one of the driving forces in shaping health care in the twenty-first century and improving the quality of life for all humankind.

REVIEW AND DISCUSSION QUESTIONS

1. What influence did early religious groups' caring for the sick have on modern nursing?
2. How did Florence Nightingale's Crimean experience affect American nursing?
3. Describe the forces leading to the establishment of training schools for nurses in the United States.
4. How was the development of nursing in the United States influenced by the medical profession?
5. What were the contributions of early African-American nurses?
6. Wars have often been the driving force in creating social change. How did wars influence the profession of nursing?
7. What are some emerging trends in health care that will impact the practice of professional nursing?

REFERENCES

Austin, A. L. (1984). Nurses in American history: Wartime volunteers—1861–1865. In *Pages from nursing history: A collection of original articles from the pages of Nursing Outlook, the American Journal of Nursing and Nursing Research.* New York: American Journal of Nursing.

Carnegie, M. E. (1986). *The path we tread: Blacks in nursing, 1854–1984.* Philadelphia: J. B. Lippincott.

Christy, T. E. (1984). Nurses in American history: The fateful decade, 1890–1900. In *Pages from nursing history: A collection of original articles from the pages of Nursing Outlook, the American Journal of Nursing, and Nursing Research.* New York: American Journal of Nursing.

Donahue, M. P. (1985). *Nursing: The finest art, An illustrated history.* St. Louis: C. V. Mosby.

Kalisch, P. A., and Kalisch, B. J. (1986). *The advance of American nursing* (2nd ed.). Boston: Little, Brown.

Kampen, N. B. (1988). Before Florence Nightingale: A prehistory of nursing in painting and sculpture. In A. H. Jones (Ed.), *Images of nurses: Perspectives from history, art, and literature*. Philadelphia: University of Pennsylvania Press.

National League for Nursing. (1990). *Nursing in America: A history of social reform* (videotape). New York: Author.

Parsons, M. E. (1984). Mothers and matrons. In *Pages from nursing history: A collection of original articles from the pages of Nursing Outlook, the American Journal of Nursing, and Nursing Research*. New York: American Journal of Nursing.

Robinson, V. (1946). *White caps: The story of nursing*. Philadelphia: J. B. Lippincott.

Selavan, I. C. (1984). Nurses in American history: The revolution. In *Pages from nursing history: A collection of original articles from the pages of Nursing Outlook, the American Journal of Nursing, and Nursing Research*. New York: American Journal of Nursing.

Smith, F. T. (1984). Florence Nightingale: Early feminist. In *Pages from nursing history: A collection of original articles from the pages of Nursing Outlook, the American Journal of Nursing, and Nursing Research*. New York: American Journal of Nursing.

Wald, L. D. (1915). *The house on Henry Street*. New York: Henry Holt.

C H A P T E R

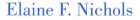

2

Elaine F. Nichols

Educational Patterns in Nursing

O B J E C T I V E S

- Trace the development of basic and graduate education in nursing.
- Discuss the influence of early nursing studies on today's nursing education.
- Discuss traditional and alternative ways of becoming a registered nurse.
- Discuss program options for registered nurses and students with baccalaureate degrees in nonnursing fields.
- Differentiate between licensed practical nurses and registered nurses.
- Explain the difference between licensure and certification.
- Define accreditation and its influence on the quality and effectiveness of nursing education programs.
- Discuss the significance of the 1965 ANA position paper to today's types of nursing programs.
- Discuss similarities and differences among three reports projecting nursing education for the twenty-first century.
- Identify current and future issues in nursing education.

V O C A B U L A R Y

accreditation
advanced degrees
advanced practice nurses
alternative educational
  programs
ANA position paper
articulation
associate degree
baccalaureate degree
basic programs
BRN

Brown Report
certification
contact hour
continuing education
  (CE)
diploma program
external degree
generic master's degree
generic nursing
  doctorate (ND)
Goldmark Report

licensure
Lysaught Report
mandatory continuing
  education
Mildred Montag
NCLEX-PN
NCLEX-RN
practical nurses
RN-to-BSN education

Diversity is the major characteristic of nursing education today. Influenced by a variety of factors—societal changes, efforts to achieve full professional status, women's issues, historical factors, public expectations, professional standards,

33

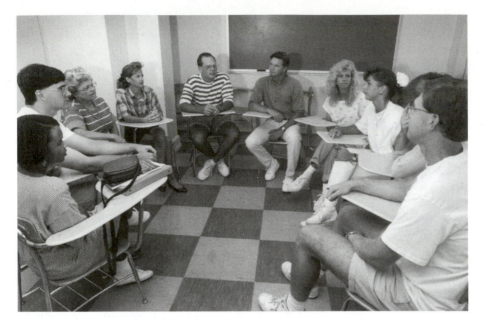

F I G U R E   2 – 1

In 1995, there were 1520 programs preparing beginning registered nurses. Students entering nursing today are widely diverse in terms of age, culture, and gender. (Photo by Fielding Freed.)

legislation, national studies, and constant changes in the health care system—many differing types of nursing education programs exist today.

In 1995, there were 1520 basic programs preparing beginning registered nurses (RNs) in the United States (Fig. 2–1). Of these, 58 percent were associate degree programs, 34 percent were baccalaureate programs, and 8 percent were diploma programs (National League for Nursing, 1995j). In addition to the basic registered nurse programs, there were also 231 accredited master's programs, 60 doctoral programs, and 1150 practical nursing programs (National League for Nursing, 1995g). Also included in the educational system of nursing are a large number of continuing education programs and advanced-practice certification programs.

This chapter provides an orientation to the multiple nursing educational patterns in existence today. It covers the history behind these educational programs, descriptions of the various programs, and trends and future issues.

DEVELOPMENT OF NURSING EDUCATION IN THE UNITED STATES

As mentioned in Chapter 1, Florence Nightingale is credited with founding modern nursing and creating the first educational system for nurses. After hospitals came into existence in western Europe and before the influence of Florence Nightingale, hospital care was given by women prisoners and prostitutes, who were held in low regard by society. These women had no formal preparation in giving care because there were no organized programs to educate nurses until the late 1800s.

Nightingale stressed that nursing was not a domestic, charitable service but a respected occupation requiring advanced education. She opened a school of nursing at St. Thomas Hospital, London, in 1860 and established the following basic principles for the school:

1. The nurse should be trained in an educational institution supported by public funds and associated with a medical school.
2. The nursing school should be affiliated with a teaching hospital but independent of it.
3. The curriculum should include both theory and practical experience.
4. Professional nurses should be in charge of administration and instruction and should be paid for their instruction.
5. Students should be carefully selected and should reside in nurses' houses that form discipline and character.
6. Students should be required to attend lectures, take quizzes, write papers, and keep diaries. Student records should be maintained (Notter and Spalding, 1976).

Nightingale also believed that the nursing schools should be separate financially and administratively from hospitals where the students trained. This was not the case, however, when nursing schools were first established in the United States.

The first training school for nurses in the United States was established in 1872. Located at the New England Hospital for Women and Children, the course of study was one year in length. In October 1873, Melinda Anne (Linda) Richards became the first "trained nurse" in the United States. During 1873, the "famous trio" of nursing schools at Bellevue Hospital in New York, in Connecticut, and in Boston opened, and by 1879 there were 11 training schools in the United States. Other schools rapidly developed, and by 1900, there were 432 hospital-owned and hospital-operated **diploma programs** in the United States (Donahue, 1985). These early training programs differed in length from six months to two years, and each school set its own standards and requirements. The primary reason for the schools' existence was to staff the hospitals. The education of students was not always the primary concern.

Early Events in Nursing Education

Nursing leaders of the early 1900s were concerned about the poor quality of the nurse training programs. They initiated studies about nursing and nursing education to prompt changes. October 1899 marked the culmination of some four years of work by the American Society of Superintendents of Training Schools for Nurses. Isabel Robb chaired a committee to investigate a means to prepare nurses better for leadership in schools of nursing. Teachers College, which had opened in New York 10 years earlier for the training of teachers, seemed the logical location for the leadership training of nurses. The program was originally designed to prepare administrators of nursing service and nursing education and began as an eight-month course in hospital economics (Donahue, 1985).

Mary Adelaide Nutting came to Teachers College in 1907 to be the "first nursing professor in the world. Under her direction, the department progressed and became a pioneer in education for nurses. The school became known as the 'Mother-House' of collegiate education because it fostered the initial movements toward undergraduate and graduate degrees for nurses" (Donahue, 1985). In 1912, Nutting conducted an investigation, "The Educational Status of Nursing," which focused on the living conditions of students, the material being taught, and the teaching methods being used (Christy, 1969).

As mentioned in Chapter 1, one of the first major studies on the status of nursing education was published in 1923. Titled "The Study of Nursing and Nursing education in the United States" and referred to as the **Goldmark Report,** it focused on the clinical learning experiences of students, hospital control of the schools, the desirability of establishing university schools of nursing, the lack of funds specifically for nursing education, and the lack of prepared teachers (Kalisch and Kalisch, 1995).

The year 1924 marked another first in nursing education when the Yale School of Nursing was opened as the first in the world to be established as a separate university department with an independent budget and its own dean, Annie W. Goodrich. The school demonstrated its effectiveness so markedly that, in 1929, the Rockefeller Foundation ensured the permanency of the school by awarding it an endowment of $1 million (Kalisch and Kalisch, 1995).

In 1934, another study entitled "Nursing Schools Today and Tomorrow" reported the number of schools in existence, gave detailed descriptions of the schools, described their currricula, and made recommendations for professional collegiate education (National League of Nursing Education, 1934). In 1937, *A Curriculum Guide for Schools of Nursing* was published outlining a three-year curriculum. This document influenced the structure of diploma schools for many years after its publication (National League of Nursing Education, 1937).

Although published over a 30-year period and undertaken by different groups, these early studies consistently made five similar recommendations:

1. Nursing education programs be established within the system of higher education.
2. Nurses be highly educated.
3. Students not be used to staff hospitals.
4. Standards be established for nursing practice.
5. All students meet certain minimum qualifications upon graduation.

These early studies set the stage for the development of the educational programs that exist today.

EDUCATIONAL PATHWAYS TO BECOMING A REGISTERED NURSE

Today, preparation for a career as an RN can begin in one of three ways: in an associate degree program, in a baccalaureate degree program, or in a hospital-based diploma program. All the programs vary in the courses offered, the length of study, and cost.

Following the completion of a basic program for registered nurses, graduates are eligible to take the National Council Licensing Examination for Registered Nurses (**NCLEX-RN**). Upon successful completion of the licensing examination, graduates may legally practice as registered nurses and use the initials *RN* after their names. Employment and career advancement vary depending on the basic program attended.

Having three different educational routes to licensure for RNs is confusing to the public and to nurses themselves. Each type of program is described with its history, unique characteristics, and special issues. The basic programs are discussed in the order in which they appeared in nursing education history.

Diploma Program

The hospital-based diploma program was the first type of nursing education begun in the United States. At the peak of diploma education in the 1920s and 1930s, approximately 2000 programs existed, with numerous programs in almost every state. Diploma programs produced many outstanding nurses, but since the peak in the first third of the century, their numbers have decreased steadily (Conley, 1973).

In the last 30 years, there has been a dramatic decline in diploma programs as nursing education moved into collegiate settings where other professionals are educated. In 1960, there were approximately 800 diploma programs in the United States. By 1980, that number had decreased to approximately 300. By 1995, there were only 122 diploma programs located in 25 states. More than half of the states had no diploma programs (National League for Nursing, 1995j).

In 1995, the largest number of diploma schools (30) remained in Pennsylvania, along with two other states, New Jersey and Ohio, having 16 and 13, respectively (National League for Nursing, 1995j). Although the number of diploma programs has significantly decreased, the majority of nurses practicing today received their basic nursing education in diploma programs.

In the late 1800s and early 1900s, diploma programs provided one of the few avenues for women to obtain formal education and jobs. Most of the early programs followed a modified apprenticeship model. Lectures were given by physicians, and clinical training was supervised by head nurses and nursing directors. Nursing courses paralleled medical areas and included surgery, obstetrics, pediatrics, and operating room experience. Students were sometimes sent to affiliated institutions where they could obtain experiences that were not available at the home hospital.

The schedule was demanding, with classes being held after patient care assignments were completed. Critics charged that students were used as inexpensive labor to staff the hospitals and that education was a lower priority. The truth of those charges varied from hospital to hospital, but there is no question that early nursing students literally ran the hospitals.

Programs lasted three years, and at graduation, students were awarded diplomas in nursing. Today, most diploma programs are about 24 months in length.

A problem that many diploma graduates have faced is that hospitals are not recognized as part of the higher education system in the United States. Most colleges and universities do not recognize the diploma in nursing as an academic credential and have often refused to give college credit for courses taken in diploma programs, regardless of the quality of the courses, students, and faculty. In recent years, diploma schools have established agreements with colleges and universities that enable diploma students to earn college credit in courses such as English, psychology, and the sciences or to move directly into advanced standing in a baccalaureate program upon completion of the diploma program.

The decline in the number of diploma programs is due to several factors: the growth of associate degree and baccalaureate degree programs in nursing; the inability of hospitals to continue to finance nursing education; accreditation standards that have made it difficult for diploma programs to attract qualified faculty; and the increasing complexity of health care, which has required nurses to have greater scientific preparation. Today, diploma programs represent only 8 percent of the total number of basic nursing education programs in the United States.

During the depths of the most recent nursing shortage, which occurred in the mid-1980s, diploma programs experienced increased enrollments. In the 1990s, however, during periods of job shortages for nurses, diploma graduates found it necessary to return to school for further education to advance within the health care system.

Baccalaureate Program

Armed with early studies of nursing education, nursing leaders wanted nursing education to move into the mainstream of higher education, that is, into colleges and universities where other professionals were educated. Their belief was that nurses needed the **baccalaureate degree** to qualify nursing as a recognized profession and to provide leadership in administration, teaching, and public health nursing roles.

By the time the first baccalaureate nursing program was established in 1909 at the University of Minnesota, diploma programs were numerous and firmly entrenched as the system for educating nurses. This first baccalaureate program was part of the School of Medicine and followed the three-year diploma program structure. Despite its many limitations, it was the start of the movement to bring nursing education into the recognized system of higher education.

Seven other baccalaureate programs in nursing were established by 1919 (Conley, 1973). Most of the early baccalaureate programs were five years in length. This structure provided for three years of nursing education and two years of liberal arts. The growth in the numbers of these programs was slow both because of the reluctance of universities to accept nursing as an academic discipline and because of the power of the diploma programs. The theoretical, scientific orientation of the baccalaureate program was in marked contrast to the "hands-on" skill and service orientation that was the hallmark of diploma education.

INFLUENCES ON THE GROWTH OF BACCALAUREATE EDUCATION

National studies of nursing and nursing education stated and restated the need for nursing education and practice to be based on knowledge from the sciences and humanities. Chief among these studies was Esther Lucille Brown's report *Nursing for the Future.* Published in 1948, the **Brown Report,** as it was called, recommended that basic schools of nursing be placed in universities and colleges and that efforts be made to recruit men and minorities into nursing education programs. This report, sponsored by the Carnegie Foundation, was widely reviewed, discussed, and debated.

Another major influence on the growth of baccalaureate education occurred in 1965, when the American Nurses Association (ANA) published a **position paper** entitled *Educational Preparation for Nurse Practitioners and Assistants to Nurses.* This paper, which created conflict and division within nursing, represented the most significant influence on the growth of baccalaureate education in nursing. In preparing the position paper, the ANA studied nursing education, nursing practice, and trends in health care. It concluded that baccalaureate education should become the basic foundation for professional practice.

The position paper made four major recommendations:

1. Education for all those who are licensed to practice nursing should take place in institutions of higher learning.
2. Minimum preparation for beginning professional nursing practice should be the baccalaureate degree in nursing.
3. Minimum preparation for beginning technical nursing practice should be the associate degree in nursing.
4. Education for assistants in the health service occupations should consist of short, intensive preservice programs in vocational education institutions rather than in on-the-job training programs (American Nurses Association, 1965).

Despite tremendous opposition from proponents of diploma and associate degree education, in 1978 the ANA further strengthened its resolve by proposing three additional positions:

1. By 1985, the minimum preparation for entry into professional nursing practice should be the baccalaureate degree in nursing.
2. Two levels of nursing practice should be identified and a mechanism to devise competencies for the two categories established by 1980.
3. There should be increased accessibility to high-quality career mobility programs that use flexible approaches for individuals seeking academic degrees in nursing (American Nurses Association, 1979).

The controversy created by the initial ANA position paper and the additional 1978 resolutions continued for many years. Practicing nurses across the United States, who were mainly diploma program graduates, as well as hospitals that supported diploma programs, vehemently protested the recommendations.

In 1970, the National Commission for the Study of Nursing and Nursing Education published its report entitled *An Abstract for Action* (Lysaught, 1970). Also known as the **Lysaught Report,** it made recommendations concerning the supply and demand for nurses, nursing roles and functions, and nursing education. Among the priorities identified by this study were (1) the need for increased research into both the practice and education for nurses and (2) enhanced educational systems and curricula (Lysaught, 1970).

In the early 1980s, the National Commission on Nursing published two reports that suggested that the major block to the advancement of nursing was the ongoing conflict within the profession about educational preparation for nurses. These studies recommend establishing a clear system of nursing education, including pathways for educational mobility and development of additional graduate education programs.

The latest major national nursing group to support the baccalaureate as the entry credential was the National League for Nursing (NLN). The organization's membership is made up of nurses, faculty members, health care agencies, all types of nursing programs, and nonnursing citizens who are supportive of nursing. In 1982, after much debate, the NLN board of directors approved the *Position Statement on Nursing Roles: Scope and Preparation*, which affirmed the nursing baccalaureate degree as the minimum educational level for professional nursing practice and the associate degree or diploma as the preparation for technical nursing practice (National League for Nursing, 1982).

BACCALAUREATE PROGRAMS TODAY

Today, baccalaureate programs provide education for both basic students who are preparing for licensure and those RNs returning to school to obtain a bachelor of science in nursing (BSN). This section focuses on the program characteristics of prelicensure baccalaureate education, sometimes called **basic programs.** Baccalaureate programs for RNs are discussed later.

Basic baccalaureate programs combine nursing courses with general education courses in a four- or five-year curriculum in a senior college or university. Students may be admitted to the nursing program as entering freshmen or after completing certain liberal arts courses. Students meet the same admission requirements to the university as other students and often must meet additional requirements to be admitted to the nursing major.

Courses in the nursing major focus on nursing science, communication, decision making, leadership, and care to persons of all ages in a wide variety of settings. Because this education takes place in senior universities, nursing students interact with the larger student population, which promotes diverse thinking, cultural awareness, and broader socialization.

Faculty qualifications in baccalaureate programs are usually higher than in other basic nursing programs. A minimum of a master's degree and often a doctorate in nursing or a related field is required. The requirement of a doctorate ensures that nursing faculty are able to meet the teaching, research, and service requirements of all faculty in universities.

Baccalaureate graduates are prepared to take the NCLEX-RN and, after **licensure,** assume beginning practice and ultimately leadership positions in any health care setting, including hospitals, community agencies, schools, clinics, and homes (National League for Nursing, 1995e). BSN graduates are also prepared to move into graduate programs in nursing and advanced practice certification programs. BSN programs are the most costly of the basic programs in terms of time and money, but the investment results in long-term professional advancement. Today, there is great demand for BSNs, and they enjoy the greatest career mobility of all basic program graduates.

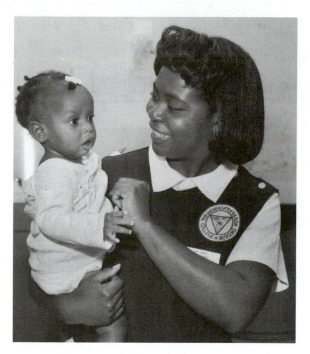

FIGURE 2–2
A nursing student enjoys working with her patient. (Courtesy of the University of Akron.)

An early criticism of baccalaureate preparation involved the perception that new BSN graduates were less skillful clinically than their diploma-educated counterparts. Contemporary BSN programs have responded to this concern by increasing students' time in clinical practice (Fig. 2–2). Additional time spent in clinical settings and preceptorships, in which students are paired with practicing RNs and work intensively in clinical settings, have been successful in strengthening the clinical skills of BSN students.

Associate Degree Program

Associate degree education in nursing represents the newest form of basic preparation for RN practice. Begun in 1952 as a result of research conducted by **Dr. Mildred Montag,** and fueled by the community college movement of the 1950s, associate degree programs are now the most common type of basic nursing education program in the United States and graduate the most RNs of all the basic programs.

In 1995, 884 (58 percent of all basic programs) programs offered the associate degree in nursing (National League for Nursing, 1995j). The popularity of this program is due to several features: accessibility of community colleges, low tuition costs, part-time and evening study opportunities, shorter length of programs, and graduates' eligibility to take the licensure examination for RNs. According to Schwirian (1984), students in associate degree programs are more likely to be older, married, and studying part-time than are students in other basic nursing programs. These characteristics, however, are also increasingly seen in diploma and baccalaureate students.

Originally, associate degree programs were designed to prepare nurse technicians to function under the supervision of professional nurses. Associate degree nurses were to work at the bedside, performing routine nursing skills for patients in acute and long-term care settings. The original associate degree program, as outlined by Montag (1951), had general education courses in the first year and nursing courses in the second year. Montag originally viewed the associate degree as a terminal degree, not a stepping stone to the baccalaureate degree in nursing.

Today, Montag's original conceptions of associative degree programs have been modified. Associate degree curricula now contain more nursing credits than she suggested. They also include content on leadership and clinical decision making, abilities that Montag did not foresee in technical nurses. Owing to additions to the curriculum, few students can complete associate degrees in only two years.

Associate degree graduates are employed in a wide variety of settings and function autonomously alongside baccalaureate and diploma graduates. In the educational system of nursing today, the associate degree can be a step in the progression to the baccalaureate degree.

In 1990, the NLN Council of Associate Degree Programs prepared a document entitled *Educational Outcomes of Associate Degree Nursing Programs: Roles and Competencies*. This document was in response to a national effort to differentiate the competencies of the associate degree nurse from the competencies of the baccalaureate nurse. The document identified associate degree competencies in three roles: provider of care, manager of care, and member within the discipline of nursing. The further development of these competencies has had a direct effect on the associate degree programs that exist today.

External Degree Programs

External degree programs in nursing are different from traditional basic nursing education in that students attend no classes and follow no prescribed methods of learning. Learning is independent and is assessed through highly standardized and validated examinations. Students are responsible for arranging their own clinical experiences in accordance with established standards.

The New York Regents External Degree Nursing Program is the most well-recognized external degree model and has both general education and nursing requirements. General education requirements include humanities, social sciences, natural sciences, and mathematics. The nursing categories represent five areas: health, commonalities of nursing care, differences in nursing care, occupational strategies, and performance. The performance examination can be taken only after successful completion of the other four categories.

The New York Regents External Degree Nursing Program received NLN accreditation in 1981 through the Council of Baccalaureate and Higher Degree Programs. In that same year, the California State University Consortium instituted a statewide external degree baccalaureate program in nursing. In contrast to the prelicensure program in New York, the California program is for RNs holding current licenses to practice in the state.

Articulated Programs

In response to the demand for educational mobility, **articulation,** or movement, between programs has become much more common in today's nursing education system. The purpose of articulation is to facilitate opportunities for nurses to move up the educational ladder. An example of a fully articulated system would be an LPN/ADN/BSN (licensed practical nurse/associate degree in nursing/bachelor of science in nursing) program in which students would spend the first year preparing to be an LPN and the second year completing the associate degree. If desired or necessary, students can "stop out" of the program at the end of the first year, take the licensure examination for practical nursing, and return to the associate degree program at a later time. Or they could continue school after the initial two years to earn a baccalaureate degree (Rapson, 1987).

Multiple-entry, multiple-exit programs are difficult to develop. A tremendous amount of joint institutional planning is needed to work out equivalent courses and to keep the programs congruent with each other. A change in one curriculum dictates changes in all the others. These challenges explain why fully articulated programs are not commonplace.

In ever-increasing numbers, however, articulation agreements between BSN and ADN programs and ADN and LPN programs are being established that facilitate student movement between programs and accept transfer credit between institutions. These requirements often result in acceleration or advanced placement within the higher-degree school.

ALTERNATIVE EDUCATIONAL PROGRAMS IN NURSING

In addition to the basic programs leading to entry-level nursing practice, several **alternative educational programs** also exist.

Baccalaureate Programs for Registered Nurses

After nursing organizations of the 1960s and 1970s publicly advocated for the baccalaureate degree as the minimum education level for professional practice, the demand for the BSN degree increased. Employers of nurses recognized that broadly educated nurses matched well with the complexities of health care. As a result, they supported the BSN as a requirement for career mobility. Diploma and associate degree graduates returned to school in increasing numbers.

RNs with diplomas and associate degrees were not always welcomed into baccalaureate programs. Many were required to take courses that they believed they had already mastered. For a number of years, it was difficult for these nurses to complete their BSNs. In the past decade, however, many baccalaureate programs have recognized the legitimacy of **RN-to-BSN education** and developed alternative tracks to accommodate the unique learning needs of the RN student. **BRN** is also used to refer to RN-to-BSN education.

Baccalaureate programs for RNs are often offered by universities that also offer a basic baccalaureate program for nonnurses. The RN students may be integrated with the basic students, or they may be in a separate or partially separate sequence. Some BSN programs for RNs are found in colleges that do not have a basic baccalaureate nursing program.

RN/BSN programs are increasingly offered owing to the demand for higher education by large numbers of associate degree nurses. In 1980–1981, 8416 RN students graduated from baccalaureate programs. There were 292 basic programs that also admitted RNs and 95 programs that admitted RNs only. By 1990, there were 12,192 RN graduates from 488 basic baccalaureate programs and 150 RN-only baccalaureate programs (U.S. Department of Health and Human Services 1990).

During the period 1990 to 1995, the number of RNs graduating from baccalaureate programs decreased because there was a shortage of nurses, and nurses were staying in their jobs rather than returning to school. In 1995, however, the job shortage for RNs in hospital settings once again began forcing nurses back to school to make themselves more marketable. A survey conducted in 1995 showed a marked increase, up 7.7 percent above a year earlier, in the numbers of RNs who were returning to school for the BSN (National League for Nursing, 1995e). In 1995, there were 509 basic baccalaureate programs that enrolled RN students and 137 BRN-only programs with graduations of 10,781 (National League for Nursing, 1995f).

Most four-year colleges and universities allow the transfer of general education credits from associate degree nursing programs. Often, some transfer credit is given for nursing courses as well, or there is the option of receiving credit for previous nursing courses through a variety of advanced placement methods.

For diploma graduates, transfer credit is usually given for previous college courses, such as English, if they were included as part of the diploma program and taught by college faculty. Options for advanced placement of diploma graduates into BSN programs are extremely variable, and prospective RN students should seek information from several BSN programs to select a program that fits individual needs and goals.

Unresolved issues surrounding BRN programs include the philosophy of some baccalaureate faculty that diploma and associate degree programs should not be stepping stones to baccalaureate degrees and that courses taken in those programs should not transfer to baccalaureate credit. There are continuing concerns about maintaining standards and protecting the integrity of the baccalaureate degree while facilitating the progression of RN students. There are also problems associated with evaluating previous learning, granting credit for that learning, and creating educational methods appropriate for the midcareer RN student.

However these issues are ultimately resolved, it is clear that the demand for the BSN by large numbers of associate degree and diploma graduates is a continuing trend. More nurses are returning to school to prepare for the wider opportunities offered by the baccalaureate degree. With broad preparation in clinical, scientific, community health, and patient education skills, the BSN nurse is well positioned to move across settings such as home health care, outpatient centers, and neighborhood clinics where opportunities are fast expanding.

Programs for Nonnursing Postbaccalaureate Students

A recent trend is a significant increase in the number of career-change students entering nursing programs with baccalaureate degrees in other fields. According to the 1994 survey *Profiles of the Newly Licensed Nurse,* close to one-fourth (25 percent) of the respondents had a college degree in another field before their nursing education (National League for Nursing, 1995h). The educational system in nursing has responded to this group of students by offering options to the traditional basic baccalaureate education. Some baccalaureate programs offer these students an accelerated sequence, which results in a second baccalaureate degree. Many individuals with one degree, however, prefer to pursue a graduate degree.

This desire for graduate degrees led to the development of an accelerated master's degree in nursing for individuals with nonnursing bachelor's degrees. These programs, known as **generic master's degree** programs, usually require about three years to complete. Graduates take the RN licensure examination after completing the generic master's program.

Another educational track for students with baccalaureate degrees in other fields is the **generic nursing doctorate (ND).** A program offering the ND as the first professional degree was begun at Case Western Reserve University in 1979. This program was based on that school's philosophy that professional nursing education should begin at the postbaccalaureate level. Following graduation, ND graduates take the RN licensure examination. Graduates are prepared to function as advanced clinical specialists or nurse practitioners and to initiate clinical research utilization studies. The generic doctorate is presently offered at three universities: Case Western Reserve in Cleveland, the University of Colorado, and Rush University in Chicago.

PRACTICAL NURSING PROGRAMS

Nursing education includes a large number of programs preparing **practical nurses.** Practical nurses are differentiated from RNs by education and licensure and have a limited scope of practice. Licensed practical nurses (LPNs), or licensed vocational nurses (LVNs), are considered technical workers in nursing.

Practical nursing programs became a significant component of the nursing field during World War II. They were created to satisfy the demand for nurses and programs that could produce nurses quickly. The first planned curriculum for practical nursing was developed in 1942. The NLN has an accrediting council for practical nursing programs, but of the 1150 LPN programs in 1994, only 179 had NLN accreditation (National League for Nursing, 1995i).

Practical nursing education is typically 12 months in length and takes place in a variety of settings: vocational/technical schools, community colleges, and high schools. Many LPN programs now offer credit for prior learning to health care workers, such as hospital aides, orderlies, paramedics, emergency medical technicians, and military corps personnel. These individuals often enter nursing through practical nursing programs.

Graduates of practical nurse programs must pass the National Council Licensing Examination for Practical Nursing (**NCLEX-PN**) to become licensed. The scope of their practice focuses on meeting basic patient needs in hospitals, long-term care facilities, and homes. They practice under the supervision of a physician or RN.

For many students enrolled in practical nurse programs, the goal is to become an RN. A significant number of newly licensed RNs were previously licensed as practical nurses. According to the *1994 Profiles of the Newly Licensed Nurse*, 17 percent of all newly licensed nurses have practiced as LPNs (National League for Nursing, 1995h).

There are increasing pressures on LPN programs to expand and upgrade. These proposals are usually discussed during times when jobs in nursing are not readily available and include phasing out practical nurse programs or converting them to associate degree programs. When the demand for nurses is greater than basic RN programs can meet, however, practical nurse programs flourish. In 1993, practical nurse programs experienced the highest number of admissions in ten years. Thirty-seven percent of those persons that applied were accepted for admission (National League for Nursing, 1995i). Currently, there are significant increases in employment opportunities for LPNs because their lower salaries fit well with the cost-containment requirements in today's health care system.

ACCREDITATION OF EDUCATIONAL PROGRAMS

The concept of **accreditation** of educational programs in nursing is important. Although all nursing programs must be approved by their respective State Boards of Nursing for graduates to take the licensure examination, nursing programs may also seek accreditation, which goes beyond minimum state approval. Accreditation refers to a voluntary review process of educational programs by a professional organization. The organization, called an accrediting agency, compares the educational quality of the program with established standards and criteria. Accrediting agencies derive their authority from the U.S. Department of Education.

Prospective nursing students should inquire about the accreditation status of any nursing program they are considering. Qualifying for certain scholarships and loans and military service usually depends on being enrolled in an accredited program. Acceptance into graduate programs in nursing is also dependent on graduation from an accredited baccalaureate program. Employers of nurses are usually interested in hiring nurses who are graduates of accredited programs.

Since 1952 the NLN has been the official professional accrediting organization for master's, baccalaureate, associate degree, diploma, and practical nursing programs in the United States. The accrediting program is conducted through four NLN councils: the Council of Associate Degree Programs, the Council of Diploma Programs, the Council of Baccalaureate and Higher Degree Programs, and the Council of Practical Nursing Programs. Each council develops its own accreditation program and criteria and revises them periodically (National League for Nursing, 1990).

Accreditation of nursing schools grew out of concern repeatedly expressed by members of the profession about the quality of and standards for nursing education. An accredited program voluntarily adheres to standards that protect the quality of education, public safety, and the profession itself. Accreditation provides both a mechanism and a stimulus for programs to initiate periodic self-examination and self-improvement. It assures students that their educational program is accountable for offering quality education.

BOX 2-1

*National League for Nursing–Established Outcome Criteria
Used to Measure the Effectiveness of Each Type
of Nursing Program.**

Baccalaureate Program
Critical thinking
Communication
Therapeutic nursing interventions
Graduation rates
Patterns of employment

Associate Degree Program
Admission, retention, graduation rates
NCLEX-RN results
Patterns of employment

Diploma Programs
Retention rates of students
Standardized testing
Graduate satisfaction
NCLEX-RN results
Employment patterns of graduates
Employer satisfaction

Practical Nurse Programs
Program satisfaction
Performance on licensing examination
Admission, retention, progression, and
   graduation
Professional growth

*Each Council established its own program outcomes.
From National League for Nursing (1992a). *Criteria and guidelines for the evaluation of baccalaureate and higher degree programs in nursing.* New York: Author; NLN (1991). *Criteria and guidelines for the evaluation of associate degree programs in nursing.* New York: Author; NLN (1992b). *Criteria and guidelines for the evaluation of diploma programs in nursing.* New York: Author; NLN (1992c). *Criteria and guidelines for the evaluation of practical nurse programs.* New York: Author.

Program areas generally reviewed during accreditation include administration and governance, finances and budget, faculty, students, program outcomes, and resources. Criteria, or standards, are established in each area.

In 1991, the NLN established outcome criteria for each type of program that are used to measure the effectiveness of each nursing program. Each council established its own program outcomes. Box 2–1 lists required program outcome criteria for each type of program.

Programs under review prepare reports, known as self-studies, that show how the school meets each criterion. The self-study is reviewed by a volunteer team composed of nursing educators from the type of program being reviewed and an on-site program review is made by the same team. Following the site visit, the visitors' report and the program's self-study are reviewed by the appropriate NLN Council, and a decision is made about the accreditation status of each nursing program.

Once accredited and in good standing, continuing accreditation reviews take place every eight years. Programs that do not meet standards may be placed on warning and given a specific time period to correct deficiencies. Accreditation can be withdrawn if deficiencies are not corrected within the specified time.

In 1994, the U.S. Department of Education revised the requirements for accrediting bodies and later notified the NLN that it did not meet the new requirements. Although the NLN made many changes, by late 1996, approval has not been granted. In the future, schools of nursing may be accredited through an agency other than the NLN.

GRADUATE EDUCATION IN NURSING

A variety of economic, educational, and professional trends are fueling the demand for RNs with **advanced degrees.** The rapidly changing health care system requires nurses to possess increasing knowledge, clinical competency, greater independence, and autonomy in clinical judgments. Trends toward community-based nursing centers, case management, complexity of home care, increasingly sophisticated technologies, and society's orientation to health and self-care are all rapidly raising the educational needs of nurses.

According to projections made by the federal government, 200,000 additional master's and doctorally prepared RNs will be needed by the year 2005 (U.S. Department of Health and Human Services, 1990). Nurses who have advanced education can become researchers, nurse practitioners, clinical specialists, educators, and administrators. Many open their own clinics where they provide direct care and serve as consultants to businesses and health care agencies. Chapter 5 describes some of the opportunities open to nurses with advanced degrees. Certainly, having highly educated nurses will further strengthen the profession.

Master's Education

The purpose of master's education is to prepare persons with advanced nursing knowledge and clinical practice skills in a specialized area of practice. Teachers College, Columbia University, is credited with initiating graduate education in nursing. Beginning in 1899, the college offered a postgraduate course in hospital economics, which prepared nurses for positions in teaching and hospital administration. From this limited beginning, there has been consistent growth in the number of master's programs in the United States.

Over the last 25 years, the growth in numbers of master's programs has been dramatic. In 1970, there were 70 programs; in 1980, 142 programs; and in 1990, 212 programs. In 1995, there were 231 accredited and 44 nonaccredited master's programs for a total of 275 programs (National League for Nursing, 1995a). Enrollment of master's degree students rose by a strong 10.7 percent during the 1994–1995 year compared with a year earlier. During the five prior years, a steady upward trend caused enrollments in master's programs to rise by an average of 2523 students annually.

Most individuals in the 1950s and 1960s viewed the master's degree in nursing as a terminal (final) degree. The master's degree was considered the highest degree nurses would ever need. Early master's programs were longer and more demanding than most other master's degrees. Master's programs in the 1950s and 1960s prepared students for careers in nursing administration and nursing education.

With the rapid development of doctoral programs in the 1970s, however, the master's could no longer be considered a terminal degree. Programs were shortened to the approximate length of master's study in most other disciplines, and clinical specialization became the emphasis. Master's programs in nursing are most often found in senior colleges and universities that have basic baccalaureate programs in nursing. These programs may also seek voluntary accreditation from the NLN's Council for the Accreditation of Baccalaureate and Higher Degree Programs.

Entrance requirements to master's programs in nursing usually include the following: a baccalaureate degree from an NLN accredited program in nursing, licensure as a registered nurse, completion of the Graduate Record Examination (GRE) or other standard aptitude test, a minimum undergraduate grade point average (GPA) of 3.0, at least one year's recent work experience as an RN in an area related to the desired area of specialization, and specific goals for graduate study.

The average program length is 12 to 18 months of full-time study. The curriculum includes theory, research, clinical applications, and courses in other disciplines related to the student's selected area of specialization and role development. Students are often required to write a comprehensive examination or to complete a thesis or research project (or both). The majority of contemporary master's students are preparing for advanced clinical practice. Almost two thirds of recent graduates surveyed had chosen concentrations in advanced clinical practice, 22 percent in administration/management, and 13 percent in teaching (National League for Nursing, 1995a). Seventy-five percent of master's students are engaged in part-time study.

Nine broad specialty areas are represented in most nursing master's curricula: adult health, child health, community/public health, gerontology, nurse anesthesia, nursing administration, nurse midwifery, and psychiatric/mental health. Newer options are being added. Recent additions include nursing informatics, oncology, early intervention, and neonatal nursing.

With the increasing demand for nurse practitioners, master's programs have expanded their practitioner tracks. Master's programs offering nurse practitioner options rose from 108 in 1992 to 136 in 1993—an increase of 126 percent. Nationwide, 51 institutions reported in 1995 that they were planning to add master's degree nurse practitioner programs to prepare advanced practice nurses. Family nurse practitioner programs were the most popular concentrations offered (National League for Nursing, 1995e). Nurse practitioners may also choose areas other than the family concentration, such as pediatric, adult, midwifery, women's health, gerontology, psychiatric/mental health, and school nurse concentrations.

The master of science (MS) and the master of science in nursing (MSN) are the two most common degrees offered. A new option in master's education is the RN/MSN track, which allows RNs prepared at the associate degree or diploma level and who meet graduate admission requirements to enter a program leading to a master's degree rather than a baccalaureate degree. Another graduate program option is the combined MSN/MBA (master of business administration) for nurse administrators. As can be seen, diversity in nursing education extends to the graduate as well as the basic level.

Doctoral Education

Doctoral programs in nursing prepare nurses to become faculty members in universities, deans of schools of nursing, administrators in large medical centers, and researchers and theorists in nursing. Doctoral programs in nursing offer several degree titles, the most common being the doctor of nursing science (DNS) and doctor of philosophy (PhD).

The DNS is viewed as a professional practice degree. Conceived as an advanced practice degree with an emphasis on clinical research, the DNS is intended to bridge the gap between practice and research (Allen, 1990). The PhD is considered the academic degree and prepares scholars for research and the development of theory.

A continuing issue is the relative merit of these two degrees. As currently structured in most universities, the two programs are more similar than different. In the major job market for nurses with doctorates, which is colleges and universities, the PhD is the more prestigious of the two degrees and therefore is favored by many doctorate-seeking nurses. Of 60 programs awarding doctoral degrees in 1995, 80 percent awarded the PhD (National League for Nursing, 1995a).

Formal doctoral education began at Columbia University's Teachers College in 1910 with the creation of the Department of Nursing and Health. The first student completed her work for the doctor of education (EdD) with a major in nursing education and was awarded her doctorate in 1932. As of 1995, Teachers College was the only doctoral program in nursing education granting the EdD.

In 1934, New York University initiated the first PhD program for nurses. The programs at Teachers College and New York University provided many of the profession's early leaders who worked over the years for improvement in nursing education (Parietti, 1990).

From 1934 to 1954, no new nursing doctoral programs were opened. In 1954, the University of Pittsburgh opened the first PhD program in clinical nursing and clinical research in the United States. The ANA's *Facts About Nursing* (1961) reported that as the 1950s drew to a close, a total of only 36 doctoral degrees had been awarded in nursing (Parietti, 1990).

Owing to the limited number of nursing doctoral programs, most nurses in the 1950s and 1960s earned doctorates in nonnursing fields, such as education, sociology, and physiology. Doctoral education for nurses moved into a new phase when the federal government initiated nurse scientist programs in 1962. These programs were created to increase the research skills of nurses and provide faculty for the development of doctoral programs in nursing. The nurse scientist programs were discontinued in 1975 after more universities began offering doctoral programs in nursing.

The 1970s saw a major increase in the number of doctoral programs in nursing. Fifteen new doctoral programs were established in that decade alone. Between 1970 and 1980, the number of programs increased to 22. Between 1980 and 1990, the number more than doubled, from 22 to 48 (Parietti, 1990). In 1995, the number of doctoral programs stood at 60 (National League for Nursing, 1995a).

Trends indicate that there is strong support for doctoral education in nursing. In the first half of the 1990s, the number of requests for admission to these programs greatly increased. This stemmed from the requirement of a doctorate for academic advancement and tenure for university nursing faculty. Nurses also desire the doctorate to become competent researchers and to advance the profession as a whole. Doctoral programs that prepare nurses predominantly for research and teaching reported 2919 students enrolled in 1994. Over the prior five years, the trend among doctoral students in nursing was continuously upward, with enrollments rising by an average of 76 students per year, and graduations rising by an average of 18 students per year (National League for Nursing, 1995f). It is projected that large numbers of doctorally prepared nurses will be needed in the future as positions requiring the doctorate expand beyond universities.

CERTIFICATION PROGRAMS

Certification is a credential that has professional but not legal status. Specialized programs developed to recognize nurses for advanced practice often lead to certification. Some certification programs are part of degree-granting programs such as a master's program; others are considered part of continuing education.

Certification means that a certificate is awarded by a professional group as validation of specific qualifications demonstrated by an RN in a defined area of practice. Certification programs that exist today include nurse practitioner preparation and programs in pediatrics, gerontology, family health, women's health care, nurse midwifery, and nurse anesthesia. These courses provide concentrated study in specific areas and last from several weeks to several months or even years. A comprehensive examination is required to become certified as well as documentation of experience, letters of reference, and other documents. Currently, more than 30 organizations offer advanced practice certification via at least 56 procedures for attaining the desired certification. Box 2–2 lists professional associations that currently grant certification.

BOX 2–2
A Sample* of Certifying Bodies in Nursing

- American Association of Critical Care Nursing (AACN)
- American Association of Nurse Anesthetists
- American Board of Post Anesthesia Nursing Certification
- American College of Nurse Midwives
- American Nurses Credentialing Center (ANCC)
- Board of Certification for Emergency Nursing
- National Certification Board of Pediatric Nurse Practitioners

- National Certification Corporation for Obstetric, Gynecologic, and Neonatal Specialties
- Oncology Nursing Certification Corporation
- Rehabilitation Nursing Certification Board

*A complete list of certifying boards and their requirements can be obtained from *The Journal of Continuing Education in Nursing*, c/o Slack, Inc., 6900 Grove Drive, Thorofare, NJ 08086. Ask for a reprint of their Annual Continuing Education Survey.

Certified nurses have greater earning potential, wider employment opportunities, status, and prestige and, in some states, are eligible for insurance reimbursement, just as physicians are. Requirements for admission to certification programs vary, with some requiring only RN licensure and others requiring either a baccalaureate or a master's degree.

The American Nurses Credentialing Center (ANCC), a subunit of the ANA, provides a number of certification programs for RNs. **Advanced practice nurses** (APNs) certified by the ANCC must have master's degrees and demonstrate successful completion of a certification examination based on nationally recognized standards of nursing practice and designed to test their special knowledge and skills. For certain specialties, APNs also must show evidence of specified clinical practice experience. Once granted, certification is effective for three to five years, whereupon the individual must apply for recertification based on either a retest or demonstration of continuing education credits.

In response to the need to be more formally organized as a national peer review program for advanced practice nursing certification bodies, the ANCC and more than a dozen other certification boards formed the American Board of Nursing Specialties (ABNS). This umbrella board, established in 1991, approves membership of those APN certifying bodies that have met the standards and principles of ABNS. One of the 12 standards that must be met is a requirement for uniform educational preparation (i.e., a master's degree in nursing).

Certification and licensure are both forms of regulation of a profession. Licensure refers to state regulation of the practice of nursing at the entry point to practice. Certification is a regulatory mechanism for advanced practice and is voluntarily pursued by individual nurses.

Nurses holding ANCC certification at the basic level can be identified by the initials *RN, C.* (registered nurse, certified) after their names. Those certified as clinical specialists use *RN, CS.* Box 2–3 lists the areas in which the ANCC offers certification.

Although certification is a desirable concept, there are many problems related to current methods of certification, such as lack of uniformity of programs, testing, and practice requirements. The questions of how to ensure certification standards and who should be responsible for certification of nurses are major issues in the nursing education system today. In October 1994, the American Association of Colleges of Nursing (AACN) issued a position statement on the certification and regulation of advanced practice nurses. The position statement emphasized that the nursing profession must develop a standardized national advanced practice nursing certification process as expeditiously as possible. The statement recommended that all advanced practice nurses should hold a graduate degree in nursing and be certified in a manner standardized by one nationally recognized certifying board. This is particularly important because professional certification validates and standardizes the qualifications and practice competencies of advanced practice nurses (American Association of Colleges of Nursing, 1994).

CONTINUING EDUCATION

Continuing education (CE) is a term used to describe informal ways in which nurses maintain clinical expertise during their professional careers. Continuing education for nurses takes place in a variety of settings: colleges, universities,

BOX 2-3

Areas of Certification Offered by the American Nurses Credentialing Center (ANCC) in 1996

Generalist Programs
- Informatics Nurse
- General Nursing Practice
- Medical-Surgical Nurse
- Gerontological Nurse
- Pediatric Nurse
- Perinatal Nurse
- College Health Nurse
- School Nurse
- Community Health Nurse
- Psychiatric and Mental Health Nurse
- Nursing Continuing Education/Staff Development
- Home Health Nurse
- Cardiac Rehabilitation Nurse

Nurse Practitioner Programs
- Adult Nurse Practitioner
- Family Nurse Practitioner
- School Nurse Practitioner
- Pediatric Nurse Practitioner
- Gerontological Nurse Practitioner
- Acute Care Nurse Practitioner

Clinical Specialist Programs
- Clinical Specialist in Medical-Surgical Nursing
- Clinical Specialist in Gerontological Nursing
- Clinical Specialist in Community Health Nursing
- Clinical Specialist in Home Health Nursing
- Clinical Specialist in Adult Psychiatric and Mental Health Nursing
- Clinical Specialist in Child and Adolescent Psychiatric and Mental Health Nursing

Nursing Administration Programs
- Nursing Administration
- Nursing Administration, Advanced

Reprinted with permission of American Nurses Credentialing Center (1996). *1996 certification catalog.* Washington, D.C.: Author.

hospitals, community agencies, professional organizations, and professional meetings. Continuing education appears in many forms, such as workshops, institutes, conferences, short courses, evening courses, telecourses, and instructional supplements in professional journals.

The ANA Council on Continuing Education was established in 1973. This council is responsible for standards of continuing education, accreditation of programs offering continuing education, transferability of CE credit from state to state, and development of guidelines for recognition systems within states.

In the 1970s, the continuing education unit (CEU) was created as a method of recognizing participation in nonacademic credit offerings. One CEU was given for every 10 hours of participation in an organized, approved, continuing education offering. Today the **contact hour** has replaced the CEU, and nurses receive one contact hour of credit for each 50 or 60 minutes they spend in a continuing education course.

A major nationwide trend currently is **mandatory continuing education.** Before renewing their licenses in states with mandatory continuing education, nurses must provide evidence that they have met that state's contact hour requirements. This requirement is the government's way of ensuring that nurses remain up-to-date in their profession. In 1994, mandatory continuing education as a prerequisite for relicensure was required in 21 states and territories with

---

B O X   2 – 4

States and Territories Requiring Continuing Education for Relicensure*

- Alabama
- Alaska
- California
- Colorado
- Delaware
- Florida
- Iowa
- Kansas
- Kentucky
- Louisiana
- Massachusetts
- Minnesota
- Nebraska
- Nevada
- New Hampshire

- New Mexico
- Ohio
- Puerto Rico
- Texas
- Virgin Islands
- West Virginia
- Wyoming

*A current list of states and territories requiring continuing education for relicensure and their requirements can be obtained from *The Journal of Continuing Education in Nursing,* c/o Slack, Inc., 6900 Grove Drive, Thorofare, NJ 08086. Ask for a reprint of their Annual Continuing Education Survey.

---

2 more expected to institute requirements in the near future. Box 2–4 lists those states.

FUTURE DIRECTIONS FOR NURSING EDUCATION

In 1993, three major organizations issued statements and reports about nursing education in the twenty-first century. Their reports addressed the new direction nursing education needed to take in the future. The reports included the NLN's "Vision for Nursing Education" (1993, 1995b), the AACN's "Nursing Education's Agenda for the 21st Century" (1993), and the Pew Health Professions Commission's "Health Professions Education for the Future: Schools in Service to the Nation" (O'Neil, 1993). Although the three organizations had somewhat different approaches and strategies, several common themes emerged in their reports. Common emphases included the following eight points:

1. Schools should recruit diverse students and faculties that reflect the multicultural nature of the larger society.
2. Curricula and learning activities should develop student's critical thinking skills.
3. Curricula should emphasize student's abilities to communicate with, form interpersonal relationships with, and make decisions collaboratively with patients, their families, and interdisciplinary colleagues.
4. The number of advanced practice nurses should be increased, and curricula should emphasize health promotion and maintenance skills for all nurses.
5. Emphasis should be placed on community-based care, increased accountability, state-of-the-art clinical skills, and increased information management skills (Fig. 2–3).

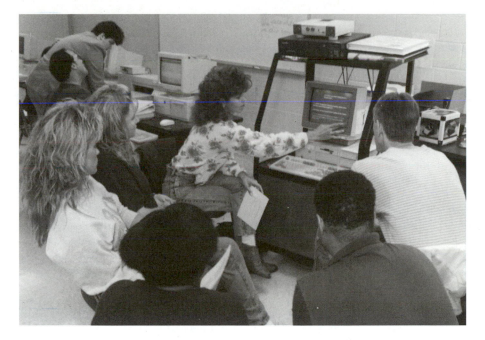

F I G U R E   2 – 3

Information management is more important than ever in nursing. These nursing students are developing their computer skills to manage the multiple sources of patient information successfully. (Courtesy of the University of Akron.)

6. Cost-effectiveness of care should be a focus in nursing curricula.
7. Faculty should develop programs that facilitate articulation and career mobility.
8. Continuing faculty development activities should support excellence in practice, teaching, and research.

PROBLEM OF REDUCED RESOURCES IN NURSING EDUCATION

Hospitals, community colleges, and universities responded to reduced applications to nursing programs during the mid-1980s by downsizing, that is, reducing the number of part-time and nontenured faculty. This resulted in an inability to meet the demand when application numbers rose again in the late 1980s and early 1990s.

Complicating the situation was the poor national economy of the early 1990s, which resulted in lower state budgets and less money for public postsecondary education. Despite enrollment increases for several consecutive years and significant demand for nursing education by qualified students, many could not be accommodated in schools of nursing owing to faculty shortages and other budgetary constraints. These changes as well as changes in the health care system had an impact on enrollments in schools of nursing. In 1995–1996, enrollments in basic baccalaureate programs fell for the first time in six years. Although the change was small, only 1 percent, it marked the end of six consecutive years of enrollment increases (Green, 1996).

Findings from the NLN's 1995 biennial census of nurse faculty show that the 10-year trend of decreasing number of full-time faculty continues unabated. In 1990–1991 alone, approximately 2292 prospective qualified baccalaureate degree students were turned away by nursing programs that did not have sufficient resources. "Admission filled" was cited by 70 percent of schools; faculty shortages were listed by more than 56 percent, followed by 54 percent with budgetary constraints, and 36 percent with insufficient clinical space (National League for Nursing, 1995d).

Compounding the problem of limited space in nursing programs in the United States is the fact that nursing faculty salaries have not kept pace with those in other settings. It is not uncommon for nursing faculty with advanced degrees and years of experience to see their former students begin their careers at higher salaries than they themselves make. This has created a situation of "faculty flight" from education to the higher-paying positions in direct practice settings.

This trend is expected to continue as colleges and universities fail to keep pace with the "market price" of nurses in direct practice today and more master's and doctorally prepared nurses reluctantly find it necessary to leave nursing education.

S U M M A R Y

The development of nursing education has been influenced by a number of factors leading to a diverse array of program offerings. First provided in hospitals, basic nursing education has evolved into three major types of programs: diploma, baccalaureate, and associate degree, each of which has positive and negative attributes. Alternatives such as baccalaureate degree programs for RNs, external degree programs, and accelerated options for postbaccalaureate students contribute to a complex RN education picture. Voluntary accreditation is designed to provide assurance of the quality of nursing education programs.

Programs in high demand in the mid-1990s include master's and doctoral preparation for nurses, specialty certification for advanced practice, and baccalaureate degree programs for RNs.

Lifelong learning through continuing education is considered essential for all professionals, particularly in practice-based disciplines such as nursing. The number of states mandating continuing education as a prerequisite for relicensure continues to increase.

The problem of reduced resources in nursing education may reach crisis proportions and weaker schools will close. This is a result of underfunding of higher education in general and, in particular, diminishing sources of federal funding for schools of nursing. Graduate programs in nursing are not preparing adequate numbers of nursing educators to meet current and future needs, and a severe faculty shortage is expected nationwide.

In response to changes in the health care system, national organizations have suggested changes in educational requirements and program emphases for the twenty-first century that will enable future RNs at all levels to meet the changing health care needs of society.

REVIEW AND DISCUSSION QUESTIONS

1. What factors did you use to determine which type of basic nursing program to enter?
2. How would you advise a high school student interested in nursing to go about selecting a program?
3. What characteristics would be needed for success in an external degree program?
4. Offering complete articulation of all levels of nursing education from practical nursing through doctoral study seems like a logical course of action. Should states mandate articulation? Why or why not?
5. Discuss the merits and drawbacks of mandatory continuing education from the viewpoints of both nurses and consumers of nursing care.
6. What unique contributions to nursing are possible by master's prepared nurses? By doctorally prepared nurses?
7. What content areas and skill preparation should be included in basic nursing programs to prepare graduates for the twenty-first century?

REFERENCES

Allen, J. (Ed.) (1990). *Consumer's guide to doctoral degree programs in nursing* (Publication No. 15–2293). New York: National League for Nursing.

American Association of Colleges of Nursing (1994). *Position statement. Certification and regulation of advanced practice nurses*. Washington, D.C.: Author.

American Association of Colleges of Nursing (1993). *Position statement. Nursing education's agenda for the 21st century*. Washington, D.C.: Author.

American Nurses Association (1979). *A case for baccalaureate preparation in nursing* (Publication No. NE-6 15M). Kansas City, MO: Author.

American Nurses Association (1965). *Educational preparation for nurse practitioners and assistants to nurses: A position paper* (Publication No. G-83). Kansas City, MO: Author.

American Nurses Credentialing Center (1995). *1995 certification catalog*. Washington, D.C.: Author.

Brown, E. L. (1948). *Nursing for the future*. New York: Russell Sage Foundation.

Christy, T. (1969). Portrait of a leader: M. Adelaide Nutting. *Nursing Outlook*, 17, 20–24.

Conley, V. (1973). *Curriculum and instruction in nursing*. Boston: Little, Brown.

Donahue, M. P. (1985). *Nursing: The finest art: An illustrated history*. St. Louis: C. V. Mosby.

Green, J. (1996). Nursing school enrollments drop. *AHA News*, 31(1), 4.

Kalisch, P., and Kalisch, B. (1995). *The advance of American nursing* (3rd ed.). Boston: Little, Brown.

Lysaught, J. (1970). *An abstract for action*. New York: McGraw-Hill.

Montag, M. (1951). *The education of nursing technicians*. New York: Putnam.

National League for Nursing (1995a). *Annual guide to graduate nursing education 1994–95* (Publication No. 19-2676). New York: Author.

National League for Nursing (1995b).

Emerging environment for nursing education and practice examined during two-year vision campaign. News from the National League for Nursing, May 11. New York: Author.

National League for Nursing (1995c). *NLN guide to undergraduate RN education* (3rd ed.) (Publication No. 41-2685). New York: Author.

National League for Nursing (1995d). *Nurse educators' findings from the RN and LPN faculty census* (Publication No. 19-6630). New York: Author.

National League for Nursing (1995e). *Nursing data review 1995* (Publication No. 19-2686). New York: Author.

National League for Nursing (1995f). *Nursing datasource 1995. Volume I—Trends in contemporary nursing education* (Publication No. 19-6649). New York: Author.

National League for Nursing (1995g). *Nursing datasource 1995. Volume II—Graduate education in nursing: Advanced practice nursing*. New York: Author.

National League for Nursing (1995h). *Profiles of the newly licensed nurse* (3rd ed.) (Publication No. 19-2700). New York: Author.

National League for Nursing (1995i). *State-approved schools of nursing LPN/LVN 1995* (Publication No. 19-2692). New York: Author.

National League for Nursing (1995j). *State-approved schools of nursing RN 1995* (Publication No. 19-2689). New York: Author.

National League for Nursing (1993). *A vision for nursing education*. New York: Author.

National League for Nursing (1992a). *Criteria and guidelines for the evaluation of baccalaureate and higher degree programs in nursing* (7th ed.) (Publication No. 15-2474). New York: Author.

National League for Nursing (1992b). *Criteria and guidelines for the evaluation of diploma programs in nursing* (8th ed.) (Publication No. 16-2444). New York: Author.

National League for Nursing (1992c). *Criteria and guidelines for the evaluation of practical nursing programs* (6th ed.) (Publication No. 38-2445). New York: Author.

National League for Nursing (1991). *Criteria and guidelines for the evaluation of associate degree programs in nursing* (7th ed.) (Publication No. 23-2439). New York: Author.

National League for Nursing (1990). *Policies and procedures of accreditation for programs in nursing education* (6th ed.) (Publication No. 18-1437). New York: Author.

National League for Nursing (1982). *Position statement on nursing roles: Scope and preparation*. New York: Author.

National League of Nursing Education (1934). *Nursing schools today and tomorrow*. New York: Author.

National League of Nursing Education (1937). *A curriculum guide for schools of nursing*. New York: Author.

Notter, L., and Spalding, E. (1976). *Professional nursing, foundations perspectives and relationships* (9th ed.). Philadelphia: J. B. Lippincott.

O'Neil, E. H. (1993). *Health professions education for the future: Schools in service to the nation*. San Francisco, CA: Pew Health Professions Commission.

Parietti, E. (1990). The development of doctoral education in nursing: A historical overview. In J. Allen (Ed.), *Consumer's guide to doctoral degree programs in nursing* (p. 1532) (Publication No. 15–2293). New York: National League for Nursing.

Rapson, M. (Ed.). (1987). *Collaboration for articulation: RN to BSN* (Publication No. 41–2182). New York: National League for Nursing.

Schwirian, P. (1984). Research on nursing students. In H. H. Werley and J. J. Fitzpatrick (Eds.), *Annual review of nursing research* (vol. 2) (pp. 211–262). New York: Springer.

U.S. Department of Health and Human Services (1990). *Seventh report to the president and congress on the status of health personnel in the United States*. Washington, D.C.: Author.

Wise, P. (Ed.) (1995). Annual CE survey: State and association/certifying boards CE requirements. *The Journal of Continuing Education in Nursing*, 26(1), 3–6.

CHAPTER

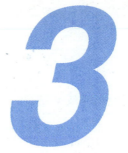

Cathy Campbell*

The Social Context for Nursing

OBJECTIVES
- Describe how individuals are socialized.
- Identify your own patterns of socialization and their effect on your personal development.
- Analyze the traditional roles of women and how these have affected the development of the nursing profession.
- Discuss social trends affecting the development of nursing as a profession.
- Explain the impact of the media on the image of nursing.
- Evaluate the continuing development of technology and the implications for nursing.
- Describe the causes of imbalances in supply and demand for nurses in the United States.

VOCABULARY

biomedical technology	information technology	role strain
caring technology	knowledge technology	sex role stereotypes
consumerism	nursing information	socialization
demographics	system	stereotypes
dominant culture	patient acuity	transcultural nursing
feminism	point of care technology	

Every profession is profoundly affected by the society it serves, and nursing is no exception. The social context has shaped nurses' attitudes, nursing practice, and the attitudes of the public toward nursing over the years. The social context also influences who chooses nursing as a career.

As you begin to read this chapter, think about what has drawn you into the profession of nursing. What is the story of your individual journey into nursing? One individual's story is found in Box 3–1. This nurse entered nursing over 20 years ago. Can you identify some of the social forces that influenced her career choice? Are any of these forces still operating today? What are some of the social

*The author wishes to acknowledge the contribution of Leslie B. Himot in the preparation of this chapter.

B O X 3 – 1
One Nurse's Journey into Nursing

"I was always interested in the sciences and did quite well in those subjects during my early years of school. In junior high I had an excellent biology teacher and thought I would like to be a biology teacher someday. In about the ninth grade, however, I questioned how I could combine my love of sciences and teaching with another goal—having a husband and children. The answer for me was to become a nurse. I believed that I could have the "best of both worlds." I wanted a career, but I also definitely wanted to get married and have children.

Another motivation was my realization that my mother had wanted to become a nurse and never did. I know I entered nursing because of an intense interest in sciences, teaching, and doing something that would help my future family. But I believe my mother's unfulfilled wish to become a nurse also entered into my career choice."

---

forces you are responding to as you enter or advance in nursing? Take a few minutes now to reflect on your own individual journey toward nursing.

Nurses need to understand how nursing is related to society as a whole. What impact does society have on the practice of nursing? Does the fact that nursing is a female-dominated profession have a bearing on the way the profession has developed? How have the women's movement and feminism influenced the practice of nursing? Since greater numbers of men are entering nursing, what issues face them, and how has society reacted to their increasing presence in a traditionally female profession? How do **demographics** (population trends) affect nursing? How does the public view nurses? Should this public image be changed? What causes periodic imbalances in supply and demand for nurses? These questions are explored in this chapter.

TRADITIONAL SOCIALIZATION OF WOMEN

Socialization is the process whereby values and expectations are transmitted from generation to generation. From birth, males and females are treated differently. Muff (1988a) asserts that:

> Little girls learn to be "feminine," meaning passive, dependent, affection-
> ate, emotional, and expressive. They learn that beauty and charm make
> one desirable to men, and that catching a man is the primary goal. Caring
> for him and his children is life's work. They learn, too, that the female role
> is less active, often less enjoyable, and certainly less valued than is the
> male role.

In Western society, women have generally been socialized to avoid risk-taking, to avoid conflict, and to acquiesce to authority. Traditionally, feminine attributes include an orientation toward security, peacekeeping, and submission (Muff, 1988b).

BOX 3–2
Common Sex Role Stereotypes of Women

Mother	**Iron Maiden**	**Superwoman**
Subrogates own needs	Is competitive vs. colla-	Demands perfection
Freely gives advice	borative	Won't delegate
Becomes the peacemaker	Possesses the ability to	Overcommits her time
Fosters dependence	"be in charge"	Assumes multiple roles
Is passive, wants recog-	Gives critical feedback	Feels isolated, not sup-
nition	Sets rigid interpersonal	ported
	boundaries	
	Can be unapproachable	

Reprinted with permission of Cummings, S. H. (1995). Attila the hun versus Attila the hen: Gender socialization of the American nurse. *Nursing Administration Quarterly,* 19(2), 25.

Women have been socialized to be self-sacrificing to parents, husbands, and children. When women subordinate their own needs for the sake of others, they can avoid dealing with unpleasantness and conflict. They also avoid the appearance of aggressiveness, for which assertive behavior has often been mistaken in the past (Muff, 1988b).

Stereotypes are prejudiced attitudes developed through interactions with family, friends, and others in an individual's social and cultural system. **Sex role stereotypes** deal with prejudiced ideas of how men and women should behave in a cultural group. Some common sex role stereotypes of women are summarized by Cummings (1995) in Box 3–2.

An outcome of this type of female socialization has been to prepare women for their primary allegiance to families, not to success in a career. The socialized female traits of dependency, passivity, and the need for approval unconsciously restrict women's choices in life to traditional family roles and certain "female" professions. Young girls have been encouraged to enter nursing because nursing was considered to be especially good training for marriage and motherhood (Muff, 1988a). This attitude was reflected by the nurse whose story appears in Box 3–1.

In the early days of modern nursing, the roles assigned to women were healer, caretaker, and nurturer, none of which was assigned high value by the larger society. The first formal schools of nursing in the United States were developed to attract "respectable women" into nursing, which could have added to nursing's value. By replacing untrained hospital "nurses" with students who worked in the hospital in return for room, board, and training, however, one powerless labor pool was simply exchanged for another. Hospitals have been described as patriarchal "families" with nurses as obedient "daughters" to administrator "daddies," helpful "wives" to physician "husbands," and loving "mothers" to patient "children" (Muff, 1988a).

For decades, middle-class American women were raised expecting to be supported financially by their husbands. This expectation freed them from the need to choose a profession that offered long-term financial security. They could make a career choice with a focus on their present needs while realizing that, with any luck at all, they would not always need to support themselves. They entered nursing with a "now-but-not-necessarily-forever" attitude. This affected both salary expectations and commitment to nursing as a career (Cummings, 1995).

Approximately 96.4 percent of nurses in the United States are women. For many reasons that are similar to other traditionally female occupations, such as teaching and social work, nursing has been historically plagued with low status, low pay, and general subordination to higher-status men. Nurses faced, and still face, a double challenge of being predominately female and operating within the stereotypic boundaries of a traditionally "female" profession (Moss, 1995).

NURSING, FEMINISM, AND THE WOMEN'S MOVEMENT

Nursing, **feminism,** and women's movements of the twentieth century have had an uneasy relationship. Contemporary feminists have often criticized nursing for failing to support women's movements. For example, the relatively young American Nurses Association (ANA) refused to endorse women's suffrage until 1915, although the fight for women's right to vote had been going on for the previous 40 years. Years later the more mature ANA chose not to endorse the passage of the Equal Rights Amendment (ERA) until the late 1970s because the ANA leadership believed that biological differences between men and women demanded special legislative attention that the more generic ERA did not address (Bunting and Campbell, 1990).

Nursing has been viewed by some feminists as a traditional and oppressive female occupation. There is some validity to this criticism because nurses have tended to build their own power bases on connections with governmental agencies and powerful, male-dominated professions such as medicine rather than on identification with other nurses and other women's groups (Bunting and Campbell, 1990).

What exactly is feminism? There are several types, but Gray's (1994) explanation is helpful: "The primary focus of feminisms is an examination of gender privilege, that is privilege that accrues or is denied because of one's biologically determined sexual characteristics" (p. 506). Gray further explained that feminisms value women, their experiences, knowledge, and ways of knowing in a **dominant culture** in which everyone lives, grows, and participates.

The women's movement that began in the 1960s had a profound effect on society that has both hurt and helped the nursing profession. As women of the 1960s and 1970s sought career opportunities beyond the traditional female ones of teaching and nursing, bright and able women who formerly might have become nurses pursued careers in accounting, architecture, engineering, computer science, and a variety of other fields. This meant that nursing faced more competition for students than it once did.

Although this hurt nursing temporarily, the pendulum has now begun to swing back as women realize how natural and good a "fit" nursing is for them. In the 1990s, when women can freely choose any professional field of study, many are again choosing nursing. Deans and directors of schools of nursing in the United States report that applications from women who were originally educated to be attorneys, computer programmers, accountants, and other "new" occupations are soaring. It seems that nursing's appeal is still strong for people who want to make a real difference in the lives of others.

The women's movement helped nursing by bringing economic issues such as low salaries and poor working conditions into the open. The movement provoked a conscious awareness that equality and autonomy for women were inherent rights, not privileges.

Nursing also benefited from the women's movement in more subtle ways. As nursing students were increasingly educated in colleges and universities, they were exposed to campus activism, protest, and organizations that were trying to effect change in the status of women. Learning informal lessons about power and how to bring about change has had a positive effect on modern students, who later use the lessons learned to improve the status of nursing.

Despite these positive effects, the nursing profession has been slow to internalize the women's movement message of self-determination and commitment. As mentioned earlier, many nurses have looked on nursing as a useful way to occupy themselves until marriage. To others, nursing was a "job" used to supplement the major breadwinner's income or pay for a family vacation, new car, or camp for the kids. Sometimes nurses worked only to tide the family over temporarily rough economic waters, returning to home and family when the family's financial situation improved. This "stepping in" and "stepping out" of the profession has meant that these nurses' energies and loyalties were split. The result is that nursing has not prospered as it might have if all of its members were committed to long-term careers.

It is unfortunate that many of the nearly 2.2 million registered nurses (RNs) have not fully accepted the necessity for long-term professional commitment, which not only enhances personal growth, but also strengthens the profession from within. Feminism and women's movements have helped nurses learn that they should be autonomous and assertive. With the firm commitment of its members to lifelong full participation, nursing can grow to its maximum potential, expand opportunities for its members, and ultimately contribute to the advancement of women and society at large.

Shea (1994) encouraged nurses to contribute to contemporary feminism in the following four areas (pp. 577–578):

1. . . . If each nurse shared her or his passionate conviction about feminism and nursing with one family member, one friend, one co-worker, and one community member, pretty soon the message would reach the powers that be, and various changes would take place. . . .
2. Nurses are getting ready to express themselves in public. Letters to the editor in professional journals and daily newspapers are on the increase. And nurses have stories to tell that the public wants and needs to hear. . . .
3. The need for good public role models is desperate. . . . The main vehicle for change in American society is television. . . . Nursing needs another "China Beach" series—updated and reflective of what nurses really do, and how they think and feel. . . . In order for these things to happen, some nurses will have to devote their full attention to "nonnursing things" such as writing scripts, performing on the stage, taking photographs, developing artwork, and making feature-length films and documentaries featuring nurses.

4. Nursing needs to care for its young. . . . Applying feminist principles, socialization into nursing has to change toward becoming a more empathic, nonhierarchial, mutually beneficial process. There must be tolerance of different learning styles and cultural values, reflecting the diversity of the population of nursing.

MEN IN NURSING

In 1992, 4.3 percent of practicing RNs in the United States were men. Enrollment of men in nursing schools had increased to 12 percent in 1994 (National League for Nursing, 1994). The male nurse, when compared with his female counterpart, is likely to be older, to be married, to have more education, and to choose nursing as a second career. Their motivations for entering nursing, however, are similar to those of their female counterparts. Most men enter nursing to help people (Villeneuve, 1994).

The American Assembly for Men in Nursing (AAMN) has developed a position statement on the role that gender should play in the nursing profession. Members of the AAMN believe that, "Every professional nurse position and every nursing educational opportunity shall be equally available to those meeting the entry qualifications regardless of gender" (Halloran and Welton, 1994, p. 690). The fact that the members of this organization thought this statement was necessary raises the question, "Have men in nursing suffered discrimination because of their gender?" Let us now examine how men have fared in a profession traditionally dominated by women.

Men are not new to the profession of nursing. They supplied much of the nursing care during the eleventh, twelfth, and thirteenth centuries. It was not until late in the nineteenth century that nursing became a predominately female profession.

Despite all the positive things she did, Florence Nightingale played a major role in excluding men from the profession by asserting that nursing was a female discipline. She worked hard to establish nursing as a worthy career for respectable women and largely ignored the historical contributions of men. She saw the male role as confined to supplying physical strength, such as lifting or moving patients, when needed.

The Industrial Revolution also influenced the exit of men from nursing. During those times, the accepted professions for men were science, technology, and business. Men chose medicine, and women chose nursing (Black and Germaine-Warner, 1995).

The first two schools of nursing for men were established in the late 1800s. They were the Mills School of Nursing for Men at New York's Bellevue Hospital and the McLean Asylum Training School. The purpose of these training programs was to prepare men for psychiatric nursing, a field that often required physical stamina and strength.

In 1901, the U.S. Congress created the Army Nurse Corps for female nurses only. The Navy Nurse Corps followed seven years later and was also restricted to women (Black and Germaine-Warner, 1995). Because of the lack of training programs and the gender restrictions placed on military nurses, it was difficult for men to enter nursing before World War II. Cummings (1995) reported that in 1941 only 68 of the 1303 schools of nursing accepted men.

After World War II, the GI bill helped to increase the number of male nursing students by providing funding for education. Military corpsmen entered nursing schools in large numbers, as they have following every major military conflict since. Nevertheless, as late as 1990, 8.3 percent of American baccalaureate nursing programs still had no male students (Villeneuve, 1995).

Why Men Enter Nursing

In a study conducted by Perkins and colleagues (1993), the top three reasons men entered the profession of nursing were job security, career opportunity, and job flexibility. These responses were followed closely by a desire to nurture and to contribute (Fig. 3–1). Traditionally, men tend to choose "aggressive" areas of nursing, such as intensive care units, cardiac care units, emergency departments, trauma units, flight nursing, or anesthesiology. These choices may also be due to a fear of being rejected in traditionally "feminine" areas of nursing, such as pediatric and obstetrical nursing (Boughn, 1994).

Men are frequently drawn to the technological aspects of acute care specialities and are challenged by the machines in those units. The typical dress in some areas may also affect the nursing choice of men. Nurses in acute care specialties typically wear "scrubs," and nurses in administrative and psychiatric settings wear street clothes. Scrubs or street clothes may be more acceptable to men than traditional white nursing uniforms.

Some men may look at nursing as a springboard to other professions. They may not stay in nursing long because of the low status and low pay (Williams,

FIGURE   3 – 1

Reasons men choose nursing and the number of respondents citing them (N = 146). (From: *Nursing & Health Care*, 4(1). Reprinted with permission. Copyright 1993 National League for Nursing.)

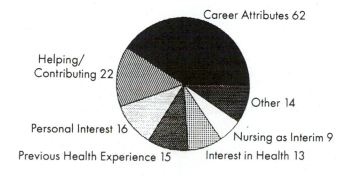

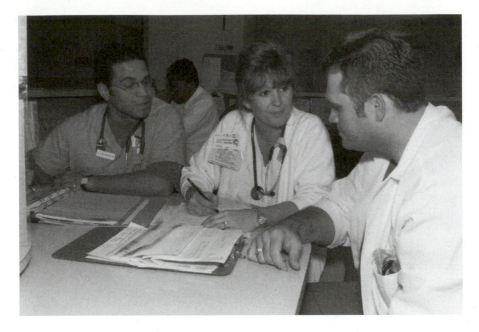

FIGURE 3 – 2
Male registered nurses are becoming more visible as their numbers increase. Photo by
Kelly Whalen.

1989). There are several issues facing the large number of men who do choose to
stay in nursing (Fig. 3–2). These men often feel **role strain,** which can be felt
by a person in a profession dominated by members of the opposite sex.

Attitudes Toward Men in Nursing

As mentioned earlier, in American society men interested in health care traditionally became physicians, whereas women became nurses. Men entering the
profession of nursing have crossed over gender lines, and their masculinity may
be questioned as a result. One negative assumption men in nursing encounter is
that all male nurses are homosexual. The pervasive homophobia in society and
the belief that nursing is strictly a feminine profession show some signs of changing; however, these attitudes are still pervasive enough to affect the decisions of
teenage boys making career choices (Villeneuve, 1994).

   Another issue men deal with is denial of the fact that men can be nurses. People commonly assume a man delivering health care is either a physician or a medical student. A male pediatric nurse commented (Williams, 1995, p. 68):

> It's very funny, working in pediatrics even today. I have 3-year-old pa-
> tients and I always introduce myself as, "I'm Bill, and I'm going to be your
> nurse." And they say, "You can't be a nurse." And I say, "Well, why?"
> [And they say,] "Well because you're a guy."

Male nursing students often face discrimination from practicing nurses, physicians, and the public. It is all too common for male students to find themselves unwelcome in prenatal clinics, delivery rooms, and other settings in which male physicians have free access.

One male obstetrician in a midsize southeastern community refused to allow a male nursing student in the delivery suite, explaining, "My patients are uncomfortable with a man in the room." The irony of one male health professional restricting the access of another male health professional student based on the student's gender did not escape the notice of the student. Unfortunately the nurse in charge of the unit chose not to advocate for the student, and the student's clinical instructor was unsuccessful in doing so. He had to transfer to a different clinical group in another hospital to complete his clinical objectives. This type of incident is not uncommon. Legal cases are being tried in the courts challenging these practices. Ketter (1994) interviewed a man involved in a recent court case who made the observation, "It makes no sense. Men doctors have been treating women for years. What's the difference if it's a doctor or a nurse?"

Williams (1995) discussed some of the "hidden advantages" for men in nursing. She claimed that men are preferred in hiring because of their strength and perceived potential for better leadership. The one exception is in the area of obstetrics and gynecology.

According to Williams, because of their "renegade status" in a female-dominated profession, men are given more respect and encouraged to increase their education and enter the most prestigious specializations. She reported that men tend to earn more money than their female counterparts in nursing and that married male nurses are viewed as the traditional breadwinners of their families and are considered more permanent, reliable employees. Physicians tend to treat male nurses better, and this, in turn, leads to greater promotions for male nurses. An exception is some older male physicians who believe men should not be nurses at all (Williams, 1989).

How can the presence of men in nursing help women? Some women believe men might help them become more assertive. A male nurse commented on what will have to happen for nursing to gain more respect (Williams, 1989, p. 126):

> Women will have to fight and stick up for who they are and what they do, and women do not do that. So many times women in nursing do not support each other, for one thing; more likely they tear each other apart. . . . I don't think women are strong enough, they're not vocal enough, they're not demanding enough. I'm sure that men are more demanding and will be over the years.

Another male nurse commented on the lack of career commitment of female nurses (Williams, 1989, p. 127):

> The reason I feel career conditions in nursing are so poor is because from the hospital's standpoint, nurses are short term employees. They come and go. They have babies. They change careers. For whatever individual reason, they're not there long enough to treat them as permanent employees. . . . Until women as a group treat it [nursing] as a career and insist upon equal benefits as they have in other careers, it's going to stay as it is.

Research by Cyr (1992) concluded that most female nurses thought of nursing as a "job." Male nurses tended to view nursing as a "professional career."

Encouraging Men to Enter Nursing

What can be done to attract more men to nursing? Boughn (1994, p. 31) recommends the following strategies:

1. Correcting public misconceptions about males' capacity for doing "caring work" such as nursing.
2. Re-educating high school guidance counselors to target appropriate populations for the rigors of nursing education and nursing practice not previously considered, such as academically capable male students.
3. Involving male nursing students in recruitment efforts and making them visible in recruitment materials.
4. Encouraging national occupation publications to present nonsexist information regarding career options for males.
5. Encouraging professional journals and other literature to portray male nurses in advertisements depicting nurses.

One thing is certain: The increasing number of men in nursing will make the profession different. This should be seen as a positive trend, for both feminine and masculine qualities and abilities are needed to treat whole human beings.

IMAGE OF NURSING

When you think of *nurse*, what image comes to mind? Is it Florence Nightingale floating down the stairs carrying her lamp to attend the wounded soldiers? Perhaps you remember a "get well" card depicting an unattractive woman carrying a bedpan under one arm and a huge hypodermic needle in the other hand? Or do you remember seeing soap opera nurses with big, blond hair and short, tight white dresses going about their work in high-heeled shoes? The image of nursing has been, and continues to be, colorfully presented and distorted in all forms of expression in society.

Why is image so important? First impressions say a lot about a particular group of people. These perceptions affect attitudes toward the profession of nursing. According to studies of public opinion, the public views nurses as nurturant and concerned for others but only moderately well educated. In the public's view, physicians cure diseases, whereas nurses are nice and caring (Campbell-Heider, Hart, and Bergren, 1994).

One problem the public has in identifying nurses is that it is difficult to know exactly who the RNs are any longer. Gone are the traditional white caps and uniforms:

> The nurse of today in many situations is unidentifiable by uniform. The
> stethoscope around the neck or tucked in a pocket serves to some degree as

identification. In most regions of the country, caps are no longer worn and school pins have been replaced by hospital identification badges that may or may not include full names and titles (Mangum, 1994, p. 54).

Many nurses, especially with the entry of more men into the profession, are glad to see the demise of the traditional caps and white uniforms. Perhaps uniforms projected a stereotypic image rather than a realistic perception of nurses as autonomous providers with a high level of education and scientific expertise (Campbell-Heider et al, 1994). Uniforms, however, did help identify RNs and differentiate them from the ever-increasing numbers of nonnursing assistive personnel.

Another area of concern for the image of nursing is the use of language and how health professionals address each other. Campbell-Heider and associates speak to this issue by noting that nurses often use their first names with patients, whereas physicians use their professional titles. These authors believe that this practice reinforces sex role stereotypes and promotes social distance and hierarchical relations between the two disciplines. If formal titles are used for physicians, they should be used for nurses. By using parallel styles of addressing each other, interdependence and mutual respect would be fostered. Campbell-Heider and associates (1994) conclude by stating, "Attention to personal symbols of language and dress advance the actuality and image of the professional nurse. Those who respect themselves will convey this attitude to their colleagues and patients" (p. 228).

Nurses cannot and should not attribute their image problems to any other group, including physicians. The nursing profession has major responsibility for improving its own image. Black and Germaine-Warner (1995) suggested a variety of things nurses can do, including recognizing that each nurse should work to improve nursing's image, participating in professional organizations, becoming politically active, writing for local media, providing technical assistance to the media, taking advantage of public speaking opportunities, and sharing positive aspects of nursing with others.

Influence of the Media on Nursing's Image

The influence of the media's portrayals of nurses is extremely powerful, and this causes great concern for nursing because the image portrayed has often been negative and demeaning.

Muff (1988b) identified six major nursing stereotypes commonly portrayed by the media:

- Angel of mercy
- Handmaiden to the physician
- Woman in white
- Sex symbol/idiot
- Battle-ax
- Torturer

Muff pointed out that almost all media depict nurses as females. They are generally portrayed as unintelligent women in traditional, even obsolete, roles. One result of this misrepresentation of nurses in the media is probably a negative impact on the recruitment of future nurses (Muff, 1988b).

Aber and Hawkins (1992) studied the portrayal of nurses in advertisements in medical and nursing journals. They found that in both profession's journals, nurses were portrayed in ways that were stereotypical and demeaning, wearing attire long outdated, as sex objects, and as handmaidens to physicians. They concluded their report with the following thoughts (p. 293):

> If we continue to accept an image of nurses as portrayed in our print media as dependent, passive and minor figures in the health care system, then that is what we will continue to be. If we demand that the image be changed to that of active participants in the delivery of care, as independent and interdependent professionals and as major figures in the health care drama, then that is what we will become.

From 1988–1991, a grant from the Pew Charitable Trusts provided support for an organization known as Nurses of America (NOA). NOA was sponsored by the four Quad-Council Organizations: the American Association of Colleges of Nursing (AACN), the ANA, the American Organization of Nurse Executives (AONE), and the National League for Nursing (NLN). NOA initiated a multimedia project designed to inform the public, legislators, and the business community about the contributions of contemporary nursing and nursing practice in the delivery of high-quality, cost-effective health care. NOA published three *Media Watch* newsletters to over 200,000 readers.

NOA also sponsored a 1991 study entitled "Who Counts and Who Doesn't in News Coverage of Health Care." The study found that nurses were "virtually silent" as sources of health care news. Even though nurses represented the largest profession in the health care system, persons in every other "occupational" category, out of 12 categories, were quoted more frequently than nurses about health care issues. Following physicians, the most frequently quoted persons were government officials, business people, patients, family members, other white-collar health professionals, and nonprofessional hospital workers.

According to the NOA report, this study has several implications for the nursing profession (Nurses of America, 1991, p. 17):

> In terms of nursing, it is difficult for a group to have influence in the development of public policy and the allocation of resources unless it can be seen and heard as part of the public discussion. The role of nursing as a contributor to the health care system is limited if the press, for whatever reason, does not consider nursing a legitimate or credible source or subject.

Another study of interest was a comparative analysis of nurse and physician characters in the entertainment media, made by Kalisch and Kalisch (1986). This study revealed that while the role of physicians was presented in an exaggerated, idealistic, and heroic light, "media nurses" were shown in substantially less desired roles (p. 185):

Even basic intelligence, rationality, problem-solving abilities and clinical skills are absent in most nurse portrayals. Nurse characters are presented as generally unimportant in health care, largely occupying the background rather than playing an instrumental role in health care. Media nurses are viewed less positively than physicians by other characters, and show little commitment to their careers. The central and diverse role the nurse actually plays in the delivery of health care to the American public is virtually absent in the entertainment media.

The Kalischs asserted that these images of nurses not only affect consumers' opinions of nurses, but also impact the images nurses hold of themselves. They called for an improvement in the manner in which nurses are portrayed in the media "even if this does require a diminishment of the intensity of the halo that the media physician has worn in recent decades" (p. 193).

Are nurses still being portrayed negatively in current popular television shows? There are mixed reviews, according to Mikulencak (1995), who wrote that nurses either love or hate television medical dramas such as "ER" and "Chicago Hope." These shows have large audiences. A Neilsen survey in the *Wall Street Journal* on January 5, 1996, reported that "ER" ranked first in the top 10 prime-time programs with a 30 percent share of the viewing audience. This means that 30 percent of all switched-on sets during that Neilsen Media Research survey period were tuned to "ER."

According to Buresh and Gordon (1995), "ER" received high positive reviews from nurses themselves. This was probably due to the fact that the past president of the Emergency Nurses Association, consisting of 24,000 members, acted as a significant advisor for the producers of "ER." She conveyed feedback from nurses, suggested story ideas, and helped construct realistic scenarios.

This type of cooperation between nurses and television producers is new. In the recent past, organized nursing has struggled with television producers over the image being portrayed. It was the unified power of nurses that launched a successful campaign to eliminate the television program "The Nightingales" in the late 1980s. This program outraged nurses by its depiction of nursing students as sex objects in demeaning situations. Pressure, in the form of a letter-writing campaign by nurses, was coordinated by NOA. This led the producers of this series to cancel the short-lived program.

Another 1980s television series, "China Beach," depicted nurses as intelligent, autonomous health professionals. This series, which received critical acclaim, was an award-winning drama about nurses in Vietnam. The program was widely praised by nursing groups, and its star became a media spokesperson and advocate for nursing. Unfortunately the series was canceled, and a letter-writing campaign by nurses calling for the renewal of the series was unsuccessful.

What can individuals do to improve the image of nursing portrayed in the media? Box 3–3 presents a checklist for monitoring media images of nurses and nursing. Use this checklist as you view television, watch movies, read books and newspapers, and look at advertisements. Then take action by writing those responsible for the negative nursing images. Nurses themselves must reinforce the positive images of nursing and, more importantly, speak out against the negative ones.

Prominence in the Plot
1. Are nurse characters seen in leading or supportive roles?
2. Are nurse characters shown taking an active part in the proceedings or are they shown primarily in the background (handing instruments, carrying trays, pushing wheelchairs)?
3. To what extent are nurse characters shown in professional roles, engaged in nursing practice?
4. Is it nurse characters or other characters who provide the actual nursing care?
5. In scenes with nonnurse professionals (physicians, hospital administrators), who does most of the talking?

Demographics
6. Does the portrayal show that men as well as women may aspire to a career in nursing?
7. Are nurse characters shown to be of varying ages?
8. Are some nurse characters single and others married?

Personality Traits
9. Are nurse characters portrayed as:

a. intelligent	e. sophisticated	i. nurturant
b. rational	f. problem solvers	j. empathic
c. confident	g. assertive	k. sincere
d. ambitious	h. powerful	l. kind

10. If other health care providers are included in the program, what differences are seen in their personality traits as compared with nurse characters?
11. When nurse characters exhibit the personality traits 9a through 9h listed above, do such portrayals show them to be abnormal in some way?

Primary Values
12. Do nurse characters exhibit values for:
    a. service to others, humanism   b. scholarship, achievement
13. If other health care providers are included in the program, what differences are seen in their primary values as compared with nurse characters?
14. When nurse characters exhibit the primary values of scholarship and achievement, do such portrayals show them to be abnormal in some way?

Sex Objects
15. Are nurse characters portrayed as sex objects?
16. Are nurse characters referred to in sexually demeaning terms?
17. Are nurse characters presented as appealing because of their physical attractiveness or cuteness as opposed to their intellectual capacity, professional commitment, or skill?

Role of the Nurse
18. Is the profession of nursing shown to be an attractive and fulfilling long-term career?
19. Is the work of the nurse characters shown to be creative and exciting?

Career Orientation
20. How important is the career of nursing to the nurse character portrayed?
21. How does this compare with other professionals depicted in the program?

(continued)

BOX 3-3 *(Continued)*

Professional Competence
22. Are nurse characters praised for their professional capabilities by other characters?
23. Do nurse characters praise other professionals?
24. Do nurse characters exhibit autonomous judgment in professional matters?
25. Is there a gratuitous message that a nurse's role in health care is a supportive rather than central one?
26. Do nurse characters positively influence patient/family welfare?
27. Are nurse characters shown harming or acting to the detriment of patients?
28. How does the professional competence of nurse characters compare with the professional competence of other health care providers?
29. When nurse characters exhibit professional competence, are they shown to be abnormal in some way?

Education
30. Who actually teaches the nursing students?
31. Who appears to be in charge of nursing education?
32. Is there evidence that the practice of nursing requires special knowledge and skills?
33. What is actually taught to nursing students?

Administration
34. Are any roles filled by nurse administrators or managers or are all nurse characters shown as staff nurses or students?
35. Is there evidence of an administrative hierarchy in nursing or are nurses shown answering to physicians or hospital administrators?
36. Are nurse characters shown turning to other nurses for assistance or are they depicted as relying on a physician or other character (generally male) for guidance, strength, or rescuing?

Overall Assessment and Comments
37. Overall, is this a positive or negative portrayal of nursing? Why or why not?

From *The Changing Image of the Nurse* by P. A. Kalisch. Copyright (©) 1987 by Addison-Wesley Publishing Company. Reprinted by permission.

GRAYING OF AMERICA

In 1990, there were approximately 32 million people 65 years of age or older in the United States. They represented 12.5 percent of the total population. There were 10,000 men and 35,000 women in 1992 over the age of 100 in the United States (U.S. Bureau of the Census, unpublished data). Demographic projections estimate that the proportion of elderly will grow rapidly in the next few decades. By the year 2030, there will be about 65 million older Americans. This phenomenon is sometimes referred to as "the graying of America."

People over 65 have fewer years of schooling and are more likely to be poor, widowed, female, living alone, and suffering from chronic disease than are younger people. As a consequence, the elderly use a disproportionately higher share of health services than other age groups.

The oldest "baby boomers," those Americans born between 1946 and 1964, will create a bulge in the aging population between the years 2010 and 2030. As these postwar babies age, their large numbers are expected to create an additional strain on the health care system. This graying of America will have a profound impact on the health care system and the nursing profession, which will stretch our already-stressed capacity to provide adequate medical and nursing care.

CONSUMER MOVEMENT

There has been a movement by consumers to make the health care system more accountable for its actions. The American public, fueled by the principles of **consumerism,** criticized the dehumanization of health care. This led to the development in 1972 of the American Hospital Association's (AHA) document "A Patient's Bill of Rights," which guaranteed certain rights and privileges to every hospitalized patient. "A Patient's Bill of Rights" was revised in 1992 (Box 3–4).

Many people believe the AHA document was the first formal declaration of its kind. A little known fact is that in 1959, 14 years before the AHA action, the NLN generated a statement about patients' rights. Until the AHA's "A Patient's Bill of Rights" was published, however, the prevailing attitude in health care was that providers knew best and good patients simply followed directions without asking questions.

The rise of consumerism in health care led to the involvement of consumers in pressing Congress for legislation protecting the public from inadequate care, experimental drugs, poor nutrition, and many other health-related issues. Consumer groups have demanded controls on spiraling health care costs and gained participation on boards of health planning agencies, accrediting bodies, and professional licensing boards. Most state boards of nursing have at least one consumer member.

The emphasis on consumerism is enhanced by the development of community partnerships designed to address health-related issues of concern to citizens. Farley (1994) stated that community partnerships are an outgrowth of an attempt to shift power from health professionals to citizens. The goal of community partnerships is not to eliminate all problems; the goal is to focus the community's energies toward those health-related problems that they are willing to work together to solve. Citizens in every community must be involved in their own health care decisions.

Nurses can play an instrumental role in taking the decision making closer to the consumer. Fagin and Binder (1994) pointed out that the traditional physician-patient relationship has been a dominant-subordinate one, and the role of consumers in the health care system has been a subordinate, passive role.

To change this traditional relationship, consumers must actively participate in the health care system, actively be responsible for their own health maintenance, and actively demand high quality and cost-effectiveness. Fagin and Binder (1994) point out that this is the nursing model of care. For change to occur, a shift in the locus of control in health matters away from the physician and to the consumer must occur. This means the development of personal accountability for one's health and medical choices. The authors further assert that (p. 458):

BOX 3 – 4
A Patient's Bill of Rights

Bill of Rights*

1. The patient has the right to considerate and respectful care.
2. The patient has the right to and is encouraged to obtain from physicians and other direct caregivers relevant, current, and understandable information concerning diagnosis, treatment, and prognosis.

   Except in emergencies when the patient lacks decision-making capacity and the need for treatment is urgent, the patient is entitled to the opportunity to discuss and request information related to the specific procedures and/or treatments, the risks involved, the possible length of recuperation, and the medically reasonable alternatives and their accompanying risks and benefits.

   Patients have the right to know the identity of physicians, nurses, and others involved in their care, as well as when those involved are students, residents, or other trainees. The patient also has the right to know the immediate and long-term financial implications of treatment choices, insofar as they are known.
3. The patient has the right to make decisions about the plan of care prior to and during the course of treatment and to refuse a recommended treatment or plan of care to the extent permitted by law and hospital policy and to be informed of the medical consequences of this action. In case of such refusal, the patient is entitled to other appropriate care and services that the hospital provides or transfer to another hospital. The hospital should notify patients of any policy that might affect patient choice within the institution.
4. The patient has the right to have an advance directive (such as a living will, health care proxy, or durable power of attorney for health care) concerning treatment or designating a surrogate decision maker with the expectation that the hospital will honor the intent of that directive to the extent permitted by law and hospital policy.

   Health care institutions must advise patients of their rights under state law and hospital policy to make informed medical choices, ask if the patient has an advance directive, and include that information in patient records. The patient has the right to timely information about hospital policy that may limit its ability to implement fully a legally valid advance directive.
5. The patient has the right to every consideration of privacy. Case discussion, consultation, examination, and treatment should be conducted so as to protect each patient's privacy.
6. The patient has the right to expect that all communications and records pertaining to his/her care will be treated as confidential by the hospital, except in cases such as suspected abuse and public health hazards when reporting is permitted or required by law. The patient has the right to expect that the hospital will emphasize the confidentiality of this information when it releases it to any other parties entitled to review information in these records.
7. The patient has the right to review the records pertaining to his/her medical care and to have the information explained or interpreted as necessary, except when restricted by law.
8. The patient has the right to expect that, within its capacity and policies, a hospital will make reasonable response to the request of a patient

(continued)

BOX 3 – 4 (Continued)
A Patient's Bill of Rights

---

for appropriate and medically indicated care and services. The hospital must provide evaluation, service, and/or referral as indicated by the urgency of the case. When medically appropriate and legally permissible, or when a patient has so requested, a patient may be transferred to another facility. The institution to which the patient is to be transferred must first have accepted the patient for transfer. The patient must also have the benefit of complete information and explanation concerning the need for, risks, benefits, and alternatives to such a transfer.

9. The patient has the right to ask and be informed of the existence of business relationships among the hospital, educational institutions, other health care providers, or payers that may influence the patient's treatment and care.

10. The patient has the right to consent to or decline to participate in proposed research studies or human experimentation affecting care and treatment or requiring direct patient involvement, and to have those studies fully explained prior to consent. A patient who declines to participate in research or experimentation is entitled to the most effective care that the hospital can otherwise provide.

11. The patient has the right to expect reasonable continuity of care when appropriate and to be informed by physicians and other caregivers of available and realistic patient care options when hospital care is no longer appropriate.

12. The patient has the right to be informed of hospital policies and practices that relate to patient care, treatment, and responsibilities. The patient has the right to be informed of available resources for resolving disputes, grievances, and conflicts, such as ethics committees, patient representatives, or other mechanisms available in the institution. The patient has the right to be informed of the hospital's charges for services and available payment methods.

A Patient's Bill of Rights was first adopted by the American Hospital Association in 1973. This revision was approved by the AHA Board of Trustees on October 21, 1992.

*These rights can be exercised on the patient's behalf by a designated surrogate or proxy decision maker if the patient lacks decision-making capacity, is legally incompetent, or is a minor.

The time is ripe for transformation in the health care system that will bring consumers into the fold as equals in the delivery of health care and leaders in the promotion of their own care. It will be up to nurses and others to couple health promotion efforts and traditional public health messages with a campaign to empower consumers within the delivery system and expose the mythology of enforced passivity that many Americans believe is endemic to receiving health services. So far only nurses have stepped forward to promote such changes in the delivery of health care.

MULTICULTURALISM IN NURSING

Since its founding, the United States has been a melting pot of people from many cultures. At one time, people new to the United States were anxious to become assimilated and assumed American names, dress, manners, and ways as soon as possible to "fit in." This is no longer the case. A more accurate description would be to call the United States a "chunky stew" (Ahmann, 1994) or a "salad bowl" (Johnson, 1994). Instead of blending together, as in a melting pot, individuals from other countries are increasingly appreciated for the uniqueness and flavor each person brings with them. This is the definition of multiculturalism, and because of it, nurses need to develop a sensitivity to and appreciation of the differences among cultures.

The population of most ethnic groups in the United States is growing. In 1980, the total white population was 188,372,000, whereas in 1990, it was 199,686,000. This represented an increase of 6 percent. The population of African-Americans in 1980 was 26,495,000, which had increased to 29,986,000 by 1990. This represented an increase of 13.2 percent. The Hispanic population totaled 14,609,000 in 1980 and grew to 22,354,000 in 1990, representing a 53 percent increase. The Native American population was 1,420,000 in 1980, and by 1990 that number had increased to 1,959,000, a 37.9 percent increase (U.S. Bureau of Census, 1992). By the year 2000, more than one-quarter of the U.S. population is expected to consist of ethnic minorities. By the year 2080, minorities will compose 51.1 percent of the total population (Andrews, 1992). Clearly the concept of a white-dominated culture is in the process of radical change.

How well are racial minorities represented in the nursing profession? Despite dramatic increases in the minority population, in 1994 minority nurses represented only 10 percent of all RNs. This 10 percent was comprised of 4 percent African-Americans, 3.4 percent Asian/Pacific Islanders, 1.4 percent Hispanics, 0.4 percent American Indian/Alaskan Natives, and 0.8 percent others (U.S. Department of Health and Human Services, 1994). As shown in Figure 3–3, the NLN (1994) reported that the percentage of minority students enrolled in basic RN programs decreased slightly from 15.8 percent in 1991 to 15.4 percent in 1992. To address the needs of a more culturally diverse society, nursing must increase its recruitment and retention of minority students.

What is nursing doing to respond to the increasing cultural diversity? The response actually began in 1955, when Dr. Madeleine Leininger, a visionary nurse sociologist, founded the field of **transcultural nursing.** She defined transcultural nursing as a:

> [H]umanistic and scientific area of formal study and practice in nursing which is focused upon differences and similarities among cultures with respect to human care, health (or well-being), and illness based upon the people's cultural values, beliefs, and practices. . . . [Nurses] use this knowledge to provide culturally specific or culturally congruent nursing care to people (Leininger, 1991, p. 60).

The Transcultural Nursing Society was legally incorporated in 1981, and the official semiannual publication of the *Journal of Transcultural Nursing* began in 1989. In 1993, a resolution by the ANA House of Delegates was adopted to

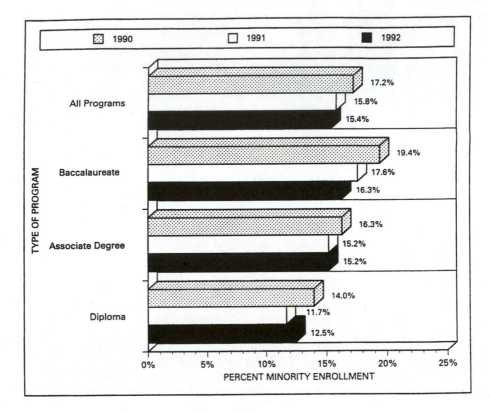

FIGURE 3-3
Minority students in basic RN programs: 1990–1992. (National League for Nursing (1994). *Nursing data review 1994* (p. 21). New York: Author.)

identify and determine strategies to promote diverse and multicultural nursing in the workforce (Kirkpatrick and Deloughery, 1995).

Leininger advocated that nurses perform cultural assessments on patients to determine their culturally specific needs. What is meant by a cultural assessment? When Toni Tripp-Reimer, RN, PhD, was asked about her views on caring for patients from other cultures, she stated (Villaire, 1994, p. 138):

> I think we often make cultural assessment a mysterious process when, in fact, it really is merely asking people their preferences, what they think, who we should talk to in making a decision, because family decision-making patterns and lines of authority are important, and they do differ.

Examples of nurses responding to culturally based challenges in a variety of situations are presented in Box 3–5.

Beginning in the early 1970s, schools of nursing began including cultural concepts as an integral part of their curricula. Increasing numbers of universities and colleges offered graduate programs in transcultural, cross-cultural, and in-

---

BOX 3-5
Culturally Based Care: Case Examples

Example 1

An emergency department nurse provided wound care for a 3-year-old Hispanic child, with Spanish-speaking parents and no insurance. Using her minimal Spanish vocabulary, the nurse asked about the family's physician and found they had none; the child had no immunizations. The nurse contacted a community agency to locate the names of Spanish-speaking pediatricians for the family and a Spanish-speaking social worker who could help the family with the financial aspects of medical care.

Example 2

The head nurse on a pediatric unit recognized that the unit was seeing an increasing number of recent immigrants from Indochina. The nurse arranged for community leaders from the immigrant community to provide in-service training for the unit nurses about common health beliefs and practices.

Example 3

A girl from Haiti was admitted to a children's hospital for a diagnostic workup and subsequent treatment related to a rare disorder. The head nurse assigned a primary nurse who spoke some French. During the girl's hospital stay, the nurse learned Creole, the girl's own language, and posted lists of common vocabulary on the girl's wall so that other staff could attempt communication as well.

Example 4

A clinic nurse worked with a first-generation Korean family with a disabled child. The nurse wanted to develop an intervention plan with the family. She began dialogue with the family by asking how families with similar children care for their children in Korea.

Adapted from *Pediatric Nursing*, 1994, Volume 20, Number 3, p. 322, 324. Reprinted with permission of the publisher, Jannetti Publications, Inc., East Holly Avenue Box 56, Pitman, NJ 08071-0056; Phone (609) 256-2300; Fax (609) 589-7463

---

ternational nursing. In 1988, the Transcultural Nursing Society began certifying nurses in transcultural nursing. By oral and written examinations and evaluation of the applicant's education background and working experiences, a qualified nurse can become a Certified Transcultural Nurse (CTN) (Andrews, 1992).

The question often arises, "Can a nonminority nurse effectively practice in transcultural settings?" According to Giger and colleagues (1994), this is definitely possible, but they insist that a structured formal course of study in transcultural nursing is necessary. This coursework helps nurses to develop the "learned objectivity" and sensitivity needed to give culturally appropriate care, not only within the United States, but also on an international level.

IMPACT OF TECHNOLOGICAL ADVANCES ON NURSING

Technological advances have had a major effect on the practice of nursing. Between 1953 and 1979, medical specialization was increasingly supported by advances in technology, and the hospital business grew into a major technologically based industry. As medicine was transformed by technology, so was the practice of nursing transformed as nurses assumed many of the responsibilities formerly performed by physicians.

Thompson and co-workers (1994) grouped health care technology into three major categories: biomedical, information, and knowledge. **Biomedical technology** involves complex machines or implantable devices used in patient care settings. This form of technology impacted nursing practice because nurses often assume responsibility for monitoring the data generated from these machines and for assessing the safety and effectiveness of the equipment itself.

Information technology refers to hardware and software used to manage and process information. Nurses assumed much of the responsibility for data entry and retrieval with the advent of this technology. Simpson (1992 p. 28) described a **nursing information system** as a:

> . . . [s]oftware system that automates the nursing process, from assessment to evaluation, including patient care documentation. It also includes a means to manage the data necessary for the delivery of patient care, e.g., patient classification, staffing, scheduling and costs. The system can be either a stand-alone system or a sub-system of a larger hospital information system.

In a survey conducted by Simpson, 37 (29 percent) of 129 chief nurses reported that their nursing information systems had bedside capabilities. This means that nurses can enter data about the patient directly from the bedside. Some of the advantages of this **point of care technology** include (1) improvement in data accuracy and timeliness of documentation, (2) increase in nursing productivity because an electronic chart is always available for ready access; and (3) easy retrieval of patient clinical information (Happ, 1994).

Knowledge technology is described as a technology of the mind. It involves the use of computer systems to transform information into knowledge and to generate new knowledge. Through the creation of "expert systems," this form of technology assists nurses with clinical judgments about patient management problems in the future. Deciding what expert knowledge to enter in these systems for clinical decision making, however, remains a challenge for nursing (Thompson, Amos, and Graves, 1994).

With so many kinds of technology, one might wonder, "Where is the patient?" One of the most widely debated issues in nursing is "high-tech" versus "high-touch" nursing. Technological advances now allow nurses to monitor their patients' conditions on computer screens at the nurses' station. Without even entering the patient's room, nurses can gather large amounts of information and make nursing decisions based on that information. Sometimes nurses seem to pay more attention to machines than to patients. They must actively guard against ignoring patients' needs for human interaction as a result of technological advances (Fig. 3–4). According to McConnell and Murphy (1990), nurses can be viewed as the "liaison between the machines" and their patients. These authors address the importance of technology in nursing by stating (p. 334):

> Nurses' knowledgeable use of technology, regardless of its sophistication, is imperative. But are nurses aware of the many opportunities being opened?

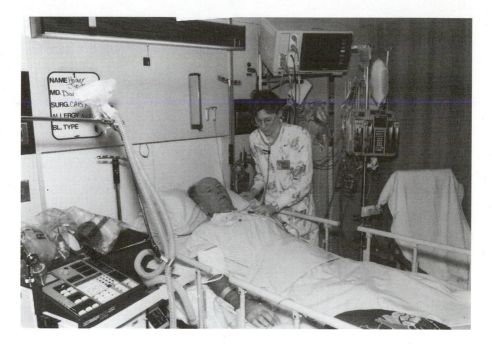

FIGURE   3–4
Nurses in high-tech environments such as this coronary care unit must remember that the patient also needs the human touch. Photo by Kelly Whalen.

> Do nurses passively accept technology or actively shape it? Do they 'react' to the transfer of technology or do they 'act' to ensure that technology and medical device use is 'appropriate'?

These are questions that bear thoughtful consideration by nurses.

Locsin (1995) described a model of **caring technology** in nursing. Technology and caring coexist in nursing practice today, and Locsin's model is an attempt to explain the interconnectedness of technology and nursing. Successfully combining technology and caring requires sensitivity to patients' physical, emotional, and spiritual needs.

The high-technology environment encountered in hospitals is now moving into the home as health care becomes more community-based. Technology can be viewed either as a "strategic opportunity" or a "strategic threat" according to Simpson (1993). His description of an innovative technological intervention that a nurse, Patricia Brennan, turned into a caring opportunity is found in Box 3–6.

IMBALANCE IN SUPPLY AND DEMAND FOR NURSES

There is nothing new about periodic imbalances between the number of nurses working and available nursing positions. Society pays far more attention to nurs-

---

BOX 3–6
Combining Technology and Caring

Patricia Brennan, PhD, RN, FAAN, associate professor of nursing and systems engineering at the Frances Payne Bolton School of Nursing at Case Western Reserve University developed a network that allowed AIDS patients and Alzheimer's disease patient caregivers to communicate with each other and their medical center. Not only did this lead to tremendous participation and acceptance, but also the 24-hour access to electronic information and support was comforting for patients facing chronic illnesses. The network was also extremely effective in educating pa-

tients about potential clinical problems. In this case, technology was used strategically to re-engineer service delivery, and not the other way around. This is as it should be. Whole new worlds can open as nursing's ability to deliver basic support, contact, and education to home-based patients is increased dramatically.

Modified with permission of Simpson, R. L. (1993). If you don't read this, you're missing out. Reproduced/adapted with permission from the September, 1993 issue of *Nursing Management*, © Springhouse Corporation.

---

ing shortages than to oversupply situations, however, because the welfare of the general public is affected more by shortages.

The generic term *nursing shortage* is misleading because actual shortages are usually confined to institutional settings such as hospitals and nursing homes. Since World War II, hospitals have been plagued with periodic nursing shortages (Abdellah, 1990). Causes of shortages may be seen as either external or internal. Internal causes include low salaries, long hours, and much responsibility with little authority. External causes include increasing demand for health care, the increasing age of the American population, and greater **patient acuity** (degree of illness) of hospitalized patients.

In the past, each time a shortage of RNs became acute, two solutions were tried: increase the supply of nurses, and create a new worker to supplement the number of nurses. Practical nursing programs, which produce graduates in only one year, were created to meet civilian and military needs of the United States during World War II. The nursing shortage of the 1950s stimulated a desire to shorten basic RN programs, and two-year associate degree programs were the result. In the 1960s, shortages led to the creation of the unit-manager role whose job was to take over certain tasks to relieve nurses, who could then concentrate on providing patient care. The 1970s produced other new workers, such as emergency medical technicians (EMTs), physician's assistants, respiratory therapists, and others who took on various aspects of patient care formerly performed by nurses. The shortage of the late 1980s witnessed a proposal by the American Medical Association to create yet another "nurse extender" called the *registered care technician*. Tired of seeing "solutions" to the nursing shortage that failed to address the real issues of low salaries and poor working conditions, nurses responded quickly and negatively, and that idea has been dropped. The registered care technician initiative is discussed more in Chapter 4.

The anticipated nursing shortage of the late 1990s will be different from previous ones and will result from a combination of internal and external factors.

One external factor is an increased demand for nurses because of the aging population. Both the population in general and RNs themselves are getting older. The average age of RNs in 1992 was 43 years. As these nurses retire and withdraw from the profession for various reasons, a projected shortage of nurses to replace them is predicted (Moses, 1992). This will occur at a time when the demand for nursing care is at an all-time high because of increasing numbers of elderly citizens, who generally use health care at a higher rate than do younger people.

Other external factors involve increased use of sophisticated technology and more educated consumers demanding better quality, affordable health care. Because nurses are identified as the ideal health care workers to provide care in a variety of settings they are increasingly employed outside hospitals. Some people believe that shortages are created by nurses leaving hospital work for non-hospital nursing positions. The fact is that hospitals employ about the same proportion of the total pool of RNs, two-thirds, as they did decades ago, but the ratio of nurses to patients is higher. This is due to two factors. First, more treatment is provided to hospitalized patients because they have illnesses and needs that demand greater attention. Less critical health problems are usually dealt with through outpatient services. Also, to control costs, patients are discharged to home care as soon as possible. There are fewer patients recuperating in the hospital. Second, technological advances, such as open heart surgery, organ transplants, and the like, have made special care units, staffed with specialized nurses, necessary. In these units, owing to the fact that patients are critically ill, one nurse cares for only one or two patients.

Despite all of the concerns about a nursing shortage, beginning in the mid-1990s, a number of areas of the United States experienced an oversupply of nurses. This was due to many factors. A downswing in the national economy in the early 1990s resulted in an increase in applications to schools of nursing nationwide. Large numbers of graduates flooded the market a few years later, just as significant downsizing and reorganization occurred in traditional employment settings such as hospitals. Although the U.S. Department of Labor forecasted in 1994 that 765,000 new RN jobs would be needed by 2005 (Fig. 3–5), a year later RN graduates in some parts of the United States were facing uncertain job prospects. According to deans in the Boston and New Jersey areas, for example, hospitals were not hiring new graduates. This downturn occurred rapidly, as mentioned by a Boston area dean: "Two years ago, at least 90% [of our new graduates] had jobs at graduation. The other 10% hadn't bothered to look. This last graduation, none had jobs. Most are placed by now, but mostly outside Boston, in hospitals in other areas, nursing homes, or rehab centers" (AJN Newsline, 1995). Most deans agreed that although new RNs often must head for rural areas or outside hospitals for their first jobs, master's prepared nurses, particularly nurse practitioners, are in demand everywhere.

There are no clear-cut answers to the problem of periodic imbalances in the supply of and demand for nurses. It should be kept in mind that periods of oversupply may actually reflect poor distribution of nurses. Nurses who are willing to relocate away from major population centers have usually been able to find work easily. With dramatic demographic and health care system changes on the horizon, however, periodic shortages and oversupplies of nurses are likely to remain a recurring theme (Abdellah, 1990).

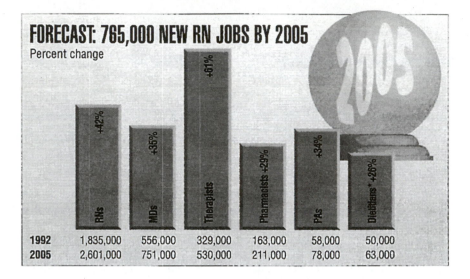

FORECAST: 765,000 NEW RN JOBS BY 2005
Percent change

	RNs	MDs	Therapists	Pharmacists	PAs	Dietitians*
	+42%	+35%	+61%	+29%	+34%	+26%
1992	1,835,000	556,000	329,000	163,000	58,000	50,000
2005	2,601,000	751,000	530,000	211,000	78,000	63,000

FIGURE   3 – 5
The health care industry will add 4.2 million jobs by the year 2005, growing at twice
the rate of the total economy, says the Labor Department in its latest projection of
employment prospects. The forecast is that registered nursing will see by far the
largest numerical growth and will continue to dwarf the other health professions with
the size of its workforce—an estimated 2,601,000 in 2005. Industry trends will also
boost employment for LPNs, aides, and techs; jobs for home health aides are expected to grow at the fastest rate—138%—to 827,000. *Includes nutritionists. (Source:
Dietetics, Nursing, Pharmacy, and Therapy Occupations. Reprinted from Occupational Outlook Handbook, 1994–95 edition. U.S. Department of Labor, Bureau of
Labor Statistics. Bulletin 2450-8, pp. 11–13. U.S. Government Printing Office.)

SUMMARY

Women have traditionally been socialized to seek security, avoid risk, and avoid
conflict. Because nursing is a female-dominated profession, the development of
nursing has been affected by the traditional socialization of women. Social trends
that have affected nursing include feminism, the women's movement, the consumer movement, the "graying of America," multiculturalism, men in nursing,
and technological advances in medicine. A powerful social influence, the media,
projects an image of nursing that is often distorted. This has led the public to
have misconceptions about nursing and nurses themselves. Imbalances in the
supply and demand for nurses arise periodically. Only by addressing basic issues
such as geographic distribution of nurses, salaries, benefits, and working conditions can these periodic imbalances be checked.

REVIEW AND DISCUSSION QUESTIONS

1. Explain how being a female-dominated profession has affected the development of the nursing profession.

2. Analyze the social influences that affected your decision to enter the nursing profession. Did the media image of nursing and nurses play a positive role or a negative role?
3. Describe your ideal nurse. What social stereotypes does your description reveal? Does your "ideal nurse" belong to a particular gender, race, or ethnic group?
4. What positive and negative impacts has the consumer movement had on health care in the United States?
5. List three social factors that have the potential to stimulate interest in nursing as a profession.
6. Describe three actions you can personally take to improve the public's image of nursing in your community.

REFERENCES

Abdellah, F. G. (1990). Reflections on a recurring theme. *Nursing Clinics of North America*, 25(3), 509–515.

Aber, C. S., and Hawkins, J. W. (1992). Portrayal of nurses in advertisements in medical and nursing journals. *IMAGE: Journal of Nursing Scholarship*, 24(4), 289–293.

Ahmann, E. (1994). "Chunky stew:" Appreciating cultural diversity while providing health care for children. *Pediatric Nursing*, 20(3), 320–322, 324.

AJN Newsline (1995). '95 RN graduates face uncertain job prospects. *American Journal of Nursing*, 95(4), 69; 72.

Andrews, M. M. (1992). Cultural perspectives on nursing in the 21st century. *Journal of Professional Nursing*, 8(1), 7–15.

Black, V. L., and Germaine-Warner, C. (1995). Image of nursing. In G. L. Deloughery (Ed.), *Issues and trends in nursing* (pp. 455–473). St. Louis: Mosby.

Boughn, S. (1994). Why do men choose nursing? *Nursing & Health Care*, 15(8), 406–411.

Bunting, S., and Campbell, J. C. (1990). Feminism and nursing: Historical perspectives. In P. L. Chinn (Ed.), *Developing the discipline: Critical studies in nursing history and professional issues* (pp. 181–195). Gaithersburg, MD: Aspen Publishers.

Buresh, B., and Gordon, S. (1995). Taking on the TV shows. *American Journal of Nursing*, 95(11), 18–20.

Campbell-Heider, N., Hart, C. A., and Bergren, M. D. (1994). Conveying professionalism: Working against the old stereotypes. In B. Bullough and V. Bullough (Eds.), *Nursing issues for the nineties and beyond* (pp. 212–231). New York: Springer.

Cummings, S. H. (1995). Attila the hun versus Attila the hen: Gender socialization of the American nurse. *Nursing Administration Quarterly*, 19(2), 19–29.

Cyr, J. (1992). Males in nursing. *Nursing Management*, 23(7), 54–55.

Fagin, C. M., and Binder, L. F. (1994). Nursing and consumerism: How can we get decision making closer to the consumer? In J. C. McCloskey and H. K. Grace (Eds.), *Current issues in nursing*, (pp. 450–459). St. Louis: Mosby.

Farley, S. (1994). Developing community partnerships: Shifting power from health professionals to citizens. In J. C. McCloskey and H. K. Grace (Eds.), *Current issues in nursing* (pp. 226–232). St. Louis: Mosby.

Flanagan, L. (1994). Staff nurses: Who are they, what do they do, and what challenges do they face? In J. C. McCloskey and H. K. Grace (Eds.), *Current issues in nursing* (pp. 15–18). St. Louis: Mosby.

Giger, J. N., Davidhizar, R. E., and Wieczorek, S. K. (1994). Transcultural nursing: Have we gone too far or not far enough? In O. L. Strickland and D. J. Fishman (Eds.), *Nursing issues in the 1990's* (pp. 491–503). Albany: Delmar.

Gray, D. P. (1994). Feminism and nursing. In O. L. Strickland and D. J. Fishman (Eds.), *Nursing issues in the 1990's* (pp. 505–527). Albany: Delmar.

Halloran, E. J., and Welton, J. M. (1994). Why aren't there more men in nursing? In J. C. McCloskey and H. K. Grace (Eds.), *Current issues in nursing* (pp. 684–691). St. Louis: Mosby.

Happ, B. (1994). Point of care technology: Does it improve the quality of patient care? In O. L. Strickland and D. J. Fishman (Eds.), *Nursing issues in the 1990's* (pp. 254–266). Albany: Delmar.

Johnson, M. H. (1994). Nursing care in a culturally diverse nation. In B. Bullough and V. Bullough (Eds.), *Nursing issues for the nineties and beyond* (pp. 187–198). New York: Springer.

Kalisch, P. A., and Kalisch, B. J. (1987). *The changing image of the nurse*. Reading, MA: Addison-Wesley.

Kalisch, P. A., and Kalisch, B. J. (1986). A comparative analysis of nurse and physician characters in the entertainment media. *Journal of Advanced Nursing*, 11(2), 179–195.

Ketter, J. (1994). Sex discrimination targets men in some hospitals. *The American Nurse*, 94(1), 24.

Kirkpatrick, S. M., and Deloughery, G. L. (1995). Cultural influences on nursing. In G. L. Deloughery (Ed.), *Issues and trends in nursing* (pp. 173–197). St. Louis: Mosby.

Leininger, M. (1991). Transcultural nursing: The study and practice field. *Imprint*, 38(2), 55–66.

Locsin, R. C. (1995). Technology and caring in nursing. In A. Boykin (Ed.), *Power, politics, and public policy: A matter of caring* (pp. 24–36). New York: National League for Nursing Press.

Mangum, S. (1994). Uniforms and caps: Do we need them? In O. L. Strickland and D. J. Fishman (Eds.), *Nursing issues in the 1990's* (pp. 46–66). Albany: Delmar.

McConnell, E. A., and Murphy, E. K. (1990). Nurses' use of technology: An international concern. *International Nursing Review*, 37(5), 331–334.

Mikulencak, M. (1995). Fact or fiction? Nursing and realism on TV's newest medical dramas. *The American Nurse*, 95(3), 31.

Moses, E. B. (1992). RN shortage seen for 21st century. *The American Nurse*, 92(7), 4.

Moss, M. T. (1995). Developing glass-breaking skills. *Nursing Administration Quarterly*, 19(2), 41–47.

Muff, J. (1988a). *Women's issues in nursing: Socialization, sexism, and stereotyping*. Prospect Height, IL: Waveland Press.

Muff, J. (1988b). Of images and ideals: A look at socialization and sexism in nursing. In A. H. Jones (Ed.), *Images of nurses: Perspectives from history, art, and literature* (pp. 197–220). Philadelphia: University of Pennsylvania Press.

National League for Nursing. (1994). *Nursing data review 1994*. New York: Author.

Neilsen Media Research. (1996). Top 10 prime-time programs. *The Wall Street Journal*, CCXXVII(3), Thursday, January 4, p. A-8.

Nurses of America (1991). *Who counts and who doesn't in news coverage of health care*. A project of the Tri-Council of Nursing Organizations. B. C. Wallace, Executive Director. Funded by the PEW Charitable Trusts, Inc.

Nurses of America (9/30/88–3/31/91). *Summary Report and Recommendations*. B. C. Wallace, Executive Director. Supported by a Grant from the PEW Charitable Trusts, Inc.

Perkins, J. L., Bennett, D. N., and Dorman, R. E. (1993). Why men choose nursing. *Nursing & Health Care*, 14(1), 34–38.

Reverby, S. M. (1993). *Ordered to care: The dilemma of American nursing, 1850–1945*. Cambridge: University Press.

Shea, C. A. (1994). Feminism: The new look in nursing. In J. C. McCloskey and H. K. Grace (Eds.), *Current issues in nursing* (pp. 572–579). St. Louis: Mosby.

Simpson, R. L. (1992). What nursing leaders are saying about technology. *Nursing Management*, 23(7), 28–30.

Simpson, R. L. (1993). If you don't read this, you're missing out. *Nursing Management*, 24(9), 18.

Talento, B. (1995). Social policy and health care delivery. In G. L. Deloughery (Ed.),

Issues and trends in nursing (pp. 129–169). St. Louis: Mosby.

Thompson, C. B., Amos, L. K., and Graves, J. R. (1994). Knowledge technology: Costs, benefits, and ethical considerations. In J. C. McCloskey and H. K. Grace (Eds.), *Current issues in nursing* (pp. 746–751). St. Louis: Mosby.

U.S. Bureau of the Census (1992). *Statistical abstract of the United States: 1992* (112th ed.). Washington, D.C.

U.S. Bureau of the Census (1994). *Statistical abstract of the United States: 1994* (114th ed.). Washington, D.C.

U.S. Department of Health and Human Services. (1994). *The registered nurse population: 1992.* Washington, D.C.: Author.

Villaire, M. (1994). Toni Tripp-Reimer: Crossing over the boundaries. *Critical Care Nurse*, 14(3), 134–141.

Villeneuve, M. J. (1994). Recruiting and retaining men in nursing: A review of the literature. *Journal of Professional Nursing*, 10(4), 217–228.

Williams, C. L. (1989). *Gender differences at work: Women and men in nontraditional occupations.* Berkeley: University of California Press.

Williams, C. L. (1995). Hidden advantages for men in nursing. *Nursing Administration Quarterly*, 19(2), 63–70.

Williams, M. B., and Cullen, K. V. (1994). Nurse shortages needn't be inevitable. *Modern Healthcare*, 24(33), 36.

4

Robert V. Piemonte
Barbara K. Redman

Professional Associations

OBJECTIVES

- Explain why professions have associations.
- Describe basic functions that nursing associations perform, both as individual organizations and in coalitions with other organizations.
- Describe a professional development program for yourself that incorporates membership in a professional association.
- Analyze organized nursing's management of select issues, according to the values they depict, and the political stances or strategies used.

VOCABULARY

certification	delegate	multiskilled worker
coalition	economic and general	professional association
Code for Nurses	welfare	professional boundary
collective action	issues management	unlicensed assistive
cross-training	lobby	personnel

Associations are organizations of persons with common interests. Merton defined a **professional association** as: "An organization of practitioners who judge one another as professionally competent and have banded together to perform social functions which they cannot perform in their separate capacity as individuals" (1958, p. 50). Associations exist in all professions and in all parts of the world. Although state governments have legal control of nursing licensure, associations' voluntary control of their members serves to assure the public of the availability and quality of services from that profession. Associations also serve their individual members through a variety of services.

WORK OF NURSING ASSOCIATIONS

Major nursing associations in Great Britain, Canada, and the United States all formed at about the same time at the turn of the century. Chapter 1 described the instrumental role played by Isabel Hampton Robb in establishing the forerunners of the American Nurses Association (ANA) and the National League for Nursing (NLN). Also mentioned was Lillian Wald's role in establishing the National Organization of Public Health Nurses.

Nursing association founders had two major concerns: (1) the need for laws to protect the public from poorly prepared nurses and (2) lack of standardization in nursing preparation. The newly formed associations won those battles first by successfully lobbying for the establishment of state licensure laws and later by promoting accreditation of schools of nursing.

As society evolves, the nursing profession must change so that it can continue to meet its responsibilities to the public. Professional associations provide a vehicle for nurses to meet present and future challenges and work toward positive, professionwide changes that keep pace with societal changes.

Whom Do Professional Associations Serve?

Nursing associations have three major constituents: the public, the profession of nursing, and individual practitioners of nursing. They serve each constituent group in different ways. They serve the public by establishing codes of ethics and standards of practice, socializing new members to these codes and standards, and enforcing codes and standards in practice. These measures, when combined with state licensure laws, assure the public that nurses are competent professionals with safe standards of practice and appropriate ethical beliefs.

Associations serve the profession by being the mechanism through which the collective interests of its members are pressed collectively and focused politically (Aydelotte, 1990). **Collective action** is a frequently misunderstood term. It simply means that activities are undertaken on behalf of a group of people who have common interests. Professional associations help nurses use collective action to push for political responses to benefit consumers of health care and members of the profession.

Associations serve individual members by providing continuing education, recognizing skill in practice through credentialing, and ensuring mechanisms for a professional workplace. They serve all of these interests by working for adequate numbers of practitioners to serve the public; by forming relationships with the public and other professions; and by ensuring that the profession's work is properly understood and supported by the public, government officials, and other health care professionals.

Examples of Professional Association Activities

One of the most important activities of professional associations is communicating information to members. Most nursing associations have either newsletters or journals, and some have both. These publications carry news stories of interest to nurses, information about pending legislation and political issues affecting nursing and health care, and editorials and articles on issues of interest to members.

The official newspaper of the ANA is *The American Nurse*, published 10 times each year. The ANA's professional journal is the *American Journal of Nursing*, which is published monthly. Other associations' publications include *Nursing and Health Care: Perspectives on Community* published bimonthly by the NLN; *Imprint,* published quarterly by the National Student Nurses Association (NSNA); and *Image, Journal of Nursing Scholarship,* published quarterly by Sigma Theta Tau. There are many others. Some journal subscriptions are included in the association's dues, and others must be subscribed to separately.

In addition to communicating with members, there are many other activities of professional associations. Examples of specific activities of the ANA are discussed. These examples of the range of issues with which professional associations deal demonstrate how there is sometimes a delicate balance between serving the public and the profession.

1. *Example A.* A hospital is threatened with closure for financial reasons. Although the hospital is in a city that is "overbedded" (has many unoccupied hospital beds that cost the community money even though unfilled), this institution serves a low-income, primarily minority community. If the hospital were to be closed, the individuals it serves would have to travel farther to obtain health care.

   Secure employment for the nurses who work at the hospital is also at stake. The hospital provides jobs for a number of nurses who are represented by the state nurses association (SNA), a constituent of the ANA, for purposes of collective bargaining. The nurses therefore would benefit personally if the hospital remained open.

   The difficulty is that the responsible resolution of this problem must serve both the public's and the nurses' needs. Through their SNA, the nurses can form a **coalition,** that is, a temporary alliance of distinct parties, with other providers of health care and consumer groups. The coalition can consider options such as obtaining a buyer for the hospital or obtaining care for patients and jobs for providers at other facilities in the city. During this process, they may work with the office of the mayor and the city council and with the corporation that owns the hospital.

2. *Example B.* As acquired immunodeficiency syndrome (AIDS) has become a full-blown epidemic, there have been concerns about protecting both health care workers and patients. Various health professions disagree about whether infected health care workers should voluntarily restrict their practices in situations in which patients could be infected. They also disagree about whether mandatory reporting of human immunodeficiency virus (HIV)–positive health care workers should be instituted.

   Although the profession's ethics require protection of patients, as of 1996 there is scanty evidence about the degree of risk to patients posed by HIV-positive workers. Meanwhile, cases are being tried, and resolution of the issue may come through the courts. The ANA has been asked to take a public position on this issue, including supporting various bills before Congress.

3. *Example C.* New technologies, such as ventilators, now keep people in comas alive even though the quality of life is no longer what they would have desired. Lifetime savings of families may be wiped out by maintaining a family member in a persistent vegetative state.

   Nurses are frequently caught in situations in which patients or their families no longer want to continue this kind of existence and yet the health

---

B O X 4 – 1
The Code for Nurses

1. The nurse provides services with respect for human dignity and the uniqueness of the client unrestricted by considerations of social or economic status, personal attributes, or the nature of health problems.
2. The nurse safeguards the client's right to privacy by judiciously protecting information of a confidential nature.
3. The nurse acts to safeguard the client and the public when health care and safety are affected by the incompetent, unethical, or illegal practice of any person.
4. The nurse assumes responsibility and accountability for individual nursing judgments and actions.
5. The nurse maintains competence in nursing.
6. The nurse exercises informed judgment and uses individual competence and qualifications as criteria in seeking consultation, accepting responsibilities, and delegating nursing activities to others.

7. The nurse participates in activities that contribute to the ongoing development of the profession's body of knowledge.
8. The nurse participates in the profession's efforts to implement and improve standards of nursing.
9. The nurse participates in the profession's efforts to establish and maintain conditions of employment conducive to high-quality nursing care.
10. The nurse participates in the profession's effort to protect the public from misinformation and misrepresentation and to maintain the integrity of nursing.
11. The nurse collaborates with members of the health professions and other citizens in promoting community and national efforts to meet the health needs of the public.

Reprinted with permission of American Nurses Association (1985). *Code for nurses with interpretive statements.* Washington, D.C.: Author.

---

care system has not developed adequate legal and decision mechanisms to deal with patients' desires. In response to the need for guidance on ethical issues, a special task force of the ANA (1985) created a document entitled the *Code for Nurses* to help nurses clarify their responsibilities. Box 4–1 contains an abbreviated form of the *Code*.

Although the *Code for Nurses* provides broad direction, the ANA also provides more specific direction on particular ethical issues. In addition to the code, the ANA has published a number of position statements on specific issues, including one on assisted suicide (Box 4–2) (American Nurses Association, 1994).

These three examples of real, yet diverse problems demonstrate several common elements related to the work of associations:

1. They are all issues in which there is no clearly right or wrong answer.
2. All the examples involve balancing the interests of individual practitioners and patients with the common good of the public nurses serve.

BOX 4–2

Summary of the American Nurses Association's Position Statement on Assisted Suicide

Nurses, individually and collectively, have an obligation to provide comprehensive and compassionate end-of-life care which includes the promotion of comfort and the relief of pain, and at times, foregoing life-sustaining treatments. The American Nurses Association (ANA) believes that the nurse should not participate in assisted suicide. Such an act is in violation of the Code for Nurses with Interpretive Statements (Code for Nurses) and the ethical traditions of the profession.

Reprinted with permission of American Nurses Association (1994). *Position statement on assisted suicide*. Washington, D.C.: Author

3. All the issues are political in that significant stakeholder groups do not agree on the right course to take.
4. From its position as a voice for experts within the area of concern, the professional association provides guidance on resolution of issues, guidance that is frequently adopted by institutions or jurisdictions.

This is the nature of the work of associations.

Joining and Using Professional Associations in Nursing

Nurses have a responsibility to belong to one or more nursing associations both as an extension of their interest in nursing and to support their fellow nurses. Chapter 6 demonstrates that having a strong professional organization is a characteristic of mature professions. Following is a discussion of how nurses can make effective decisions about which nursing association(s) to join and learn how to use these groups to meet their needs for professional growth and stimulate activities on behalf of the members of the group (otherwise known as collective action).

TYPES OF ASSOCIATIONS

A list (not comprehensive) of nursing associations in the United States appears in Box 4–3. This list dramatically demonstrates the number and variety of associations that nurses may choose to join. Understandably, individual nurses often express confusion about which association(s) to join.

In general, the associations listed can be classified as one of three main types:

1. Broad purpose professional associations.
2. Specialty practice associations.
3. Special interest associations.

BOX 4-3
Nursing Organizations in the United States

- American Nurses Association
- American Academy of Ambulatory Nursing Administration
- American Academy of Nurse Practitioners
- American Assembly for Men in Nursing
- American Association for Continuity of Care
- American Association for the History of Nursing
- American Association of Colleges of Nursing
- American Association of Critical-Care Nurses
- American Association of Neuroscience Nurses
- American Association of Nurse Anesthetists
- American Association of Nurse Attorneys
- American Association of Occupational Health Nurses
- American Association of Office Nurses
- American Association of Spinal Cord Injury Nurses
- American College of Nurse-Midwives
- American Holistic Nurses' Association
- American Nephrology Nurses' Association
- American Organization of Nurse Executives
- American Psychiatric Nurses' Association
- American Radiological Nurses Association
- American Society of Plastic and Reconstructive Surgical Nurses
- American Society of Post Anesthesia Nurses
- Association of Black Nursing Faculty in Higher Education
- Association of Community Health Nursing Educators
- Association of Nurses in AIDS Care
- Association of Operating Room Nurses
- Association of Pediatric Oncology Nurses
- Association of Rehabilitation Nurses
- Association of Women's Health, Obstetric and Neonatal Nurses
- Chi Eta Phi
- Dermatology Nurses Association
- Drug and Alcohol Nursing Association
- Emergency Nurses Association
- Hospice Nurses Association
- Intravenous Nurses Society
- National Alliance of Nurse Practitioners
- National Association of Hispanic Nurses
- National Association of Neonatal Nurses
- National Association of Orthopedic Nurses
- National Association of Pediatric Nurse Practitioners and Associates
- National Association of School Nurses
- National Black Nurses Association
- National Flight Nurses Association
- National Gerontological Nurses Association
- National League for Nursing
- National Nurses Society on Addictions
- National Organization for the Advancement of Associate Degree Nursing
- National Student Nurses Association
- Nurses Organization of the Veterans Administration
- Oncology Nursing Society
- Sigma Theta Tau
- Society for Peripheral Vascular Nursing
- Society of Nursing History
- Transcultural Nursing Society

Reprinted with permission of *American Journal of Nursing*, 1993 Directory of Nursing Organizations, vol. 93. April 1993.

The ANA is the broad purpose association in nursing. Individual nurses belong to SNAs, and SNAs compose the ANA. The ANA is a federation made up of 53 state and territorial nurses associations. Its purposes are threefold:

1. To work for the improvement of health standards and the availability of health care services for all people.
2. To foster high standards for nursing.
3. To stimulate and promote the professional development of nurses and advance their **economic and general welfare.**

As the nursing profession grew and diversified, many nurses limited their practices to specialty areas, such as maternal/infant health, school health, community health, critical care, perioperative nursing, or emergency/trauma nursing. Members of specialty nursing associations frequently choose to belong to an SNA also because specialty associations focus on standards of practice in that specialty only and on the particular professional needs of that group of nurses only.

Examples of special purpose organizations include Sigma Theta Tau, the international nursing honor society, which one must be invited to join, and the Transcultural Nursing Society, which focuses on a particular area of study in nursing. A comprehensive updated list of nursing organizations is available through *AJN Net*, the *American Journal of Nursing*'s online service.

BENEFITS OF BELONGING TO PROFESSIONAL ASSOCIATIONS

A variety of benefits result from membership in professional associations. Most nurses were drawn to their profession because it exemplifies caring for others; because it makes a difference in others' lives; and because it demands full use of their intellectual, interpersonal, and emotional talents. Once in nursing, however, both students and practicing nurses have many needs.

Developing Leadership Skills.   Students usually want to socialize with, and learn from, other nursing students on both state and national levels. They need to develop leadership and organizational skills to help them in many phases of their professional and personal lives. They need to learn how associations function and how to participate as active, effective members. The NSNA, which has local and state chapters in addition to the national organization, provides all of these opportunities and more.

The mission of the NSNA (1995) is to:

- Organize, represent, and mentor students preparing for initial licensure as registered nurses (RNs) as well as those nurses enrolled in baccalaureate completion programs.
- Promote development of the skills that students will need as responsible and accountable members of the nursing profession.
- Advocate for high-quality health care.

Recognition Through Certification.   Practicing nurses want to be recognized, both by salary and by position, for their level of professional expertise.

They may seek recognition for their expertise through certification in a specialty area, which is granted by professional associations. **Certification** is a formal but voluntary process of demonstrating expertise in a particular area of nursing. Certified nurses often receive salary supplements and special opportunities.

Legislative Lobbying Power. As their careers develop, nurses may obtain master's level preparation or become nurse practitioners and practice independently outside an institution. These nurses desire and deserve direct reimbursement for their work. They need state laws that mandate direct reimbursement of nurses. Others work in nursing homes and may be concerned that there are not enough RNs available to provide the quality of care the residents need. They need state laws that regulate nurse-to-patient ratios and control educational requirements for unlicensed assistive personnel.

Some nurses work in settings in which they have little voice in the quality of care in that institution, are paid poorly, and are required to "float" to cover specialized units for which they have not been trained. These nurses may wish to be represented for purposes of collective bargaining so they can negotiate for improved salary and work conditions.

In each of these instances, nursing's general purpose association, the ANA, is involved in vital work supporting nurses as they fulfill their roles as professionals. SNAs **lobby** the government to influence laws affecting nursing, such as those that mandate that insurance companies reimburse nurse practitioners for the services they provide. They also influence laws determining how many RNs are required to staff nursing homes and educational requirements for nurse aides, for whom nurses are legally responsible. If invited to do so, many SNAs assist nurses in dealing with workplace issues, such as salaries, working conditions, and patient care issues such as staffing ratios.

Other Benefits. These examples—developing leadership skills, achieving recognition through certification, and banding together for legislative lobbying power—represent major benefits of association membership. There are many others, such as publications; eligibility for group health and life insurance; continuing education offerings; and discounts on travel, eyeglasses, and other goods and services.

DECIDING WHICH ASSOCIATION(S) TO JOIN

In making a decision about joining an association, nurses should ask several questions:

1. What are the purposes of this association?
2. Are the association's purposes compatible with my own?
3. How many members are there nationally, statewide, and locally?
4. What activities does the association undertake?
5. How active is the local chapter?
6. What are the benefits of membership?
7. Does this organization lobby for improved health care legislation? How successful is it?

8. Is membership in this association cost-effective?

Answering these questions should provide nurses with adequate information to make reasoned membership decisions.

BECOMING A PRODUCTIVE ASSOCIATION MEMBER

Nurses get involved with a nursing association by joining as members, attending meetings, volunteering for committees, and participating in the association's activities. Members directly influence the association's priorities, and they provide the volunteer labor that makes the association function. By becoming active participants in professional associations, nurses become part of something bigger than their present work situation, something central to their professional role, and something through which they can make a difference throughout their professional lives.

PERSPECTIVES OF NURSING LEADERS ABOUT PROFESSIONAL ASSOCIATIONS

To present readers a personal view of what organizations do and mean to nurses, the presidents of four major nursing organizations were asked to describe the benefits members receive from belonging to their organizations and what they personally have attained by involvement with their organizations.

Dr. Melanie C. Dreher, President, Sigma Theta Tau International

Sigma Theta Tau International is the honor society of the nursing profession and exists to promote the development, dissemination, and utilization of nursing knowledge. The Society is committed to improving the health of people worldwide through increasing the scientific base of nursing practice. In support of this mission, Sigma Theta Tau International advances nursing leadership and scholarship and furthers the use of nursing research in health care and health policy.

The honor society is organized into chapters within accredited Schools of Nursing that grant baccalaureate and higher degrees. There currently are 346 chapters at 391 colleges and universities with over 115,000 active members, representing over 60 countries worldwide. As members of Sigma Theta Tau International, inductees join the company of nurses throughout the world who have been identified as scholars and leaders. Participation in the Society provides members with opportunities for career development through exposure to more senior members of the profession, meeting new colleagues, and through exchange and mentoring.

The Society replenishes leadership and scholarship in the profession through various initiatives, including continuing education; the Leadership Extern Program; funding for nursing research; and sponsorship of local, regional, national, and international research conferences. It also houses the Virginia Henderson Electronic Library and On Line Journal of Nursing Knowledge, both of which provide students and practicing nurses affordable access to the most current and ready to use knowledge. *Image*, the Society's research journal, and *Reflections*, the Society's magazine, are included in the membership and link individual members to nurses throughout the world.

In summary, induction into Sigma Theta Tau International is an honor, and active membership in the Society is highly regarded by employers and other influentials in the profession. Participation in Sigma Theta Tau International provides opportunities for career development, continuing education and the enhancement of nursing practice, thus placing members at the forefront of the profession (Dreher, 1995, personal communication).

Kathryn E. Sexson, President, National Student Nurses Association

At the time of this communication, Sexson was a nursing student at The University of Alaska in Anchorage.

The primary purpose of the NSNA is to socialize the nursing student into the profession (Fig. 4–1). This is accomplished through interaction between students, faculty, future colleagues, and nursing leaders. In this environment students are afforded the opportunity to develop their leadership expertise, gain insight into the rights as well as the responsibilities of the nursing profession, and develop the skills that will enable them to advocate effectively for the clients they wish to serve. These opportunities not only facilitate the development of a proactive professional nurse, but also lead to an increased marketability in a competitive health care market.

F I G U R E   4 – 1

Students attending a National Student Nurses Association convention learn leadership and political skills while having fun and meeting others from around the United States. (Courtesy of National Student Nurses Association.)

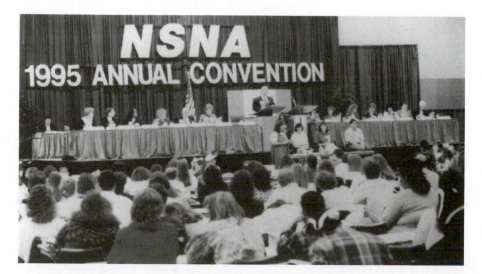

NSNA seeks to achieve this purpose through a series of publications, leadership workshops, career development symposiums, conferences, and conventions. Additionally, it offers licensing review courses, discounts on educational materials, group health insurance, and other benefits to help defray student costs.

Personally, I have gained much from my involvement in the Association. It has enabled me to put theory into practice, interact with individuals whose research I have studied, and develop my leadership potential. But, most of all, it has allowed me to come to the realization that every nurse is a leader who strives to empower his or her clients and the profession to achieve their full potential.

I would strongly encourage students to participate in their local, state, and national associations. Not only does it provide an avenue for professional development, but also it offers an unparalleled support system as you aspire to accomplish your endeavor. As you stand next to each other, the future of nursing, you will develop great pride in who and what you are about to become (Sexson, 1995, personal communication).

Dr. M. Jean Watson, Immediate Past President, National League for Nursing

The League is a coalition of nurses, other health professionals, and consumers. The League works to advance the health of diverse communities through nursing. Its mission is to improve education and health outcome by linking communities and information. The League's goals and objectives include assuring the quality of nursing education and improving the quality of health care through accreditation, continuing education programs, test services, research, publications, videos, and lobbying efforts.

Benefits of NLN membership include a subscription to *Nursing and Health Care: Perspectives on Community*; discounts on all NLN programs, conventions, and publications; and networking, which is so important to professional development. Membership also provides direct involvement in policies affecting nurses, patients, and the profession. It gives you an opportunity to see nursing's and nurses' efforts accomplished. And you interact with tremendous people and exchange ideas and work on solutions.

The League acts from the belief that the most pressing issues facing nursing today include ensuring access to primary health care and advancing the World Health Organization's goal of "Health For All," advancing and monitoring the highest standards of nursing care and nursing education, and finding new ways of working with other professions and community groups.

My advice to students is to learn about your profession and be involved. Get to know other professionals early to learn what their contributions are to the health delivery system. Network, network, network! Share your talents with others (Watson, 1995, personal communication).

Virginia Trotter Betts, MSN, JD, Immediate Past President, American Nurses Association

The ANA is the comprehensive, multipurpose professional organization that speaks for the profession and all nurses on matters of ethics, clinical

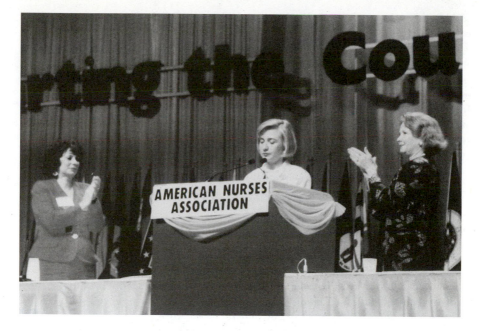

FIGURE 4–2
Hillary Rodham Clinton addresses the 1994 ANA convention as ANA President Virginia Trotter Betts (*right*) looks on. (Courtesy of American Nurses Association.)

standards, public policy, and economic and general welfare. The Association serves as the spokesperson for the profession (Fig. 4–2). ANA focuses its resources and energies on issues of nursing practice and nursing economics and is organized through the membership of individual nurses in SNAs and the SNAs in the ANA federation. ANA represents the United States on the International Council of Nurses.

Individual nurses, both novice and expert, have much to gain from SNA/ANA membership. Up-to-the-minute information on nursing and health care issues is available through ANA publications of *The American Nurse* and the *American Journal of Nursing*, and ANA is now offering SNA members online information through the *Nurse Forum*. A range of products such as malpractice insurance, travel cards, and financial services are offered to members at a competitive price.

SNAs have regular local and state meetings to enhance collegiality and channel each individual's input into local nursing issues. The SNAs work vigorously to expand practice, career, and economic opportunities for all nurses, and it is the SNA nurse members who develop the direction for the entire organization.

However, individual gain is not what ANA is singularly about. Rather, ANA, as the voice and advocate for the profession, needs the membership, support, and commitment of each nurse. Membership in your SNA and ANA should be a part of demonstrating professionalism for it is *the* means through which nursing's public policy and practice goals can be realized (Betts, 1995, personal communication).

ANALYSIS OF SELECTED ISSUES NURSING ASSOCIATIONS ADDRESS

Several issues of critical importance to the future of the nursing profession required collective action by organized nursing in coalition with other stakeholders. One involved a threat from organized medicine to nursing's **professional boundary** (dividing line between two professions), and the other involved constructing a new boundary made necessary because of predicted massive change in the health care system. Neither initiative would have been possible without associations, and each issue directly impacted nurses working in all settings.

Registered Care Technologists and Other Assistive Personnel

As discussed in Chapter 3, for some time nursing has been plagued with periodic imbalances in supply and demand. Shortages have an impact on health care settings, particularly hospitals, which sometimes have to close beds because there are not enough nurses to staff them. Shortages also have an impact on physicians, who may not be able to admit nonemergency patients because staffed beds are not available. Closing hospital beds and restricting admissions create adverse economic conditions for both hospitals and physicians.

From time to time, when the pressure from this kind of economic impact has been strong, various groups have suggested that nurse substitutes be trained. In the midst of a nursing shortage that peaked in 1988, the American Medical Association (AMA) introduced a proposal for a new health care worker they called the *registered care technologist* (RCT).

Despite nursing's opposition, the AMA attempted to find hospitals in which the RCT proposal could be pilot tested. In each potential site, nurses protested so effectively that plans were dropped. Next, the AMA attempted to find test sites in nursing homes, but the same thing occurred. At state and local levels, nurses formed coalitions with sympathetic physicians and medical societies to persuade these colleagues, with whom they frequently worked closely, that this was not a good idea. Two years after the original proposal, the AMA's House of Delegates essentially barred further active promotion of the RCT. The curriculum plan for training such workers, however, remains available to those who wish to purchase it.

Although the RCT is less a threat now than it was a few years ago, new threats have arisen. In an attempt to downsize hospitals and curtail costs, institutions have begun a process called **cross training** personnel. Unlicensed individuals are being taught a variety of skills that heretofore were not part of their job. **Multiskilled worker** is the term associated with this new category of unlicensed provider. As these individuals assume tasks that have traditionally been performed by nurses, there is an attempt to reduce the number of professional nurses required to staff the institution. Of concern to professional nursing is the question of quality as well as safety.

It is the assumption of the ANA that the provision of safe, accessible, and affordable nursing care for the public may include the appropriate use of **unlicensed assistive personnel** and that the changes in the health care environment have and will continue to alter the activities delegated to them.

In delegating, it is the RN who uses professional judgment to determine the appropriate activities to **delegate.** The determination is based on the concept of protection of the public and includes consideration of the needs of patients, the education and training of the nursing and assistive staff, the extent of supervision required, and the staff workload. Any nursing intervention that requires independent, specialized nursing knowledge, skill, or judgment cannot be delegated. Box 4–4 provides a summary of the ANA *Basic Guide to Safe Delegation* (1995).

BOX 4–4
American Nurses Association Basic Guide to Safe Delegation

Delegation: Defining the Term

The ANA defines delegation as "The transfer of responsibility for the performance of an activity from one individual to another, with the former retaining accountability for the outcome." Delegation can also be differentiated as direct or indirect.

- Direct delegation comes about when the nurse determines which tasks can be delegated and to whom to delegate.
- Indirect delegation provides that tasks or activities from an approved list contained within the policies and procedures of the facility can be carried out by the LPN/LVN or unlicensed assistive worker.

In either case, the nurse is still obligated to assess the competence of the individual carrying out the assignment.

Delegation: Determining the Appropriate Delegate

Key issues must be addressed in determining when, and to whom, to delegate. In addition to state laws and institutional policies that guide the nurse, the following steps help to reinforce the decision-making process about delegation:

- Assess the patient's status and needs and the appropriateness of delegating tasks to another caregiver. Then evaluate available staff for skills and competence before determining the delegate—the person receiving the delegation.
- Educate the delegate about what is to be done. It is vital that the nurse demonstrate the task or procedure and then observe the delegate's ability to perform safely and appropriately. The nurse must document the training, observations, and competence of the delegate and keep the documentation available and updated for legal protection.
- Communicate expectations of both performance and outcomes as well as receptivity to questions and concerns. Be certain also to inform the delegate which situations require asking for immediate assistance.
- Observe the delegate directly the first time any task or procedure is done. In addition, make certain to reassess competencies from time to time. Most important of all, the nurse must always be available to assist the delegate should the need arise.

Development of Nursing's Agenda for Health Care Reform

There are many indicators that the U.S. health care system is not working well and needs reform. Although the United States has the most technologically sophisticated system in the world, millions of Americans must overcome enormous obstacles to get even the most elementary services. For example, increasing numbers of children are not receiving immunizations, and there is a resulting resurgence of diseases, such as measles, that are preventable.

Nurses see people daily who are denied or delayed in obtaining appropriate care because of inability to pay or lack of adequate health insurance. These people often delay seeking help until they appear in hospital emergency departments in advanced stages of illness. Often, they have problems that could have been treated in less costly settings or prevented altogether with earlier treatment or prevention services.

Organized nursing felt a professional responsibility to contribute its expertise to the national debate about how health care will be financed and how people, especially those who cannot pay, can gain access to practitioners. In essence, the problems are:

1. Inequitable and limited access to health care providers.
2. Soaring costs.
3. Inconsistencies in quality of care.

Because the *Code for Nurses* (see Box 4–1), in points 1 and 11, directs nurses to be advocates for their clients, it is clearly nursing's responsibility to participate actively in seeking solutions for health care problems in the United States.

Realizing that public demand for changes in the health care system was building, the ANA and the NLN each began to design a reformed health care system. In spring 1991, their efforts were merged into a single plan, and 65 other nursing organizations endorsed the resulting document, known as *Nursing's Agenda for Health Care Reform* (1991).

Many of the elements of nursing's plan reflect the profession's values. Examples of nursing's values expressed in the agenda include:

1. Special attention to the unique needs of population groups whose health care needs have been neglected—vulnerable groups such as the poor, minorities, and persons with AIDS.
2. A core of federally defined essential health services available to all citizens and residents, regardless of income level or existing health conditions.
3. A major change in the focus of health care—from current practice, which emphasizes acute care only after a patient becomes ill, to a balance of illness and wellness care.
4. Expanded direct consumer access to a range of qualified health care providers, including nurses, in familiar, accessible, and convenient community settings such as schools, the workplace, the home, and community clinics.

Developing such a comprehensive proposal and following through on it requires a considerable commitment of time, money, and political clout. This kind of effort is uniquely appropriate for associations and is impossible without them. What was developed in the process of generating *Nursing's Agenda* was a coalition of more than 65 nursing professional associations representing a total of 700,000 nurses. There is tremendous strength in numbers of this magnitude.

Although federal legislation to reform the health care system in the United States has not yet been passed, the need for reform remains a paramount concern of nursing professionals. Even in the absence of federal mandates, changes in the delivery system are occurring at the state level through initiatives led by the private sector.

Managed care, a form of cost control, is becoming the watchword in most communities, with physicians having the "gatekeeper" role in most plans. Nurses are not usually included in provider panels of managed care plans. The ANA, however, is working to position nursing for full participation in the reformed delivery system, including managed care plans. At ANA's 1995 House of Delegates assembly, delegates voted to endorse a single-payer mechanism as one of the most desirable options for financing health care. At the same meeting, the House voted to direct that ANA communicate the unique contributions of professional RNs in health promotion, prevention, and maintenance services in all facets of the managed care delivery systems and to promote multiple strategies to establish full participation of nursing in managed care plans. The interests of American nurses are being safeguarded through these efforts.

Nursing's Agenda for Health Care Reform remains a valuable document, and elements of the Agenda continue to be used by grass roots political networks in educating senators and representatives. Total reform, not just tinkering, is the goal of organized nursing and is crucial to ensure access to care for all U.S. citizens. Meanwhile, the debate about health care reform continues, with nursing playing a vital role in shaping the future delivery system.

Nursing's Agenda for Health Care Reform and the activities designed to promote it are examples of **issues management** by professional associations. Issues management involves assisting a group to resolve a particular question on which there are significant differences of opinion. Through its agenda, organized nursing is attempting to assist the United States to resolve its health care crisis. This process offers many opportunities for nurses to be involved in reforming the system that impacts the welfare of their patients and their own professional practices. How nurses can influence the political process is discussed further in Chapter 21.

S U M M A R Y

Professional associations are the vehicle through which nursing takes collective action to improve health care and nursing. There are many nursing associations from which to choose, and they offer a variety of benefits to the public, to the nursing profession as a whole, and to individual members. Membership in professional associations is considered essential for true professionals, but selecting which association(s) to join can be a challenge. Prospective members can ask several key questions to help them select wisely. The ANA, which represents all nurses, is at the forefront in addressing issues of importance to all nurses, including the use of assistive personnel and the enactment of legislative proposals that address health care reform. The NSNA develops leaders whose future membership in their state nurses associations will strengthen the profession.

REVIEW AND DISCUSSION QUESTIONS

1. Look in the local newspaper for articles about the health care system, especially its costs and problems with lack of access for the poor. How does *Nursing's Agenda for Health Care Reform* address these problems? Could you sell this plan to a group of consumers, other students, or health professionals?
2. Find out if there is a student nurses association on your campus. If there is, learn all you can about it and consider joining. If there isn't one, consider establishing one.
3. Based on what you now know about associations, how will you personally be involved with them? Establish goals for participation while you are a student, for the first two years after graduation, and for five years after that. Share your goals with a classmate.
4. From the list of associations, contact one that interests you. Ask how one becomes a member and what the association offers its members. Would you want to join? Why or why not? At what stage of your career? Does the cost seem to equal the benefits? What three major issues is that association now addressing, and what has been its effectiveness?
5. Interview a nurse who is active in a professional association. Ask what he or she sees as the benefits of membership. Find out how he or she decided which association(s) to join.
6. Request a copy of your state nurses association's legislative platform for the current year. How will their initiatives affect your professional future?

REFERENCES

American Nurses Association (1995). *Basic guide to safe delegation.* Washington, D.C.: Author.

American Nurses Association (1994). *Position statement on Assisted Suicide.* Washington, D.C.: Author.

American Nurses Association (1985). *Code for nurses with interpretive statements.* Kansas City, MO: Author.

Aydelotte, M. K. (1990). The evolving profession: The role of the professional organization. In N. L. Chaska (Ed.), *The nursing profession: Turning points.* St. Louis: Mosby.

Merton, R. K. (1958). The functions of the professional association. *American Journal of Nursing,* 58(1), 50–54.

National Student Nurses Association (1995). *Mission statement.* New York: Author.

Nursing's agenda for health care reform. (1991). Washington, D.C.: American Nurses Association.

Cathy Campbell*

Nursing Today

OBJECTIVES

- Describe the "typical" registered nurse of today.
- Identify the broad range of settings in which registered nurses practice.
- Cite examples of nursing roles in various practice settings.
- Explain the roles of advanced practice nurses and the preparation required to assume them.
- Identify issues facing advanced practice nurses.

VOCABULARY

advanced practice nurse (APN)
ambulatory care
autonomy
case manager
certified nurse-midwife (CNM)
certified registered nurse anesthetist (CRNA)

clinical coordinator
clinical ladder
clinical nurse specialist (CNS)
entrepreneur
extended care
flexible staffing
home health nursing
moonlighting

nurse manager
nurse practitioner (NP)
occupational health nurse
private practice
salary compression
school nurse
staff nurse

Far-reaching economic and social changes in the United States have profoundly changed the way health care is delivered. Many of the changes outlined in Chapter 3 have opened avenues to new and exciting employment opportunities for nurses. This chapter provides an overview of the registered nurse (RN) population in the United States and briefly presents a selection of employment options available to nurses today both within and outside of hospitals. Integrated into the chapter are interviews with several nurses who describe their work and tell what they find are the rewards and challenges of their positions.

*The author wishes to acknowledge the contribution of Leslie B. Himot in the preparation of this chapter.

CURRENT STATUS OF NURSING IN THE UNITED STATES

What is the profile of nurses today? Is there a "typical" RN of the 1990s? Where do nurses work? What incomes do they earn in today's market? Are there enough jobs to provide employment for all nurses?

Every few years since 1977, the federal government has conducted a national survey of RNs in the United States. The most recent survey was conducted in 1992. These data were published by the U.S. Department of Health and Human Services in a document entitled *The Registered Nurse Population: 1992* (1994). This document and other data provided by the American Nurses Association (ANA) describe many of the characteristics of RNs today.

Characteristics of Registered Nurses

More than 2.2 million individuals held licenses as RNs in 1992, with nearly 1.9 million of that number actively working in nursing. The remainder of the RN population were either not working or working in fields other than nursing.

According to the 1992 survey, almost one-third of employed RNs worked part-time. Hospitals were the primary work site reported by more than two-thirds of employed RNs. In addition, 8 percent worked in **ambulatory care** settings, most of them physicians' offices; 10 percent worked in community or public health settings such as health departments or visiting nurse services; and 7 percent worked in nursing homes or **extended care** facilities based in and out of hospitals.

Of the RNs surveyed in 1992, 66 percent listed their position title as **staff nurse.** Staff nurses are first-line direct patient care providers who work in many settings both in and out of hospitals.

RNs who worked for temporary employment services as their primary work source constituted 2 percent of all employed RNs. In 1994, the U.S. Department of Labor reported the average hourly earnings of temporary RNs was $21.98 (U.S. Department of Labor, 1995). Nurses often hold more than one position. Referred to as **"moonlighting,"** the practice of holding more than one position is not uncommon in nursing.

The Department of Labor's 1992 figures also showed that most RNs were women. Among employed RNs, 4.3 percent were men, up from 3.3 percent in 1988. The historic trend of nursing as a female-dominated occupation is slowly changing. The admission of men into all basic nursing programs increased to 12 percent in 1992, compared to 10.7 percent in 1991 (Fig. 5–1) (National League for Nursing, 1994).

White RNs represent 90 percent of the population. The distribution by ethnic/racial backgrounds of the 10 percent nonwhite employed RN population includes African-American, 4 percent; Asian/Pacific Islander, 3.4 percent; Hispanic, 1.4 percent; and Native American/Alaskan Native, 0.4 percent (National League for Nursing, 1994).

As shown in Figure 3–3, the National League for Nursing (NLN) (1994) reported a 13.3 percent graduation rate of minority students from all basic RN programs in 1991–1992. To achieve a more culturally diverse professional population, an identified need exists both to recruit and to retain minority groups in the practice of nursing.

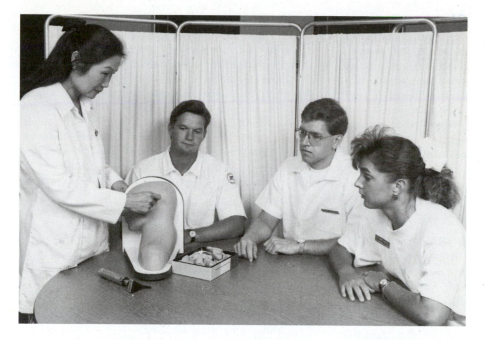

FIGURE   5–1

The number of men in basic nursing programs is increasing. Photo by Fielding Freed.

Similar to the rest of American society, the RN population is getting older. This "graying" of the work force was revealed in 1992 statistics, which showed more than 60 percent of RNs were 30 to 49 years old. The average age of RNs in 1992 was 43 years, and only 11 percent were under 30. Seventy-two percent were married, and the majority of married nurses (55 percent) had children at home (U.S. Department of Labor, 1992).

Employment Opportunities for Nurses

RNs are the largest health care profession in the United States serving in diverse settings such as hospitals, homes, schools, workplaces, community centers, children's camps, homeless shelters, and migrant camps. Some RNs even work in **private practice.** Nurses in private practice—whether they are consultants or counselors or are providing hands-on care—must have advanced degrees or specialized education, training, and certification.

Not all nurses provide direct patient care as a primary part of their roles. Nurses conduct research, teach undergraduate and graduate students, are chief executives of companies, and serve as consultants to health care organizations. Nurses who have advanced education, such as master's and doctoral degrees, are prepared to become researchers, educators, administrators, and advanced practice nurses (APNs), including nurse practitioners (NPs), clinical nurse specialists (CNSs), certified nurse-midwives (CNMs), and certified registered nurse anesthetists (CRNAs). These advanced nurse practice roles are discussed in greater detail later.

In deciding which of the many available options to select, nurses should consider their special talents, their likes and dislikes, and whether their talents and preferences are a good match with the employment opportunity under consideration. Although two-thirds of nurses are employed in hospitals, many others are pursuing challenges elsewhere. Numerous new opportunities and roles are being developed that use nurses' skills in different and exciting ways. What follows are descriptions of a sampling of the broad range of settings in which nurses now practice. In some instances, nurses actually practicing in these settings are interviewed. It must be stressed that these represent only a few of the opportunities available.

RURAL NURSING

Are you independent, intolerant of red tape, and dedicated to the needs of others? Are you from or interested in living far from the maddening crowd? If so, rural nursing may be for you. Today, rural Americans are increasingly elderly and poor. These are the two populations frequently characterized by chronic illness and frailty and thereby most in need of health care.

A complicating factor in providing health care to people in rural areas is the scarcity of physicians. The fact that many rural hospitals are closing means even fewer physicians will choose rural areas. Yet the predominantly elderly, poor rural population remains to be served.

In South Dakota, it is common for patients to drive 100 miles each way for routine health care. South Dakota nurses, similar to rural nurses in other states, believe that RNs are prepared to meet the rural health care challenge. A South Dakota RN had this to say about her job in a rural hospital: "A smaller hospital offers nurses the opportunity to be more autonomous and to use all their nursing education and interpersonal skills. We do it all here." This nurse clearly is an independent thinker who enjoys her practice freedom.

In 1991, the ANA was successful in supporting legislature to require Medicare, a federally funded insurance program for the elderly, to reimburse NPs directly for services they provide in rural areas (American Nurses Association, 1991). This action by the ANA is an example of the power of collective action through professional associations (see Chapter 4). The result is good for nursing and provides rural patients with better access to health care.

Nurses are experts at assessing the whole person. Nurses are also experts in illness prevention and patient education, both of which can greatly improve the quality of health care and keep health care costs low. Because nurses are often the only health professionals in remote rural areas, this expertise is critical in assisting rural patients to develop their personal self-care abilities and independence.

For many nurses the advantages of living in a rural area outweigh the benefits of working in a big-city facility. On the personal side, they prefer to raise their families away from cities and enjoy the atmosphere of country living. In a professional sense, having a lot of **autonomy**, or freedom from the influence of others, is a plus. The ability to form close relationships with their patients, who are also their neighbors and friends, is a major reason nurses like working in rural areas.

HOME HEALTH NURSING

Are you creative? Can you improvise? Do you like to deal with people in the context of the family, rather than strictly as individuals? If so, you may find your niche in **home health nursing.**

Lillian Wald is credited with initiating public health nursing when she established the Henry Street Settlement in New York City. Home health care, which includes visiting nurses and hospice nurses, is an outgrowth of public health nursing. Today, nurses employed by health departments work in clinics, where patients come to them, and also go into the patients' home to deliver care.

Since 1980, there has been a tremendous increase in the number of private agencies providing home health services. In fact, home health care is a fast-growing segment of the health care industry (Fig. 5–2). Many home health nurses predict that most health care services in the future will be provided in the home. This is especially true as patients are being discharged earlier from the hospital.

FIGURE   5 – 2
Home health nursing is a fast-growing segment of the health care industry. (Photo by Kelly Whalen.)

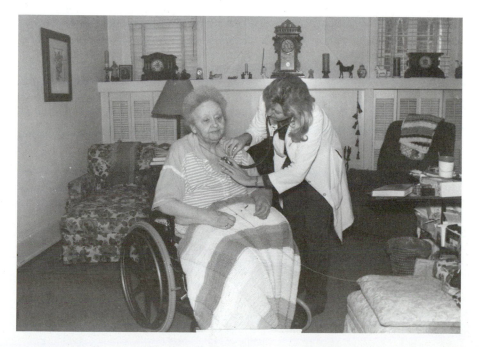

Home health care has traditionally been, and will continue to be, nursing's "turf." Home health nurses across the United States provide quality care in the most cost-effective and, for patients, the most comfortable setting possible—the home. Patients cared for at home today are sicker than ever. Therefore, more high-technology equipment is being used in the home. Equipment and procedures formerly unheard of outside of hospital settings, such as intravenous pumps and chemotherapy administration, are routinely encountered in home care today.

Home health nurses must possess up-to-date nursing knowledge and be secure in their own nursing skills. They do not have the backup of physicians or more experienced nurses as they might in a hospital. They must have good assessment skills, make independent judgments, recognize patients' and families' teaching needs, and have good communication skills. They must also know what their limits are and seek help when the patient's needs are beyond the scope of their abilities.

An RN working in home health in Atlanta, Georgia, relates:

> I have always found a tremendous reward in working with the terminally ill and the elderly, and I get a great deal of contact with this particular population working in home health. One patient I cared for developed a pressure ulcer while at home. I was able to assess the patient's physiological needs as well as teach the family how to care for their loved one to prevent future skin breakdown. Within a few weeks the skin looked good, and the family felt important and involved. To me this is real nursing.

NURSE ENTREPRENEURS

Are you a self-starter? Are you a risk-taker? Can you make independent decisions? Can you lead others? If you answer yes to all of these questions, you may want the challenge of being a nurse **entrepreneur.** A nurse entrepreneur identifies a need and creates a service to meet the identified need. Some nurses are creative and energetic people who like the idea of new forms of expression. They are good candidates for entrepreneurship.

Nurse entrepreneurs enjoy the autonomy that is derived from owning and operating their own health-related businesses. Groups of nurses, some of whom are faculty in schools of nursing, have opened nurse-managed centers to provide direct care to clients. Nurse entrepreneurs are self-employed as consultants to hospitals, nursing homes, and schools of nursing. Others have started private practices and carry their own caseloads of patients with physical or emotional needs. They are sometimes involved in presenting educational workshops and seminars. Some nurses establish their own creative apparel businesses, which provide articles of clothing for premature babies or handicapped people. Others own and operate their own health equipment companies and home health agencies.

Here are a few comments from one such entrepreneur, the chief executive officer of a privately owned home health agency:

> I like working for myself. I know that my success or failure in my business is up to me. Having your own home health agency is a lot of work. You have to be very organized and have excellent communication skills. You cannot be afraid to say no to people. There is nothing better than the feel-

ing you get from a family calling to say our nurses have made a difference in their loved one's life, but I also have to take the calls of complaint about my agency. Those are tough.

A number of nurses are taking the business of health care into their own hands. They seem to agree that the opportunity to create their own businesses has never been better. One such business, based in Columbus, Ohio, offers nursing care for mothers, babies, and children. The emphasis is the care of women whose pregnancies may be complicated by diabetes, hypertension, or multiple births. "Our main specialty is managing high-risk pregnancies and high-risk newborns," reports the RN founder. She continued:

> Home care for these individuals is a boon not only to the patients themselves, but also to hospitals, insurance companies, and doctors. With the trend toward shorter hospital stays, risks are minimized if skilled maternity nurses are on hand to provide patients with specialty care in their homes.

As with almost any endeavor, there are disadvantages that come with owning a small business. There is the risk of losing your investment if the business is unsuccessful. Fluctuations in income are common, especially in the early months, and regular paychecks may become a memory, at least at first. A certain amount of pressure is created because of the total responsibility for meeting deadlines and paying bills, salaries, and taxes. But there is great opportunity, too.

Aspiring entrepreneurs can eliminate much of the risk involved in small business ownership by completing four preliminary steps:

1. Conduct a thorough needs assessment to determine if the service or product is needed and wanted by consumers.
2. Develop a detailed business plan complete with short-term and long-term goals, marketing plans, and schedules for business development.
3. Have enough capital to carry the business for at least a year, even if there is no profit, and keep overhead low.
4. Prepare appropriately by learning about effective business practices, for example, budgeting, accounting, personnel policies, and legal aspects of small business.

In addition to financial incentives, there are also intangible rewards in entrepreneurship. For some people, the autonomy and freedom to control one's own practice are more than enough to compensate them for increased pressure and initial uncertainty.

With rapid changes occurring daily in the health care system, there are always new and exciting horizons. Alert nurses who possess creativity, initiative, and business savvy have tremendous opportunities as entrepreneurs.

NURSES IN OFFICE SETTINGS

Nurses who are employed in office settings work directly with physicians and their patients. Nursing activities include performing health assessments, drawing blood, giving immunizations, administering medications, and providing health teaching. Nurses in office settings also act as liaisons between patients and physicians. They amplify and clarify orders for patients as well as provide emotional support to anxious patients. They may visit hospitalized patients, and some assist the employing physician in surgery. Often, they supervise other office workers, such as practical nurses, nurse aides, scheduling clerks, and record clerks. Educational requirements, hours of work, and specific responsibilities vary, depending on the preferences of the employer.

An RN who works for a group of three nephrologists in Atlanta, Georgia, describes a typical day:

> I first make rounds independently on patients in the dialysis center, making sure that they are tolerating the dialysis procedure and answering questions regarding their treatments and diets. I then make rounds with one of the physicians in the hospital as he visits patients and orders new treatments. The afternoon is spent in the office assessing patients as they come for their physician's visit. I may draw blood for a diagnostic test on one patient and do patient teaching regarding diet to another. No two days are alike, and that is what I love about this position. I have a sense of independence but still have daily patient contact.

RNs considering employment in office settings need good communication skills because a large part of their responsibilities includes communicating with patients, families, physicians, pharmacists, and hospital admitting clerks. They should inquire about the specifics of the position because office nursing roles range from performing only routine tasks to the multifaceted functions described by the nurse interviewed.

NURSES IN OCCUPATIONAL HEALTH SETTINGS

Would you enjoy working in a large company or manufacturing plant with adults who work there? Are you wellness oriented? Do you enjoy teaching people how to live healthy lifestyles? These are some of the characteristics needed by **occupational health nurses.**

Many large companies today employ nurses to deliver basic health care services, health education, screenings, and emergency treatment to company employees. Corporate executives have long known that good employee health reduces absenteeism, insurance costs, and worker errors, thereby improving company profitability. Occupational health nurses represent an important investment by companies. They are often asked to serve as consultants on health matters within the company. They may participate in health-related policy development, such as policies governing employee smoking or family leaves (formerly known as maternity leaves). Depending on the size of the company, the nurse may be the only health professional employed and therefore could have a good deal of autonomy.

The usual educational requirement for nurses in occupational health roles is licensure. Some positions call for a baccalaureate degree in nursing. These nurses must possess knowledge and skills that enable them to perform routine physical assessments, including vision and hearing screenings for all employees. Good interpersonal skills to provide counseling and referrals for lifestyle problems, such as stress or substance abuse, are a plus for these nurses. They must also have first-aid and cardiopulmonary resuscitation (CPR) skills. If employed in a heavy manufacturing setting where burns or traumas are a risk, they must have special training in those medical emergencies.

The responsibilities of occupational health nurses extend to the entire work environment. They must be able to assess the environment for potential safety hazards and work with management to eliminate or reduce them. They need a working knowledge of governmental regulations, such as the requirements of the Occupational Safety and Health Administration (OSHA), and must ensure that the company is complying with them. They also need to understand worker's compensation regulations and coordinate the care of injured workers with the treating physician.

Nurses in occupational settings have to be confident in their nursing skills, be effective communicators with both employees and management, motivate employees to adopt healthier habits, and be able to function independently in delivering care.

SCHOOL NURSING

Nurses choosing school nursing must love to work with children, their families, and teachers. Although some states have well-developed **school nurse** programs, others do not. In 1995 only six states—Alaska, Connecticut, Delaware, Maine, New Hampshire, and Vermont—had the recommended minimum number of school nurses of 1 nurse per 750 students. States with the most students per school nurse were Tennessee, with 10,814 students per nurse; Georgia, with 8800 students per nurse; North Dakota, with 6404 students per nurse; Alabama, with 5315 students per nurse; and Utah, with 4317 students per nurse (Carey and Mullins, 1995). With such high ratios, it is difficult to imagine how children in these states can be deriving any true benefit from the school nurse program.

Health care futurists believe that school nursing is the wave of the future (Moccia, 1992). The role of school nurse has expanded to include members of the school child's immediate family. It will require many more school nurses as well as a willingness by states and local school boards to pay them to support the expansion of school nurse programs.

Most school systems require nurses to have a minimum of a baccalaureate degree in nursing, whereas some school districts have higher educational requirements. Prior experience working with children is also usually required. School health has become a specialty in its own right, and in states where school health is a priority, graduate programs in school health nursing have been established.

School nurses need a working knowledge of human growth and development to detect developmental problems early. First aid for minor injuries and emergency care for more severe ones are additional skills school nurses use. Counseling skills are important because many children turn to the school nurse as counselor. School nurses keep records of children's immunizations and are responsible for seeing that immunizations are current. When an outbreak of a childhood communicable disease occurs, school nurses educate parents, teachers, and students about treatment and prevention of transmission.

Legislation requiring mainstreaming of children has brought many physically challenged children into regular school classrooms. School nurses must work closely with parents and teachers to provide these children with the special care they need while at school.

School nurses work closely with teachers to incorporate health concepts into the curriculum. They conduct vision and hearing screenings. Parents expect school nurses to make referrals to qualified physicians and other health care providers when routine screenings identify problems outside the nurses' scope of practice.

School nurses must be prepared to handle both routine illnesses of children and adolescents and emergencies. One of their major concerns is safety. Accidents are the leading cause of death in children of all ages, yet accidents are preventable. Preventive aspects of child health are a major focus of school health nurses. In terms of safety, prevention requires both protection from obvious hazards and education of teachers, parents, and students about how to avoid accidents. School nurses practice safety, are alert to safety needs in the school and surrounding environment, and recognize the need for safety education in contributing to accident reduction.

School nursing is a complex and multifaceted field that is constantly expanding. It represents a challenge for those nurses who choose it as a career.

CASE MANAGERS

Are you organized? Do you like to get a bargain for your money and also appreciate quality? A nursing **case manager** is a recently developed role you might be interested in pursuing as a challenging career.

Case management is a process of following an individual patient's health care to ensure maximum positive outcomes while containing costs. The case manager is the person responsible for this process, and RNs are the most common professional group to act as case managers. A nursing case manager may follow the patient from the diagnostic phase through hospitalization, rehabilitation, and back to home care. Through careful planning, every step of the patient's care is coordinated in a timely manner.

The key to making case management work is the development of critical paths that include specific timelines and standard treatment protocols. A critical path is an abbreviated version of the case management plan that is used for daily decision making about patient care. It lists key nursing and medical interventions that should occur within a certain timeline to ensure positive patient outcomes. Case management is considered successful if the patient is well enough for discharge within the DRG (Diagnostic-Related Grouping)-directed length of stay. Figure 5–3 shows a CareMap for Sickle Cell Anemia. CareMaps are a trademarked concept of The Center for Case Management, South Natick, Massachusetts. They are a clinical system similar to critical paths being used in many institutions across the United States.

Case management involves collaboration with other health care disciplines, so nursing case managers must possess good interpersonal skills. Because of nurs-

Initiated by _____ Date: ____ /____ /____ Time: _____

Notify Case Manager Craford Long Hospital
          The Emory University System of Health Care
          Sickle Cell Care Map

Target LOS: 7.0 days

Only initiate CareMap for patients after notifying primary physician or Clinical Case Manager.

Pre-existing Medical Conditions (check applicable):

☐ **Fever**
  –Intermediate outcome: Basic culture results should be obtained within 48–72 hours—antibiotic prescribed should match pathogen identified.
  –Discharge outcome: Maintains temperature of <38.3°C unless other explanation for temperature has been determined.

☐ **Bone Infarction**
  –Intermediate outcome: Maintains pre-existing level of function.
  –Discharge outcome: Patient should express comfort with pain management on oral medications.

☐ **Aplastic Anemia**
  –Intermediate outcome: Hematocrit stabilized within 4 days.
  –Discharge outcome: If reticulocyte count <10, appropriate follow-up plan is in place.

☐ **Septicemia**
  –Intermediate outcome: Basic culture results should be obtained within 48–72 hours—antibiotic prescribed should match pathogen identified.
  –Discharge outcomes: Temperature <38.3°C.
                   Negative blood cultures.
                   Off antibiotics.

☐ **Nausea/Vomiting**
  –Intermediate outcome: Patient able to tolerate oral fluids.
  –Discharge outcome: Usual diet pattern re-established.

☐ **Pneumonia/Pulmonary Infarcts/Dyspnea**
  –Discharge outcome: Ambulates 50 ft. with no more than 2 on dyspnea scale, or, return to baseline level of dyspnea on exertion.

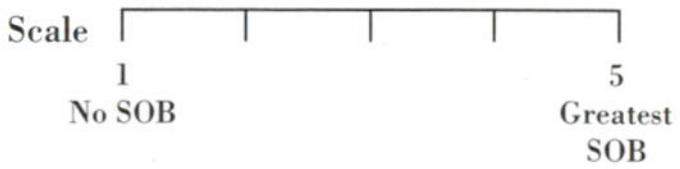

          Scale   ⌐————|————|————|————⌐
                   1   5
                No SOB   Greatest
                                SOB

☐ **Sickle Chest Syndrome**
  –Discharge outcomes: Pulse oximetry >92% or, consistently stable. Tolerates increased activity.

☐ **Catheter Sepsis**
  –Intermediate outcome: Identify organism by culture and begin antibiotic therapy. Remove catheter if unable to treat.
  –Discharge outcome: No positive culture from catheter site for (3) days.

FIGURE 5–3
CareMap: Sickle cell anemia. (Courtesy of Crawford Long Hospital, The Emory University System of Health Care.)

(continued)

Interdis-ciplinary Action Plan	CareMap Day 1 Date ____ /____ /____	Initials			Time	Interdisciplinary Progress Notes
		N	D	E		
Consults/ Other Therapies	Case manager Nutrition Respiratory therapy Social services Other					
Tests	Routine Orders: If ABG ordered results called _____ (time called) If O_2 ordered (check appropriate): ☐ pulse ox 1 hour later _____% (results) ☐ ABG 1 hour later & call report ____ (time called)					
Treatments	TENS (if ordered) Warm packs prn Whirlpool (if ordered) O_2 @ ____ via ____ Strict I & O q shift Weight on admission					
Medications	Routine Orders Review MAR					
Nutrition	Diet (type) _____ Circle amount consumed: Breakfast: all ¾ ½ ¼ 0 NPO Lunch: all ¾ ½ ¼ 0 NPO Dinner: all ¾ ½ ¼ 0 NPO					
Activity/ Safety	Report continued discomfort to physician Bedrest/Bathroom privileges					
Assessment	Pain assessment form completed					
Teaching/ DC Planning	Intravenous line care precautions Social services notified					
Expected Patient Outcomes (explain variations to expected outcomes on Variation Record)	0.1 Verbalizes satisfaction with pain management 0.2 Verbalizes improvement with activity level					
No nursing initials required in gray shaded areas	Initials/Signature ____ /_____ ____ /_____			Initials/Signature ____ /_____ ____ /_____		

* = Variance ■ = Key intermediate goals

F I G U R E   5 – 3 *(Continued)*

ing's holistic view of patients, nurses are uniquely qualified to provide direction to the multidisciplinary team caring for each patient.

Both patient and nurse satisfaction are high with the one-on-one relationship fostered with case management. Patients like the security of having one familiar person coordinating their care, and a nursing case manager has the satisfaction of coordinating a patient's care from beginning to end (McKenzie, Torkelson, and Holt, 1989).

HOSPITAL NURSING

As reviewed in Chapter 1, nursing care originated in the home setting and moved into hospitals only within the last century. In 1992, 66 percent of employed RNs worked in hospital settings. Hospitals vary widely in size, services offered, and geographic location. In general, nurses in hospitals work with patients who have medical or surgical conditions, with children, with women and their newborns, with cancer patients, with people who have had severe traumas or burns, in operating rooms or emergency departments, and in many other capacities. In 1992, hospital nurses worked in the following areas:

Area	Number of RNs
General units	449,000
Intensive care units	203,000
Operating/recovery rooms	128,000
Stepdown units	70,000
Emergency departments	76,000
Labor and delivery units	63,000
Outpatient units	62,000

The median salary of a staff nurse working full-time in hospitals in 1992 was $33,278 (U.S. Department of Labor, 1992).

In addition to direct patient care roles, nurses in hospitals serve as educators, managers, and administrators who teach or supervise others and establish the direction of nursing hospitalwide. There is perhaps no other setting that offers so much variety within the same organization as do hospitals.

The educational credentials required of RNs practicing in hospitals can range from associate degrees and diplomas to doctoral degrees. Generally, entry-level positions require only a license. Many hospitals require nurses to hold baccalaureate degrees to move up the clinical ladder or to move into management. **Clinical coordinators,** who are responsible for the management of more than one unit, are generally expected to hold master's degrees.

Most new nurses choose to work in acute care hospitals initially to gain experience in organizing and delivering patient care. For some, staff nursing is extremely enjoyable, and they continue in this role for their entire careers.

Others pursue additional education, often provided by the hospital, and move into specialty units such as coronary care. Although specialty units usually require experience and advanced training, some hospitals do allow exceptional new graduates to work in these units.

Some nurses find that management is their strength. Head nurses, often called **nurse managers,** are in charge of all activities on their units, including patient care, continuous quality improvement, personnel selection and evaluation, and resource management. Being a nurse manager in a hospital today is somewhat like running a business, and nurses need an entrepreneurial spirit to be effective in this role. Nurse managers earned a median salary of $47,335 in 1992 (U.S. Department of Labor, 1992).

Most nurses in hospitals provide direct patient care. In the past, it was necessary for nurses to move into administrative or management roles to be promoted or receive salary increases. This took them away from the bedside. Today, **clinical ladder** programs allow nurses to progress while staying in direct patient care roles.

A clinical ladder is a multiple-step program that begins with entry-level staff nurse positions. As nurses gain experience, participate in continuing education, demonstrate clinical competence, pursue formal education, and become certified, they are eligible to move up the rungs of the ladder.

At the top of most clinical ladders are CNSs. **Clinical nurse specialists** are nurses with master's degrees in specialized areas of nursing, such as oncology. The role varies but generally includes responsibility for serving as a clinical mentor and role model for other nurses as well as setting standards for nursing care on the particular unit. The oncology clinical specialist, for example, works with the nursing staff on the oncology unit to help them stay abreast of the latest research in the care of cancer patients. The clinical specialist is a resource person for the unit and often provides direct care to patients or families with particularly difficult or complex problems. The CNS establishes nursing protocols and is responsible for seeing that nurses adhere to high standards of care.

Salaries and responsibilities increase at the higher levels of clinical ladders. The clinical ladder concept benefits nurses by allowing them to advance while still working directly with patients. Hospitals also benefit by retaining experienced clinical nurses in direct care roles, thus improving the quality of nursing care throughout the hospital.

One of the greatest drawbacks to hospital nursing in the past was the necessity for nurses to work rigid schedules, which usually included evenings, nights, and weekends. Although nurses still must work a fair share of undesirable times, **flexible staffing** is becoming the norm. Sometimes nurses on a particular unit negotiate with each other and establish their own schedules that meet personal needs while ensuring that appropriate patient care is provided.

Each hospital nursing role has its own unique characteristics. In the following profile, an RN discusses his role as a bedside nurse in a burn unit:

> A burn nurse has to be gentle, strong, and patient enough to go slow. You must be confident enough to work alone; you must believe that what you're doing is in the patient's best interest because some of the procedures hurt far worse than anyone can imagine. Every burn is unique and a challenge. Fifteen years ago, the prognosis for surviving an intensive burn was not good, but with today's techniques for fluid replacement and the development of effective antibiotics, many patients are surviving the first few criti-

cal days. During the long hours of one-on-one care you really get to know your patient. There is nothing more rewarding.

When the "fit" between nurses and their role requirements is good, nursing is a gratifying profession. An oncology nurse demonstrated that gratification as she discussed her role:

Being an oncology nurse and working with people with potentially terminal illnesses brings you close to patients and their families (Fig. 5–4). The family room for our patients and their families is very homelike. Families bring food in and have dinner with their loved one right here. Working with dying patients is a tall order. You must be able to support the family and the patient through many stages of the dying process including anger and depression. Experiencing cancer is always traumatic with the diagnosis, the treatment, and the struggle to cope. But today's statistics show that more people experience cancer and live. Because of research and early detection, being diagnosed with cancer is no longer the automatic death sentence it used to be. I love getting involved with patients and their families

FIGURE   5–4

Hospital nurses work closely with the families of patients as well as with the patients themselves. (Photo by Kelly Whalen.)

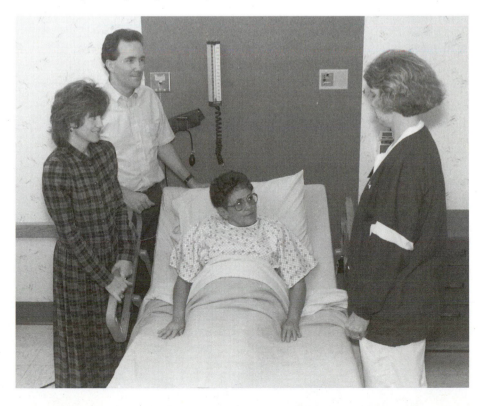

and feel that I can contribute to their positive mental attitude, which can impact their disease process, or hold their hand and help them to die with dignity. They cry, I cry—it is part of my nursing, and I would have it no other way.

These are only two of the many possible roles nurses in hospital settings may choose. Although brief, these descriptions convey a flavor of the responsibility, complexity, and fulfillment to be found in hospital-based nursing today.

SALARIES OF NURSES PRACTICING IN HOSPITAL SETTINGS

The latest survey of *The Registered Nurse Population: 1992* (U.S. Department of Health and Human Services, 1994) shows positive signs in terms of salaries for RNs. Salaries are up nationwide, but discussing salaries from a national perspective is often misleading. Salary figures in major cities are much higher than those in smaller communities. Readers should bear this in mind when reviewing these figures. The 1992 average annual salary of a full-time RN in a staff position was $35,212 (U.S. Department of Health and Human Services, 1994). Figure 5–5 shows the average annual salaries of staff nurses in each geographical area of the United States.

FIGURE   5–5
Average annual salaries of full-time registered nurses in staff positions by geographic region, March 1992. (From U.S. Department of Health and Human Services (1994). *The registered nurse population: 1992*. Washington, D.C.)

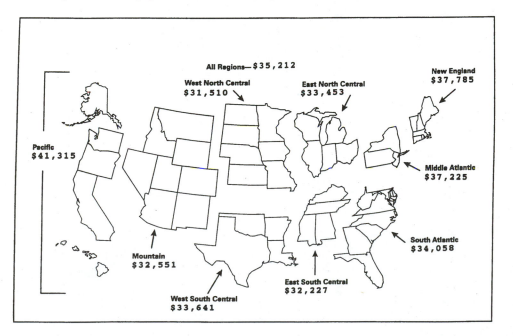

TABLE 5–1
Nursing Salary Comparison to Other Professions

Profession	Average Beginning	Average Maximum	Salary Comparison of Registered Nurse to Other Professions' Average Maximum
Accountants	$24,809	$75,347	154.0%
Accounting clerks	14,639	24,787	49.3%
Chemists	27,162	88,749	181.4%
Computer programmers	26,103	42,533	115.0%
Engineers	32,459	95,058	194.0%
Personnel directors	45,618	101,922	208.3%
Registered nurses	27,225	48,924	
Secretaries	19,844	34,085	69.6%

From U.S. Department of Labor, Bureau of Labor Statistics (1992). Occupational wage survey: Hospitals. Bulletin 2392, p. 128.

An important issue to RNs is the problem of **salary compression.** Salary compression means that pay increases are limited during a typical career. Nurses "top out" early in their careers, and nurses with years of experience sometime make little, if any, more than their younger counterparts. No differential pay for experience and no allowances for administrative responsibilities contribute to the typically "compressed" nature of a nurse's salary.

The effect of salary compression on RNs' salaries when compared with other professions' average maximum salaries can be seen in Table 5–1. This issue is certainly one of concern to nurses, and much work remains to be done in this important area. Changes will occur as nurses educate others about inequities, introduce legal remedies in courts and state legislatures, and promote changes in the workplace.

NURSING OPPORTUNITIES REQUIRING HIGHER DEGREES

Many RNs choose to pursue roles that require a master's degree, doctoral degree, or specialized education in a specific area. Already mentioned in this chapter are CNSs, nurse managers, and nurse executives in hospital settings. Nurse educators, whether in clinical or academic settings, also are required to hold advanced degrees. In 1992, 2 percent of RNs worked in nursing education.

Nurse educators in accredited schools of nursing must hold a minimum of a master's degree in nursing, and many have doctoral degrees in nursing or other fields. In 1992, 21.4 percent of nursing faculty were doctorally prepared, a favorable improvement when compared with only 3% in 1972 and 10.6% in 1984 (Anderson, 1994).

Most nursing faculty are women, 8.5 percent are members of minority groups, and 49.2 percent of faculty teaching in colleges and universities are untenured (Anderson, 1994). In 1992, fewer than 10 percent of graduate students chose nursing education and prepared for a teaching role. This trend seems to be continuing and contributes to anxiety about a shortage of nursing faculty in the future.

Approximately 140,000 RNs in 1992 reported having the education and credentials to work as APNs. **Advanced practice nurse** is an umbrella term applied to an RN who has met advanced educational and clinical practice requirements beyond the 2 to 4 years of basic nursing education required of all RNs. There are four categories of advanced practice nurses: NP, CNS, CNM, and CRNA.

Nurse Practitioner

Nurse practitioners (NP) work in clinics, nursing homes, hospitals, or their own offices. Most NPs choose a specialty area such as adult, family, or pediatric health care. They are qualified to handle a wide range of basic health problems. These nurses can perform physical examinations, take medical histories, diagnose and treat common acute minor illnesses or injuries, order and interpret laboratory tests and x-ray films, and counsel and educate clients (Fig. 5–6). In 1992, NPs could legally write prescriptions in 48 states but generally require physician supervision to do so. Some NPs are independent practitioners and can be reimbursed by Medicare or Medicaid for their work. Others work for hospitals, health maintenance organizations (HMOs), or private industry.

There were 150 NP education programs in 1992. These programs grant master's degrees and prepare nurses to sit for national certification examinations. Approximately 36 states require NPs to be nationally certified by the ANA or other nursing specialty organizations. By 1992, approximately 58 percent of the 48,237 NPs in the United States were nationally certified. The average salary of an NP in 1992 was $43,636, but this varies widely according to specialty and geographic area (American Nurses Association, 1994).

Clinical Nurse Specialist

Similar to NPs, CNSs work in a variety of settings, including hospitals, clinics, nursing homes, their own offices, private industry, home care, and HMOs. CNSs hold advanced nursing degrees—master's or doctoral—and are qualified to handle a wide range of physical and mental health problems. CNSs are experts in a particular field of clinical practice, such as mental health, gerontology, cardiac care, cancer care, community health, or neonatal health. They perform health assessments, make diagnoses, deliver treatment, and develop quality control methods. Additionally, CNSs also work in consultation, research, education, and administration. Direct reimbursement to some CNSs is possible through Medicare, Medicaid, Champus, and private insurers. In 1992, there were 58,185 CNSs in the United States. Their average salary was $41,226 (American Nurses Association, 1994).

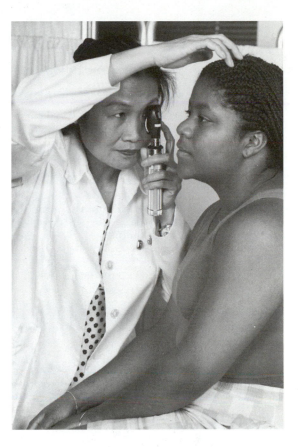

FIGURE   5–6
A nurse practitioner examines her patient. (Photo by Fielding Freed.)

Certified Nurse-Midwife

A **certified nurse-midwife** (CNM) provides well-woman care and attends to or assists in childbirth in various settings, including hospitals, birthing centers, and homes. The ANA reported (1993a) that in 1990, CNMs delivered 148,728 babies, or about 3.6 percent of all U.S. births that year. Births attended by CNMs had fewer episiotomies, fewer forceps deliveries, and fewer low-birth-weight and premature infants according to an ANA study. CNMs are able to prescribe medications in more than 33 states (ANA, 1993a). Increasingly educated at the master's level, CNMs receive an average of 1.5 years of specialized education beyond basic nursing school. The average salary of the 7400 CNMs in 1992 was $43,636 (American Nurses Association, 1994).

Because of patient acceptance and a good safety record, CNMs are expected to increase in the future. The accompanying *News Note* summarizes a report by Ralph Nader, the consumer advocate, describing the value of CNMs in a reformed health care system.

NEWS NOTE

"Nader Group Sees CNMs Replacing OBs in 'Majority of American Births'"

Washington, D.C.—If Ralph Nader and his Public Citizen advocacy group have anything to say about it, the majority of American births, "not too long from now," will be attended by certified nurse-midwives [CNMs].

Releasing his Health Research Group's latest findings, Nader called the press to his Washington headquarters in November to explain why CNMs are a "better alternative" for birthing and maternity care and why they should outnumber obstetricians in a rational health care system. The research group is publishing a survey supporting that argument together with a national *Consumer's Guide to Nurse-Midwifery*, a 252-page directory that the researchers compiled with detailed descriptions of the services offered by 414 hospital-based practices and 41 freestanding birth centers.

"The 4000-plus CNMs in the U.S. offer . . . sensible, woman-oriented, old-fashioned care along with the latest medical and scientific expertise," said Public Citizen's head health researcher, physician Sidney Wolfe.

A group of new mothers told reporters about their contrasting experiences with OBs and CNMs. Johns Hopkins CNM Lisa Summers pointed out that healthy women are most in need of providers who don't answer questions "with our hand on the doorknob." Ruth Watson Lubic, founder of New York's Maternity Center Association, called on insurers to pay for prenatal and follow-up care, "rather than another 24 hours in an institution."

"Get the Message Out"

The powerful consumer group announced that it's pushing state and federal officials to loosen restrictive laws and to fund expanded education programs. It's urging consumers to choose a CNM as a primary care provider and spread the message: "Talk to your friends . . . Write to your legislators . . . Ask your insurance company to cover nurse-midwifery . . . Let the administrator of your local hospital know that you would like to see nurse-midwives given admitting privileges."

Wolfe stressed that CNMs should play a major role in cutting health care costs and curbing infant mortality rates. Assistant Secretary for Health Philip Lee endorsed the campaign and pledged continued federal support.

The $3000-plus cost of cesarean births was spotlighted as an example of what's wrong with the current delivery system. While nearly one in four U.S. babies are now born by cesarean section, Public Citizen's data on 127,000 births showed a rate of only 11.6% for hospital births attended by CNMs. At freestanding birth centers, the rate dropped to 6.7%.

The CNMs who were surveyed also averaged a 68.9% rate of vaginal birth after cesarean—2.8 times higher (better) than the national average. The rates can't be explained away by risk profiles; most of the CNMs surveyed care for moderate- and high-risk as well as low-risk women.

Resurgence Seen in U.S.

As recently as 1975, fewer than 1% of American births in-hospital were attended by CNMs. By contrast, midwives supply much of the prenatal and labor and delivery care in many countries with better mortality records. But the past two decades have seen a steady rise that in 1993 reached 178,537—4.4% of U.S. hospital births.

The 460 practices that answered Public Citizen's questions are responsible for an estimated 50% to 60% of CNMs' childbirth activity.

"Nurse-midwifery is not assembly-line care," the survey found. Over 90% of the practices reported that they offer 11 of 14 "options" in care, from oral fluids, room to ambulate, and use of a bath, shower, or hot tub to encouragement of alternative positions.

(continued)

NEWS NOTE *(Continued)*

Besides comparable outcomes and control over their childbirth experience, CNMs' clients "can look forward to longer prenatal visits, greater emphasis on education and birth preparation, and greater emotional support," the Nader group concluded.

Yet the responses showed CNMs still struggling for acceptance. Over 60% were coping with some kind of restriction: limits on prescribing and reimbursement, refusal of admitting privileges, and hospital policies that assume a medical model of care.

Reprinted with permission of *American Journal of Nursing* (1996). Nader group sees CNMs replacing OBs in "majority of American births." 96(1): 62, 65. Used with permission of Lippincott-Raven Publishers, Philadelphia, PA.

Certified Registered Nurse Anesthetist

Certified registered nurse anesthetists (CRNA) administer anesthetic agents to patients undergoing operative procedures. CRNAs administer more than 65 percent of all anesthetics given to patients each year. In rural hospitals, CRNAs provide 85 percent of anesthetics. Working with physician anesthesiologists or frequently independently, CRNAs are found in a variety of settings—operating rooms, dentist's offices, and ambulatory surgical settings.

Two to 3 years of specialized education in master's or certification programs is required beyond the required 4-year bachelor's degree. The accrediting body for schools of anesthesia in the United States has required that by 1998 all accredited programs in nurse anesthesia will offer master's preparation. CRNAs must also meet national certification and recertification requirements. There were 25,238 CRNAs in 1992, and their average salary was $76,053 (American Nurses Association, 1994).

Issues in Advanced Practice Nursing

Some nursing leaders (Jones, 1994; Sparacino, 1993) believe that the boundaries between the roles of CNSs and NPs are increasingly blurred, and nursing might benefit from having a common educational base and common titling for these two advanced practice roles. Pearson (1995) claimed that it is clear to insurance companies what physicians, hospitals, and dentists do. She stated that it is often not as clear, however, what APNs do, and this impedes progress toward direct reimbursement for services for these highly qualified professionals. Nurses are challenged to be clear to the public about the services they are qualified to provide.

Pearson addressed another challenge in the January 1995 issue of *The Nurse Practitioner.* She asserted that although there has been some progress in state legislation to improve the scope of practice of APNs, there is little to celebrate regarding national legislation. Until the U.S. Congress approves legislation to provide primary health care for all U.S. citizens and makes provisions for APNs to share fully in the provision of that care, the role of APNs is at the mercy of the various state legislatures.

Currently, more than 100,000 APNs provide primary health care services, often to underserved populations in rural and inner-city areas. These nurses frequently find, however, that they must navigate a patchwork of laws and regulations that vary from state to state and within the Medicare program. Their hands are often tied, with legislative and administrative barriers preventing them from providing services to a broader segment of the public.

There are substantial barriers to the practice of APNs because of the overlap between traditional medical and nursing functions. "The independent practice of nurses is a politically charged arena, with organized medicine firmly against all efforts of nurses to be recognized as independent health care providers who receive direct reimbursement for their services" (Stafford and Appleyard, 1994, p. 24). What nursing needs is more understanding of the political process and power. Pearson (1995) states that APNs need to be clear about these three things:

1. There are large crossover areas of expertise and overlapping competencies between APNs and physicians.
2. There are many medical and health care problems that do not require the experience or expertise of a physician.
3. When physicians and NPs work together collaboratively, the patients receive the best standard of care because each profession has its own unique qualities—the NP listens better, manages the care in a broader and more efficient way, and is more available, whereas the physician has specialized knowledge for more serious and complicated care situations.

Pearson further insists that when explaining their roles, APNs must use concrete words everyone can understand: *APNs diagnose, treat, and prescribe in ways that are cost-effective.*

Based on the relative cost and time of educating NPs and CNSs compared with the basic education of physicians, four or five NPs could be educated for the price of producing a single physician (*American Journal of Nursing*, 1993). Even though there is an oversupply of physicians and an undersupply of nurses nationally, federal funding for graduate medical education continues to be allocated disproportionately—$4.8 billion goes to physician education, whereas only $300 million is directed to educating future nurses (American Nurses Association, 1993b). In 1992, the average net income for physicians was $170,600, and the average salary of a nurse practitioner was $43,600 (*The American Nurse*, 1994). The public needs this information to decide who the most cost-effective providers of primary care are.

SUMMARY

There are more than 2.2 million RNs in the United States, and nearly 1.9 million are actively practicing. Two-thirds of working nurses are employed in hospitals, a traditional setting for nursing practice, but a setting that should see dramatic changes as health care in the United States becomes more community-based. An exciting trend is toward practice settings in home health, school nursing, and small health-related businesses. APNs are one solution to the U.S. health care crisis. APNs are capable of delivering high-quality care to many segments of the population not currently receiving health care. Barriers to APNs must be removed in the future through political action of organized nursing and politically active nurses.

REVIEW AND DISCUSSION QUESTIONS

1. What characteristics do nurses of today have in common, and how do they differ?
2. Think of the areas of nursing that interest you most. How do your personal and professional qualifications compare with the characteristics needed in the roles discussed in this chapter?
3. Interview nurses in various practice settings. Find out how they prepared for their positions, what their daily activities are, and what they enjoy most and least about their work.
4. Call the nurse recruiter or personnel office of a nearby hospital and inquire about salaries and other benefits for entry-level and advanced nursing practice positions. How do they compare with those listed in this chapter?
5. Interview an advanced practice nurse working in your community. What does he or she see as the major impediments to practice? Find out what is being done about these barriers in your state.

REFERENCES

American Journal of Nursing (1996). Nader group sees CNMs replacing OBs in "majority of American births." 96(1), 62, 65.

American Journal of Nursing (1993). Nurse practitioners emerge as key players in the debate over reform; MDs will fight inroads on practice, 93(7), 69, 72.

American Nurses Association (1994). *Today's registered nurse—numbers and demographics.* Kansas City, MO: Author.

American Nurses Association (1993a). *Advanced practice nursing: A new age in health care.* Kansas City, MO: Author.

American Nurses Association (1993b). *Primary health care: The nurse solution.* Kansas City, MO: Author.

American Nurses Association (1991). *Nursing and the American Nurses Association.* Kansas City, MO: Author.

Anderson, C. A. (1994). Nursing faculty: Who are they, what do they do, and what challenges do they face? In J. C. McCloskey and H. K. Grace (Eds.), *Current issues in nursing* (pp. 32–37). St. Louis: Mosby.

Carey, A. R., and Mullins, M. E. (1995). Schools lack enough nurses. *USA Today* (Source: Asthma Zero Mortality Coalition).

Jones, D. A. (1994). Advanced practice: Merging the roles of the nurse practitioner and clinical specialist. In O. L. Strickland and D. J. Fishman (Eds.), *Nursing issues in the 1990's* (pp. 126–132). Albany: Delmar.

McKenzie, C. B., Torkelson, N. G., and Holt, M. A. (1989). Care and cost: Nursing case management improves both. *Nursing management*, 20(10), 30–34.

Moccia, P. (1992). In 1992: A nurse in every school. *Nursing & Health Care*, 13(1), 14–18.

National League for Nursing (1994). *Nursing data review 1994.* New York: Author.

Pearson, L. J. (1995). Annual update of how each state stands on legislative issues affecting advanced nursing practice, *The Nurse Practitioner*, 20(1), 13–18.

Sparacino, P. S. A. (1993). The advanced practice nurse: Is the time right for a singular title? *Clinical Nurse Specialist*, 7(1), 3.

Stafford, M., and Appleyard, J. (1994). Clinical nurse specialists and nurse practitioners: Who are they, what do they do, and what challenges do they face? In J. C. McCloskey and H. K. Grace (Eds.), *Current issues in nursing* (pp. 32–37). St. Louis: Mosby.

The American Nurse (1994, January). ANA expresses disappointment over AMA opposition to APN autonomy. Washington, D.C.: American Nurses Association.

U.S. Department of Health and Human Services (1994). *The registered nurse population: 1992*. Washington, D.C.: Author.

U.S. Department of Labor, Bureau of Labor Statistics (1992). *Occupational wage survey: Hospitals*. Washington, D.C.: Author.

U.S. Department of Labor, Bureau of Labor Statistics (1995). *Occupational compensation survey: Temporary help supply services United States and selected metropolitan areas, November 1994*. Bulletin 2392. Washington, D.C.: Author.

6

Kay K. Chitty

Defining Profession

OBJECTIVES

- Identify the characteristics of a profession.
- Distinguish between the characteristics of professions and occupations.
- Evaluate nursing's current status as a profession.
- Recognize characteristic behaviors of professional nurses.

VOCABULARY

accountability	cognitive	occupation
altruism	Flexner Report	profession
autonomy	helping profession	professional
code of ethics	nursing process	professionalism

What is a **profession,** and who can be called a professional? These terms are used loosely in everyday conversation. Historically, only medicine, law, and the ministry were accepted as professions. Today, however, **professional** is a term commonly used to identify many types of people ranging from wrestlers and rock stars to college professors and archaeologists. Are all these individuals professionals? The answer to that question depends on how profession is defined.

In sports, a professional is distinguished from an amateur by being paid. Amateur golfers, for example, cannot accept money; professional golfers compete for it. So in sports, making money is one characteristic of being a professional. Professionals are generally better at what they do than are others. Therefore, in most fields, expertise is also a part of being a professional. Being paid and having expertise, however, are not the only criteria for being professional.

CHARACTERISTICS OF A PROFESSION

Over the years, many thoughtful people have grappled with the meaning of **professionalism.** In the early 1900s, the Carnegie Foundation issued a series of papers about professional schools. The first of these reports was based on sociologist Abraham Flexner's 1910 study of medical education (Flexner, 1910). The

Flexner Report, as it became known, is a classic piece of educational literature that provided the impetus for the much-needed reform of medical education.

Flexner went on to study other disciplines and later, in a paper about social work, published a list of criteria that he believed were characteristic of all true professions (Flexner, 1915). Since Flexner's original criteria were published, they have been widely used as a benchmark for determining the status of various occupations in terms of professionalism and have had a profound influence on professional education in several disciplines, including nursing.

Flexner's Criteria

Flexner believed that professional work:

1. Is basically intellectual (as opposed to physical) and is accompanied by a high degree of individual responsibility.
2. Is based on a body of knowledge that can be learned and is refreshed and refined through research.
3. Is practical, in addition to being theoretical.
4. Can be taught through a process of highly specialized professional education.
5. Has a strong internal organization of members and a well-developed group consciousness.
6. Has practitioners who are motivated by **altruism** (the desire to help others) and who are responsive to public interests (Figure 6–1).

Since 1915, a number of other authorities have also identified criteria for professions, which built on and vary slightly from Flexner's.

Bixler and Bixler's Criteria

Genevieve and Roy Bixler, a husband and wife team of nonnurses who were nevertheless advocates and supporters of nursing, first wrote about the status of nursing as a profession in 1945. In 1959, they again appraised nursing according to their original seven criteria, noting the progress made (Bixler and Bixler, 1959). Their criteria included the following:

1. "A profession utilizes in its practice a well-defined and well-organized body of specialized knowledge which is on the intellectual level of the higher learning" (p. 1142).
2. "A profession constantly enlarges the body of knowledge it uses and improves its techniques of education and service by the use of the scientific method" (p. 1143).
3. "A profession entrusts the education of its practitioners to institutions of higher education" (p. 1144).
4. "A profession applies its body of knowledge in practical services which are vital to human and social welfare" (p. 1145).
5. "A profession functions autonomously in the formulation of professional policy and in the control of professional activity thereby" (p. 1145).

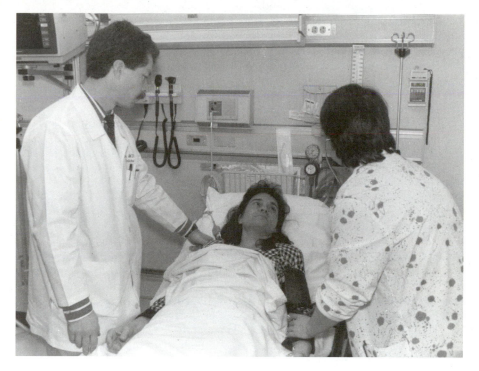

F I G U R E   6 – 1

According to Flexner, professionals are motivated by a desire to help others. (Photo by Kelly Whalen.)

6. "A profession attracts individuals of intellectual and personal qualities who exalt service above personal gain and who recognize their chosen occupation as a life work" (p. 1146).
7. "A profession strives to compensate its practitioners by providing freedom of action, opportunity for continuous professional growth, and economic security" (p. 1146).

A comparison of Flexner's and Bixler and Bixler's criteria reveals many similarities. General agreement exists about what constitutes a profession, but not all people agree about which occupations are professional. How contemporary nursing stacks up as a profession is discussed later.

DIFFERENCES IN PROFESSION AND OCCUPATION

Professions usually evolve from occupations that originally consisted of tasks but developed more specialized educational pathways and publicly legitimized status. The established professions, such as law, medicine, and the ministry, generally followed a typical developmental pattern. First, practitioners performed full-time work in the discipline. They then determined work standards and established training programs. Next, they promoted organizing into effective occupational associations. Then they worked toward legal protection that limited practice of their unique skills by outsiders. Finally, they established codes of ethics (Carr-Saunders and Wilson, 1933).

Occupation is often used interchangeably with *profession*, but their definitions differ. Webster defines *occupation* as "what occupies, or engages, one's time; business; employment." *Profession* is defined as "a vocation requiring advanced training . . . , and usually involving mental rather than manual work, as teaching, engineering, etc.; especially, medicine, law, or theology (formerly called the learned professions)" (*Webster's*, 1989). There is widespread overall agreement that a profession is different from an occupation in at least two major ways—preparation and commitment.

Preparation

Professional preparation usually takes place in a college or university setting. Preparation is prolonged to include instruction in the specialized body of knowledge and techniques of the profession. Professional preparation includes more than knowledge and skills, however. It also includes orientation to the beliefs, values, and attitudes expected of the members of the profession. Standards of practice and ethical considerations are also included. These components of professional education are part of the process of socialization into a profession. They are discussed in Chapter 8.

Commitment

Professionals' commitment to their profession is strong. They derive much of their personal identification from their work and consider it an integral part of their lives. People engaging in a profession often consider it their "calling." Although people may readily change occupations, it is less common for people to change professions. Several critical differences between occupations and professions are summarized in Table 6–1.

TABLE 6–1
Comparison of Characteristics of Occupations and Professions

Occupation	Profession
Training may occur on the job	Education takes place in a college or university
Length of training varies	Education is prolonged
Values, beliefs, and ethics are not prominent features of preparation	Values, beliefs, and ethics are an integral part of preparation
Commitment and personal identification vary	Commitment and personal identification are strong
Workers are supervised	Workers are autonomous
People often change jobs	People unlikely to change professions
Accountability rests with employer	Accountability rests with individual

HELPING PROFESSIONS

Historically, nursing has been considered one of the helping professions. Groups in this category include, among others, social workers, teachers, counselors, probation officers, and youth workers. A **helping profession** is primarily committed to assisting clients. Personalized care of clients is central to a helping profession's practice, and their needs take precedence above all else. There is a selfless dedication to duty and putting the needs of others first. Making a substantial salary is not usually the most important factor to those in the helping professions.

The helping professions are imbued with a service ideology and a sense of vocation. Helping professionals often see their role as the regulation and control of problematical areas of social life.

The concept of caring is a central part of the helping professions. Helping professionals demonstrate their particular type of caring through their professional expertise. A challenge for nursing and the other helping professions is attempting to care in a society that, by and large, does not value caring but instead values material goods and money as measures of success.

NURSING AS A PROFESSION

An ongoing subject for discussion in nursing circles has been the question: "Is nursing a profession?" Much has been written on both sides of this issue over the years. Nursing sociologists do not all agree that nursing *is* a profession. Some believe that it is, at best, an *emerging profession*. Others cite the progress nursing has made toward meeting the commonly accepted criteria for full-fledged professional status.

Kelly's Criteria

Kelly (1981, p. 157) reiterated and expanded Flexner's criteria in her 1981 listing of characteristics of a profession:

1. The services provided are vital to humanity and the welfare of society.
2. There is a special body of knowledge that is continually enlarged through research.
3. The services involve intellectual activities; individual responsibility (**accountability**) is a strong feature.
4. Practitioners are educated in institutions of higher learning.
5. Practitioners are relatively independent and control their own policies and activities (**autonomy**).
6. Practitioners are motivated by service (**altruism**) and consider their work an important component of their lives.
7. There is a **code of ethics** to guide the decisions and conduct of practitioners.
8. There is an organization (association) that encourages and supports high standards of practice.

Let us examine how well contemporary nursing fulfills these criteria.

"The Services Provided Are Vital to Humanity and the Welfare of Society."   If 10 students were asked why they chose nursing, most would reply, "To help people." Certainly nursing is a service that is essential to the well-being of people and to society as a whole. Nursing promotes the maintenance and restoration of health of individuals, groups, and communities. Assisting others to attain the highest level of wellness of which they are capable is the goal of nursing. Caring, meaning nurturing and helping others, is a basic component of professional nursing.

"There Is a Special Body of Knowledge That Is Continually Enlarged Through Research."   In the past, nursing was based on principles borrowed from the physical and social sciences and other disciplines. Today, however, there is a body of knowledge that is uniquely nursing's. Although this was not always so, the amount of investigation and analysis of nursing care has expanded rapidly in the past 20 years. Nursing theory development is also proceeding swiftly. Nursing is no longer based on task orientation, intuition, or trial and error but increasingly relies on research as a basis for practice. Several theoretical models of nursing are discussed in Chapter 11, and issues in research are discussed in Chapter 12.

"The Services Involve Intellectual Activities; Individual Responsibility (Accountability) Is a Strong Feature."   Nursing has developed and refined its own unique approach to practice, called the **nursing process.** The nursing process is essentially a **cognitive** (mental) activity that requires both critical and creative thinking and serves as the basis for providing nursing care. There is more about the nursing process in Chapter 17.

Individual accountability in nursing has become the hallmark of practice. Accountability, according to the American Nurses Association's (ANA) *Code for Nurses* (1985, p. 10), is "being answerable to someone for something one has done. It means providing an explanation to self, to the client, to the employing agency, and to the nursing profession." Organized nursing has also demonstrated a commitment to accountability in the ANA's *Standards of Nursing Practice* (1973). Through legal opinions and court cases, society has demonstrated that it, too, holds nurses individually responsible for their actions as well as for those of personnel under their supervision.

Shared governance describes a model of shifting accountability from the hospital nursing administration suite to the "front lines," where the individual provider of nursing care functions. Shared governance is discussed further in Chapter 13.

"Practitioners Are Educated in Institutions of Higher Learning."   As presented in Chapter 2, the first university-based nursing program began in 1909 at the University of Minnesota. Several studies, including Esther Lucille Brown's 1948 report *Nursing for the Future*, called for nursing education to be based in universities and colleges. Recall that another milestone was the 1965 position paper of the ANA, which called for all nursing education to take place in institutions of higher education (American Nurses Association, 1965).

The majority of programs offering basic nursing education are now associate degree and baccalaureate programs located in colleges and universities. There are master's and doctoral programs in nursing, although the number of graduates is small compared with other health professions. Because professional status and power increase with postgraduate education, a legitimate question is: "How can nursing take its place as a peer among the professions when most nurses currently in practice hold less than a baccalaureate degree?" The differentiation between professional nursing and technical nursing is a challenging issue that nursing has not yet resolved. Diversity within the ranks of nursing has slowed the progress toward acceptance of the baccalaureate or higher degree as the prerequisite for professional practice. Lack of resolution of these differences threatens to undermine nursing's development as a profession.

"Practitioners Are Relatively Independent and Control Their Own Policies and Activities (Autonomy)." Autonomy, or control over one's practice, is another controversial area for nursing. Although many nursing actions are independent, most nurses are employed in hospitals, where authority resides in one's position. One's place in the hierarchy, rather than expertise, confers or denies power and status. Physicians are widely regarded as gatekeepers, and their authorization or supervision is required before many activities can occur. Nurse practice acts in most states reinforce nursing's lack of self-determination by requiring that nurses perform certain actions only when authorized by supervising physicians or hospital protocols.

There are at least three groups who wish to control nursing practice: organized medicine, health service administration, and organized nursing. Both the medical profession and health service administration are attempting to maintain control of nursing because they believe it is in their best interest to keep nurses dependent on them. Both are well organized and have powerful lobbies at state and national levels. Organized nursing promotes independence and autonomy, but its power is fragmented by subgroups and dissension. Rivalry between diploma-educated, associate degree-educated, and baccalaureate-educated nurses saps the energy of the profession. The proliferation of nursing organizations (see Box 4–2 for a partial list of nursing organizations) and competition among them also diminish nursing's potential. Only 10 percent of the 2.2 million registered nurses in the United States are members of the ANA (Little, 1992). The fact that most nurses are not members of any professional organization impairs nursing's ability to lobby effectively. These are major challenges for nursing if it is to realize its potential collective professional power and autonomy.

"Practitioners Are Motivated by Service (Altruism) and Consider Their Work an Important Component of Their Lives." As a group, nurses are dedicated to the ideal of service to others, which is also known as altruism. This ideal has sometimes become intertwined with economic issues and historically has been exploited by employers of nurses. No one questions the right of other professionals to charge reasonable fees for the services they render; when nurses want higher salaries, however, others sometimes call their altruism into question. Nurses must take responsibility for their own financial well-being and for the health of the profession. This will, in turn, ensure its continued attractiveness to those who might choose nursing as a career. If there are to be adequate numbers

---

B O X   6 – 1
The Florence Nightingale Pledge

I solemnly pledge myself before God and in the presence of this assembly to pass my life in purity and to practice my profession faithfully.

I will abstain from whatever is deleterious and mischievous, and will not take or knowingly administer any harmful drug. I will do all in my power to maintain and elevate the standard of my profession, and will hold in confidence all personal matters committed to my keeping and all family affairs coming to my knowledge in the practice of my calling.

With loyalty will I endeavor to aid the physician in his work and devote myself to the welfare of those committed to my care.

Reprinted with permission of Pillitteri, A. (1991). Documenting Lystra Gretter's student experiences in nursing. *Nursing Outlook*, 39(6), 273–279.

---

of nurses to meet society's needs, salaries must be comparable with those in competing disciplines. Being concerned with salary issues does nothing to diminish a nurse's altruism.

Another issue, consideration of work as a primary component of life, has been a thornier problem for nurses. Commitment to a career is not a value equally shared by all nurses. Some still regard nursing as a job and drop in and out of practice depending on economic and family needs. This approach, although appealing to many female nurses and conducive to traditional family management, has retarded the development of professional attitudes and behaviors for the profession as a whole.

"There Is a Code of Ethics to Guide the Decisions and Conduct of Practitioners."

An ethical code does not stipulate how an individual should act in a specific situation; rather, it provides professional standards and a framework for decision making. The trust placed in the nursing profession by the public requires that nurses act with integrity. To aid them in doing so, both the International Council of Nurses (ICN) and the ANA have established codes of nursing ethics through which standards of practice are established, promoted, and refined. Chapter 4 contains the ANA's *Code for Nurses*, and Chapter 20 contains the *International Council of Nurses Code for Nurses*.

In 1893, long before these codes were written, "The Florence Nightingale Pledge" (Box 6–1) was created by a committee headed by Lystra Eggert Gretter and presented to the Farrand Training School for Nurses located at Harper Hospital in Detroit, Michigan (Pillitteri, 1991). The Nightingale pledge can be considered nursing's first code of ethics.

"There Is an Organization (Association) That Encourages and Supports High Standards of Practice."

As shown in Chapter 4, nursing has a number of professional associations that were formed to promote the improvement of the profession. Foremost among these is the ANA, the purposes of which are to foster high standards of nursing practice, promote professional and educational ad-

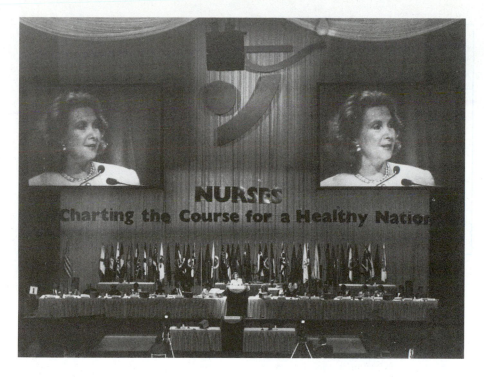

FIGURE 6–2
Professionals belong to associations that encourage and support ethical standards of practice. (Courtesy of American Nurses Association.)

vancement of nurses, and promote the welfare of nurses to the end that all people have better nursing care (Fig. 6–2) (American Nurses Association, 1970). The ANA is also the official voice of nursing and therefore is the primary advocate for nursing interests in general. Unfortunately, fewer than 1 out of 10 nurses belongs to the official professional organization. The political power that could be derived from the unified efforts of 2.2 million registered nurses nationwide would be impressive; that goal has not yet been realized.

CHARACTERISTIC BEHAVIORS OF PROFESSIONAL NURSES

If being a professional nurse is different from practicing the occupation of nursing, there must be certain behaviors that differentiate the two. As students develop their ideas of how they want to function as nursing professionals, it may help to have an ideal in mind. Many students already know a nurse they consider to be a role model of professionalism. If not, there may be interest in hearing about Joan, the subject of the following case study.

Joan: A Case Study

Joan is a 32-year-old married mother of two. She graduated from River City College of Nursing at the age of 26 and has been practicing since her graduation. Her first position was as a staff nurse at Providence Hospital, a 300-bed private hospital. Nursing administration at Providence encourages nurses to provide individualized nursing care while protecting the dignity and autonomy of each patient and family. She chose Providence because the philosophy of nursing there paralleled her own. Another reason for selecting this hospital was that Joan wanted to practice oncology (cancer) nursing, and there is an oncology unit at Providence.

Each day Joan uses the nursing process in caring for her patients and in dealing with their families. That means she assesses their condition, plans and implements their care, and evaluates the care she has given. Then she writes what she has done in each patient's chart in the accepted format. She communicates clearly to the other members of the nursing staff and to the other health care professionals involved in the care of the patients on her unit.

After two years as a staff nurse, Joan accepted a position as a team leader. This means that now she takes responsibility not only for her own practice, but also for supervising licensed practical nurses and nursing assistants on her team. To do this effectively, she stays abreast of changes in her state's nursing practice act and Providence Hospital's policies and procedures. In addition, she updates her knowledge by reading current journals and research periodicals. She makes it a policy to attend at least two nursing conferences each year to stay on top of trends. She belongs to her professional organization and participates as an active member. She finds that this is another source of the latest information on professional issues.

Joan looks forward to working with the nursing students at Providence Hospital. She remembers when she was a student and how a word from a practicing nurse could make or break her day. Of course, students do mean extra work, but she sees this as a part of her role and patiently provides the guidance they need, even when she is busy.

In the course of her daily work, Joan sometimes has a question about certain procedures. She is not embarrassed to seek help from more experienced nurses, from textbooks, or from other health pro-

Professional Behavior Demonstrated

Has developed own philosophy of nursing

Self-determination

Uses critical thinking

Collaborates and communicates with other health professionals

Demonstrates accountability for self and others

Committed to lifelong learning

Active in professional organization

Mentors aspiring professionals

Recognizes own limits; seeks help when needed

fessionals. Sometimes she offers suggestions to the head nurse and the oncology clinical nurse specialist about possible research questions and participates in gathering data when the unit takes on a research study.

Contributes to expansion of nursing's body of knowledge

Providence Hospital uses a shared governance model, which means nurses serve on committees that develop and interpret nursing policies and procedures. Joan serves on two committees and chairs another. Right now the hospital is preparing a self-study for an upcoming accreditation, so the meetings are frequent. Instead of complaining about the meetings, Joan prepares and organizes her portion of the meeting so that everyone's time is used most effectively. She has to delegate some of her patient care responsibilities to others while she is attending meetings. Because she has taken the time to know the other workers' skills and abilities, she does not worry about what happens while she is gone.

Provides leadership

Uses principles of time management

Delegates responsibility wisely

At the end of the day when Joan goes home, she occasionally gets a call from a friend with a health-related question or a request to give a neighbor's child an allergy injection. Although she is tired, she recognizes that in the eyes of others, she represents the nursing profession. She is proud to be trusted and respected for her knowledge, skills, and dedication. Helping others through nursing care is something Joan has wanted to do since she was small, and she finds it very fulfilling.

Represents profession to the public

Models altruism

Lately Joan has recognized in herself some troubling signs: She has been irritable, impatient with family and co-workers, and generally out of sorts. She has gained weight and is exercising less than usual. She wonders if working with terminally ill patients and their families is the source of her stress. Joan's husband suggested that she take "a break" from nursing and stay home with the children, but after talking it over with her head nurse, she decided to ask for assignment to different nursing responsibilities for a while. She knows that she needs to be her own advocate and take care of herself. Next week she will begin a 3-month stint in outpatient surgery, where the emotional intensity will be a bit less.

Possesses self-awareness

Demonstrates commitment to nursing

Models healthy coping behavior

This brief description illustrates more than 18 characteristic behaviors exhibited by professional nurses. Nursing is clearly much more than an occupation to Joan and to many others like her. The Research Note (Holl, 1994) describes several factors that are related to the development of professionalism in nurses.

RESEARCH NOTE

Rita M. Holl conducted a study of RNs to determine which characteristics influenced professional beliefs and decision making. The characteristics she was interested in included age, years of practice, area of practice, level of education, certification, and membership in professional organizations.

She developed an instrument and asked 133 RN subjects how they would deal with real-life nurse-patient situations. Results were analyzed according to the degree of independence required, the degree to which they met the patient's needs, and their professional standards.

Holl found that professional beliefs and decision making were related to level of education, membership in professional organizations, and certification. Critical care nurses demonstrated higher levels of independent decision making than did nurses in other areas of practice. The results of this study supported, in general, the notion that nurses who continue their education and belong to professional organizations are more likely to be independent thinkers and to participate in creative problem solving.

Adapted with permission of Holl, R. M. (1994). Characteristics of the registered nurse and professional beliefs and decision making, *Critical Care Nursing Quarterly*, 17(3), 60–66.

SUMMARY

Commitment to a profession is different from commitment to a job or an occupation. People who have studied professions agree that there are several characteristics that all true professions have in common. A body of knowledge, specialized education, service to society, accountability, autonomy, and ethical standards are a few of the hallmarks of professions. Although nursing has a briefer history than some traditional professions and is still dealing with autonomy, preparation, and commitment issues, great progress has been made in moving nursing toward full professional status. An awareness of the characteristics of professions and professional behavior helps nurses assume leadership in continuing that progress.

It is important to remember that being a professional is a dynamic process, not a condition or state of being. Professional growth evolves throughout the different stages of nurses' careers.

REVIEW AND DISCUSSION QUESTIONS

1. How might nursing be different today if all its practitioners viewed it as their profession rather than a job?
2. What impact might the traditional male orientation to work as a lifelong career commitment have on the potential for success of men in nursing?
3. What is the relationship between training and education?
4. On a scale of 1 to 10, rate nursing on each of Flexner's, Bixler and Bixler's, and Kelly's criteria for professions.

CHAPTER

7

Kay K. Chitty

Defining Nursing

OBJECTIVES
- Recognize the evolutionary nature of definitions.
- Compare early definitions of nursing with contemporary ones.
- Identify themes in existing definitions of nursing.
- Develop personal definitions of nursing.

VOCABULARY

active collaborator	high-tech nursing	maximum health
caring	high-touch nursing	potential
educative instrument	holism	milieu
health maintenance	humanistic nursing care	nursing practice act
health promotion		scientific discipline

It may be surprising to learn that finding a universally acceptable definition of nursing has been an elusive goal. It seems that even nurses themselves have been unable to agree on one definition. Individuals, including the venerable Nightingale, and organizations, such as the International Council of Nurses (ICN) and the American Nurses Association (ANA), have made attempts to achieve consensus, and some have been more successful than others. Despite the inability of those in the profession to agree on one definition, most of the definitions reviewed in this chapter have similar themes. Considering the variations in knowledge and technology during the different points in history when these definitions were written, the similarities are remarkable. All the definitions were affected by significant political and social events of the day that shaped the form of nursing as it is now known.

WHY DEFINE NURSING?

Why is it important for people to spend time trying to define nursing? Having an accepted definition of nursing is helpful in a variety of ways and provides a framework for nursing practice. It establishes the parameters, or boundaries, of

5. Discuss technical versus professional education.
6. Describe at least five characteristic behaviors of professional nurses.

REFERENCES

American Nurses Association (1985). *Code for nurses with interpretive statements.* Kansas City, MO: Author.

American Nurses Association (1973). *Standards of nursing practice.* Kansas City, MO: Author.

American Nurses Association (1970). *Association bylaws.* Kansas City, MO: Author.

American Nurses Association (1965). *Educational preparation for nurse practitioners and assistants to nurses: A position paper.* Kansas City, MO: Author.

Bixler, G. K., and Bixler, R. W. (1959). The professional status of nursing. *American Journal of Nursing*, 59(8), 1142–1147.

Brown, E. L. (1948). *Nursing for the future.* New York: Russell Sage Foundation.

Carr-Saunders, A. M., and Wilson, P. A. (1933). *The professions.* Oxford: Clarendon Press.

Flexner, A. (1915). Is social work a profession? *School Society,* 1(26), 901.

Flexner, A. (1910). *Medical education in the United States and Canada: A report to the Carnegie Foundation for the advancement of teaching.* Bethesda, MD: Science & Health Publications.

Holl, R. M. (1994). Characteristics of the registered nurse and professional beliefs and decision making. *Critical Care Nursing Quarterly,* 17(3), 60–66.

Kelly, L. (1981). *Dimensions of professional nursing* (4th ed.). New York: Macmillan.

Little, M. (1992). Sprout growers unite! *Tennessee Nursing Matters,* 1(3), 7.

Pillitteri, A. (1991). Documenting Lystra Gretter's student experiences in nursing. *Nursing Outlook*, 39(6), 273–279.

Webster's new collegiate dictionary (9th ed.). (1989). Springfield, MA: Merriam-Webster.

the profession; identifies the purposes and functions of the work; and guides the educational preparation of aspiring practitioners.

To illustrate the importance of defining human activity, suppose a person was told that he had been selected to play on a major league baseball team, but he did not know how to play. So he asked the team owner, "What is important for me to know about baseball?" And she said, "Just win games!" Then he went to a pitcher, who showed him a fast ball, a curve ball, and a slider. From there he went to a batting coach, who showed him how to hit fast balls, slow balls, and sliders. When he went to a fielding coach, he was told how to cover the bases and catch balls. Next, he consulted a trainer who showed him how to condition his body to avoid injuries. He has spent a great deal of time and still does not have an overall picture of baseball. Now, suppose he had been told initially, "Baseball is a game played with a ball and a bat on a large field on which there are three bases and a home plate. There are two nine-member teams, one at bat and one in the field. The object of the game is for a member of the batting team to hit a pitched ball and to run around the bases to home plate without being called out. The team with the most runs at the end of nine turns at bat wins." Although this description leaves out a lot of detail, it succinctly states the boundaries of the game, the purpose of the game, and gives guidance on how to play the game. Therefore, it would be more useful as a first step in an attempt to master baseball than the unorganized approach of talking to owners, players, and coaches.

So it is with definitions. They are a good place to begin in attempting to understand any complex enterprise such as nursing.

Nightingale Defines Nursing

Considering how relatively undeveloped nursing was during her time, Florence Nightingale's definitions contain contemporary concepts. Remember that during Nightingale's day, formal schooling in nursing was just beginning. In writing *Notes on Nursing: What It Is and What It Is Not* in 1859, she became the first person to attempt a definition of nursing. She wrote, "And what nursing has to do . . . is put the patient in the best condition for nature to act upon him" (Nightingale, 1946, p. 75). She also wrote:

> I use the word nursing for want of a better. It has been limited to signify little more than the administration of medicines and the application of poultices. It ought to signify the proper use of fresh air, light, warmth, cleanliness, quiet, and the proper selection and administration of diet—all at the least expense of vital power to the patient (p. 6).

Although Nightingale lived in a time when little was known about disease processes and available treatments were extremely limited, these definitions foreshadowed contemporary nursing's focus on the therapeutic **milieu** (environment) as well as the modern emphasis on **health promotion** and **health maintenance.** Nightingale was also the first person to differentiate between nursing provided by a professional nurse using a unique body of knowledge and nursing care such as a mother would perform for an ill child.

EVOLUTION OF DEFINITIONS OF NURSING

In the decades since Nightingale thought about, practiced, wrote about, and transformed nursing, many others have attempted to distill into one definition the essence of nursing. This section reviews a number of definitions that evolved over the years.

Early Twentieth-Century Definitions

Fifty years after Nightingale, the search for a definition began in earnest. Following the English model, many schools of nursing had been established in the United States, and numbers of "trained nurses" were in practice. They sought to develop a professional identity for their rapidly expanding discipline. Shaw's *Textbook of Nursing* (1907, pp. 1–2) defined nursing as an art: "It properly includes as well as the execution of specific orders, the administration of food and medicine, the personal care of the patient." Harmer's *Textbook of the Principles and Practice of Nursing* (1922) elaborated on Shaw's bare-bones definition: "The object of nursing is not only to cure the sick . . . but to bring health and ease, rest and comfort to mind and body. Its object is to prevent disease and to preserve health" (p. 3). The fourth edition of the Harmer text, which showed the influence of coauthor and nursing notable Virginia Henderson, redefined nursing: "Nursing may be defined as that service to an individual that helps him to attain or maintain a healthy state of mind or body" (Harmer and Henderson 1939, p. 2).

Post–World War II Definitions

World War II, similar to all wars, helped advance the technologies available to treat people, which, in turn, influenced nursing. The war also made nurses aware of the influential role emotions play in health, illness, and nursing care. Hildegard Peplau (1952), widely regarded as a pioneer among contemporary nursing theorists and herself a psychiatric nurse, defined nursing in interpersonal terms: "Nursing is a significant, therapeutic, interpersonal process. . . . Nursing is an **educative instrument** . . . that aims to promote forward movement of personality in the direction of creative, constructive, productive, personal and community living" (p. 16). She reinforced the idea of the patient as an **active collaborator** in his own care.

During the late 1950s and early 1960s, the number of master's programs in nursing increased. As more nurses were educated at the graduate level and learned about the research process, they were anxious to test new ideas about nursing. Nursing theory was born. (See Chapter 11 for a fuller discussion of nursing theory.)

One of the theorists who began work during this period was Orem. Her 1959 definition of nursing captures the flavor of her later, more completely elaborated self-care theory of nursing: "Nursing is perhaps best described as the giving of direct assistance to a person, as required, because of the person's specific inabilities in self-care resulting from a situation of personal health" (Orem, 1959,

p. 5). Orem's belief, that nurses should do for a person only those things the person cannot do without assistance, also emphasized the patient's active role.

By 1960, Henderson's earlier definition had evolved into a statement that had such universal appeal that it was adopted by the ICN:

> The unique function of the nurse is to assist the individual, sick or well, in the performance of those activities contributing to health or its recovery (or to a peaceful death) that he would perform unaided if he had the necessary strength, will or knowledge. And to do this in such a way as to help him gain independence as rapidly as possible (Henderson, 1960, p. 3).

Never before or since has one definition of nursing been so widely accepted both in the United States and worldwide. Many believe it is still the most comprehensive and appropriate definition of nursing in existence.

Another pioneer nursing theorist, Martha Rogers, included the concept of the nursing process in her definition: "Nursing aims to assist people in achieving their **maximum health potential.** Maintenance and promotion of health, prevention of disease, nursing diagnosis, intervention, and rehabilitation encompass the scope of nursing's goals" (Rogers, 1961, p. 86).

A Controversial Definition Emerges

Definitions are not usually considered controversial, but in 1980, the ANA issued a statement of beliefs called *Nursing: A Social Policy Statement* that contained perhaps the most controversial definition of nursing to date. It stated: "Nursing is the diagnosis and treatment of human responses to actual and potential health problems" (p. 9). This definition was criticized for a number of reasons, a chief one being that it failed to identify health as a goal of nursing. The emphasis on diagnosis and treatment ignored the health promotion and maintenance aspects that others defined as the essence of nursing.

Terming the ANA definition "incomplete and in part illogical," prominent nurse educator Rozella Schlotfeldt (1987) went so far as to assert that the definition, by its incompleteness, "may delay or deter progress in theory development" (p. 6). She suggested that a more accurate and appropriate definition, and one that can inform and guide current and future practitioners, would be: "Nursing is the appraisal and the enhancement of the health status, health assets, and health potentials of human beings" (p. 67).

The ANA responded to the criticisms, and the 1995 revision of what is now named *Nursing's Social Policy Statement* defined nursing much more comprehensively. The new definition included four essential features of contemporary nursing practice (American Nurses Association, 1995, p. 6):

- Attention to the full range of human experiences and responses to health and illness without restriction to a problem-focused orientation.
- Integration of objective data with knowledge gained from an understanding of the patient or group's subjective experience.
- Application of scientific knowledge to the processes of diagnosis and treatment.
- Provision of a caring relationship that facilitates health and healing.

A Focus on Caring, Humanism, and Holism

After a period of intense interest in **high-tech nursing** during the late 1960s and 1970s, modern nursing returned to its **high-touch** roots, so to speak, in the late 1970s with a renewed interest and public recognition as the health discipline that "cares." That trend has continued to the present.

A **caring** professional is one who watches over, attends to, and provides for the needs of others. Contemporary nursing stresses **humanistic nursing care,** that is, viewing professional relationships as human to human rather than nurse to patient. The meaning of the patient's experience is an important aspect of humanistic nursing. **Holism** is also receiving emphasis in modern definitions of nursing. Holism is a system of comprehensive care that takes the physical, emotional, social, economic, and spiritual needs of the person into consideration (Fig. 7–1).

Jean Watson, a nursing theorist, illustrated the return to caring and humanism in 1979, when she wrote, "Nursing is both scientific and artistic. I seek to combine science with humanism. . . . Nursing is a therapeutic interpersonal process. . . . Nursing is a **scientific discipline** that derives . . . its practice base from scientific research" (p. xvii). Nurses can expect to hear more about the caring aspects of nursing as a counterbalance to the dizzying array of technologies anticipated in the future.

This brief review of selected definitions of nursing in vogue during the past 150 years is summarized in Box 7–1.

F I G U R E   7 – 1
Holistic nursing practice takes the physical, emotional, social, economic, and spiritual needs of the person into consideration. (Photo by Kelly Whalen.)

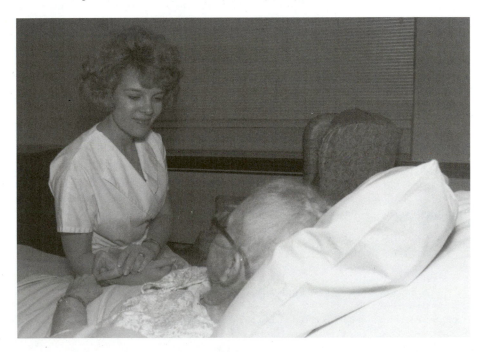

BOX 7-1
Themes in the Evolution of Definitions of Nursing, 1859–1987

Nightingale, 1859 (1946)

". . . nursing . . . ought to signify the proper use of fresh air, light, warmth, cleanliness, quiet, and the proper selection and administration of diet—all at the least expense of vital power to the patient" (p. 6).

"And what nursing has to do . . . is put the patient in the best condition for nature to act upon him" (p. 75).

- The nurse's center of concern is the patient.
- Nature and a healthful, restful environment are the nurse's allies.
- Health maintenance and restoration are the nurse's goals.

Shaw, 1907

"Nursing is an art. . . . It properly includes as well as the execution of specific orders, the administration of food and medicine, the personal care of the patient. . . . To fill such a position requires certain physical and mental attributes as well as special training" (pp. 1–2).

- More than knowledge and skills are needed by nurses. The attribute of personal caring is also required.

Harmer, 1922

"Nursing is rooted in the needs of humanity. . . . Its object is not only to cure the sick . . . but to bring health and ease, rest and comfort to mind and body. Its object is to prevent disease and to preserve health" (p. 3).

- Disease prevention and health promotion are the focus.
- Nursing is based on human needs.

Harmer and Henderson, 1939

"Nursing may be defined as that service to an individual that helps him to attain or maintain a healthy state of mind or body" (p. 2).

- Nursing deals with the health of both psyche (mind) and soma (body).

Peplau, 1952

"Nursing is a significant, therapeutic, interpersonal process. . . . Nursing is an educative instrument . . . that aims to promote forward movement of personality in the direction of creative, constructive, productive, personal and community living" (p. 16).

- Effective nursing results from a therapeutic relationship between nurse and patient.

Orem, 1959

"Nursing is . . . described as the giving of direct assistance to a person, as required, because of the person's specific inabilities in self-care resulting from a situation of personal health" (p. 5).

- Nursing is doing for a person what he cannot do at this time because of health-related limitations. Return to self-care is the goal.

Henderson, 1960

"The unique function of the nurse is to assist the individual, sick or well, in the performance of those activities contributing to health or its recovery (or to a peaceful death) that he would perform unaided if he had the necessary strength, will or knowledge. And to do this in such a way as to help him gain independence as rapidly as possible" (p. 3).

- Both well and ill people are the focus of nursing.
- Responsibility for care is shared by nurse and patient.
- The goal is independence of the patient.

(continued)

BOX 7–1 (continued)
Themes in the Evolution of Definitions of Nursing, 1859–1987

Rogers, 1961
"Nursing aims to assist people in achieving their maximum health potential. Maintenance and promotion of health, prevention of disease, nursing diagnosis, intervention, and rehabilitation encompass the scope of nursing's goals" (p. 86).

- Each person has a personal maximum health potential. Nursing seeks to strengthen each human being's capacity to achieve that potential.

American Nurses Association, 1980
"Nursing is the diagnosis and treatment of human responses to actual and potential health problems" (p. 9).

- Nursing focuses on human responses to illness or the threat of illness.

Watson, 1979
"Nursing is both scientific and artistic. I seek to combine science with human-

ism. . . . Nursing is a therapeutic interpersonal process. . . . Nursing is a scientific discipline that derives . . . its practice base from scientific research" (p. xvii).

- Nursing represents a balance between science and humanism.
- The interpersonal features of nursing are paramount.
- Nurses care for people with a holistic approach even while using the scientific approach.

Schlotfeldt, 1987
"Nursing is the appraisal and the enhancement of the health status, health assets, and health potentials of human beings" (p. 67).

- Regardless of where a person is on the continuum of wellness to illness, nursing focuses on enhancing that person's health care status.

DEVELOPING PERSONAL DEFINITIONS OF NURSING

Students may not realize that faculties of accredited schools of nursing are encouraged to develop definitions of nursing as part of the school's statement of philosophy. Some of the most spirited discussions during faculty meetings center around what one or another faculty member believes nursing really is. A description of nursing that combines humanistic and holistic values can be found in the University of Rochester School of Nursing's thoughtful and comprehensive philosophy statement:

> We believe that the profession of nursing has as its essence, assisting people to attain and maintain optimal health and to cope with illness and disability. Nursing derives its rights and responsibilities from society and is, therefore, accountable to society as well as to the individuals who comprise it. The nurse functions as a caring professional in both autonomous and collaborative professional roles, using critical thinking, ethical principles, effective communication, and deliberative action to render holistic care, facilitate access to health care, and aid consumers in making decisions about their health (Radke et al, 1991, p. 12).

All nursing students and practicing nurses, whether or not they realize it, are in the process of developing and refining their own definitions of nursing. From time to time, it is helpful to write down just what your personal definition is and compare it with those developed by nursing scholars over the years.

On a practical note, it is important to keep in mind that the most significant definition of nursing for every nurse is contained in the **nursing practice act** of the state in which that nurse practices. Regardless of how restrictive or permissive it may be, this definition constitutes the legal definition of nursing in that state, and the wise nurse maintains familiarity with the latest version of the act. The current nursing practice act in each state can be obtained by calling or writing the state board of nursing. The addresses of the boards of nursing are found in Box 7–2.

SUMMARY

Although attempting to define nursing has been an interesting activity since the days of Nightingale, all attempts have fallen short of capturing the scope, diversity, and richness that is nursing. Storlie struck a chord of truth when she wrote, "The glorious thing about nursing is that it cannot be defined. The irony is that we never give up trying. . . . Nursing will resist being reduced to so-called facts no matter how precise the researcher" (Storlie, 1970, pp. 254–255).

Note that the definitions reviewed in this chapter have more similarities than differences. Review some of their major themes highlighted in Box 7–1. Notice how the definitions have evolved over time even though many themes are constant. It is possible to find definitions by some of the same authors that are different from the ones given in this chapter. This is because definitions change over time as both society and nursing change and as each individual's perceptions about, and experiences in, nursing change. Although nursing may wish for one, succinct definition, the dynamic nature of the nursing profession, society, and health care will likely prevent us from ever developing one eternal, universally accepted definition of nursing.

REVIEW AND DISCUSSION QUESTIONS

1. From the definitions of nursing presented in this chapter, select the one you most prefer and explain your choice.
2. Using your thoughts as well as elements of others' definitions, write your own definition of nursing. Explain it to a classmate, giving your rationale for what you included and excluded.
3. How might new developments and practice options for nurses affect future definitions of nursing?
4. How has your personal definition of nursing changed over time?
5. Using the appropriate address from Box 7–2, obtain a copy of the nursing practice act for your state. Find the legal definition of nursing and compare it with other definitions found in this chapter. How are they alike, and how are they different?

BOX 7–2
State Boards of Nursing

ALABAMA. Board of Nursing
RSA Plaza, Suite 250
770 Washington Avenue
Montgomery, AL 36130-3900
(334) 242-4060

ALASKA. Board of Nursing
Division of Occupational Licensing
Frontier Building
3601 C Street, Suite 722
Anchorage, AK 99503
(907) 269-8160

ARIZONA. State Board of Nursing
1651 East Morten Avenue, Suite 150
Phoenix, AZ 85020
(602) 255-5092

ARKANSAS. State Board of Nursing
Suite 800, University Tower Building
1123 South University Avenue
Little Rock, AR 72204
(501) 686-2700

CALIFORNIA. Board of Registered
   Nursing
P.O. Box 944210
Sacramento, CA 94244-2100
(916) 322-3350

COLORODO. State Board of Nursing
1560 Broadway, Suite 670
Denver, CO 80202
(303) 894-2430

CONNECTICUT. Dept. of Public Health
Nurse Licensure
410 Capitol Avenue, MS#12APP
Hartford, CT 06134
(203) 566-1032

DELAWARE. Board of Nursing
Cannon Building, Suite 203
P.O. Box 1401
Dover, DE 19903
(302) 739-4522 ext. 217

DISTRICT OF COLUMBIA. Board of
   Nursing
614 H Street N.W., Room 904
Washington, DC 20001
(202) 727-7454

FLORIDA. Board of Nursing
Suite 202, 4080 Woodcock Drive
Jacksonville, FL 32207
(904) 858-6940

GEORGIA. Board of Nursing
166 Pryor Street S.W.
Atlanta, GA 30303
(404) 656-3943

HAWAII. Board of Nursing
Box 3469
Honolulu, HI 96801
(808) 586-3000

IDAHO. State Board of Nursing
P.O. Box 83720
Boise, ID 83720-0061
(208) 334-3110

ILLINOIS. Department of Professional
   Regulation
320 West Washington Street, 3rd Floor
Springfield, IL 62786
(217) 782-8556

INDIANA. State Board of Nursing
Indiana Government Center South
402 West Washington Street, Room 041
Indianapolis, IN 46204
(317) 232-1105

IOWA. Board of Nursing
State Capitol Complex
1223 East Court Avenue
Des Moines, IA 50319
(515) 281-3256

(continued)

B O X   7 – 2   (continued)

KANSAS. State Board of Nursing
Landon State Office Building
900 S.W. Jackson, Suite 551-S
Topeka, KS 66612-1230
(913) 296-4929

KENTUCKY. Board of Nursing
312 Whittington Parkway, Suite 300
Louisville, KY 40222-5172
(502) 329-7000

LOUISIANA. State Board of Nursing
3510 North Causeway Boulevard
Suite 501
Metairie, LA 70005
(504) 838-5332

MAINE. State Board of Nursing
35 Anthony Avenue
State House Station 158
Augusta, ME 04333-0158
(207) 624-5275

MARYLAND. Board of Nursing
4140 Patterson Avenue
Baltimore, MD 21215
(410) 764-5124

MASSACHUSETTS. Board of
   Registration in Nursing
100 Cambridge Street, Room 1519
Boston, MA 02202
(617) 727-9961

MICHIGAN. Board of Nursing
Department of Commerce/BOPR
Ottawa Towers North
611 West Ottawa, Box 30018
Lansing, MI 48909
(517) 373-1600

MINNESOTA. Board of Nursing
2700 University Avenue West, #108
St. Paul, MN 55114
(612) 642-0572

MISSISSIPPI. Board of Nursing
239 North Lamar Street, Suite 401
Jackson, MS 39201
(601) 359-6170

MISSOURI. State Board of Nursing
P.O. Box 656
Jefferson City, MO 65102
(314) 751-0681

MONTANA. Board of Nursing
111 North Jackson
Arcade Building
P.O. Box 200513
Helena, MT 59620-0513
(406) 444-2071

NEBRASKA. Board of Nursing
Department of Health, Professional &
   Occupational Licensure Division
P.O. Box 95007
Lincoln, NE 68509
(402) 471-0317

NEVADA. Board of Nursing
P.O. Box 46886
Las Vegas, NV 89114
(702) 739-1575

NEW HAMPSHIRE. Board of Nursing
Health and Welfare Building
6 Hazen Drive
Concord, NH 03301-6527
(603) 271-2323

NEW JERSEY. Board of Nursing
P.O. Box 45010
Newark, NJ 07101
(201) 504-6430

NEW MEXICO. Board of Nursing
4206 Louisiana N.E., Suite A
Albuquerque, NM 87109
(505) 841-8340

(continued)

B O X 7 – 2 *(continued)*
State Boards of Nursing

NEW YORK. State Education
    Department
Division of Professional Licensing
    Services, Cultural Education Center
Empire State Plaza
Albany, NY 12230
(518) 474-3845

NORTH CAROLINA. Board of Nursing
P.O. Box 2129
Raleigh, NC 27602
(919) 782-3211

NORTH DAKOTA. Board of Nursing
Suite 504, 919 South 7th Street
Bismarck, ND 58504
(701) 328-9777

OHIO. Board of Nursing
77 South High Street, 17th Floor
Columbus, OH 43266-0316
(614) 466-3947

OKLAHOMA. Board of Nursing
2915 North Classen Boulevard, Suite 524
Oklahoma City, OK 73106
(405) 525-2076

OREGON. State Board of Nursing
Suite 465, 800 N.E. Oregon Street
Portland, OR 97232
(503) 731-4745

PENNSYLVANIA. State Board of
    Nursing
Department of State
Box 2649
Harrisburg, PA 17105-2649
(717) 783-7142

PUERTO RICO. Office of Regulations
    and Certification of Health
    Professionals
ATTN: Board of Nurse Examiners
Call Box 10200
San Juan, PR 00908
(809) 725-7904

RHODE ISLAND. Board of Nurse
    Registration and Nursing Education
3 Capitol Hill, Room 104
Providence, RI 02908
(401) 277-2827

SOUTH CAROLINA. State Board of
    Nursing
220 Executive Center Drive, Suite 220
P.O. Box 12367
Columbia, SC 29210
(803) 731-1648

SOUTH DAKOTA. Board of Nursing
3307 South Lincoln Avenue
Sioux Falls, SD 57105-5224
(605) 367-5940

TENNESSEE. Board of Nursing
283 Plus Park Boulevard
Nashville, TN 37247-1010
(615) 367-6232

TEXAS. Board of Nurse Examiners
Box 140466
Austin, TX 78714
(512) 835-4880

UTAH. Division of Occupational and
    Professional Licensing
Board of Nursing
160 East 300 South
P.O. Box 45805
Salt Lake City, UT 84145-0805
(801) 530-6628

VERMONT. Board of Nursing
109 State Street
Montpelier, VT 05609-1106
(802) 828-2396

VIRGINIA. Board of Nursing
Department of Health Professions
6606 West Broad Street, 4th Floor
Richmond, VA 23230-1717
(804) 662-9909

(continued)

B O X   7 – 2   (continued)

WASHINGTON. State Nursing Care
Quality Assurance Commission
1300 Quince Street
P.O. Box 47864
Olympia, WA 98504-7864
(360) 753-2686

WEST VIRGINIA. Board of Examiners
for Registered Professional Nurses
101 Dee Drive
Charleston, WV 25311-1620
(304) 558-3596

WISCONSIN. Bureau of Health Service
Professions
Box 8935
Madison, WI 53708-8935
(608) 266-0257

WYOMING. Board of Nursing
2020 Carey Avenue, Suite 110
Cheyenne, WY 82002
(307) 777-7601

Reprinted with permission of Mattera, M. D.
(Ed.). (1992). *RN presents: Nursing opportunities for 1992* (23rd ed.). Montvale, NJ: Medical Economics.

REFERENCES

American Nurses Association (1995). Nursing's social policy statement. Washington, D.C.: Author.

American Nurses Association (1980). *Nursing: A social policy statement.* Kansas City, MO: Author.

Harmer, B. (1922). *Textbook of the principles and practice of nursing.* New York: Macmillan.

Harmer, B., and Henderson, V. (1939). *Textbook of the principles and practice of nursing* (4th ed.). New York: Macmillan.

Henderson, V. (1960). *Basic principles of nursing care.* London: International Council of Nurses.

Mattera, M. D. (Ed.). (1992). *RN presents: Nursing opportunities for 1992* (23rd ed.). Montvale, NJ: Medical Economics.

Nightingale, F. (1946 facsimile of 1859 edition). *Notes on nursing: What it is and what it is not.* Philadelphia: J.B. Lippincott.

Orem, D. (1959). *Guidelines for developing curricula for the education of practical nurses.* Washington, D.C.: Government Printing Office.

Peplau, H. (1952). *Interpersonal relations in nursing: A conceptual frame of reference for psychodynamic nursing.* New York: G.P. Putnam's Sons.

Radke, K. J., et al. (1991). Curriculum blueprints for the future: The process of blending beliefs. *Nurse Educator,* 16(2), 9–13.

Rogers, M. (1961). *Educational revolution in nursing.* New York: Macmillan.

Schlotfeldt, R. M. (1987). Defining nursing: A historic controversy. *Nursing Research,* 36(1), 64–67.

Shaw, C. W. (1907). *Textbook of nursing* (3rd ed.). New York: Appleton.

Storlie, F. (1970). Nursing need never be defined. *International Nursing Review,* 70(17), 255–258.

Watson, J. (1979). *The philosophy and science of caring.* Boston: Little, Brown.

CHAPTER 8

Kay K. Chitty

Professional Socialization

OBJECTIVES

- Discuss how students' initial images of nursing are modified by professional education.
- Differentiate between formal and informal socialization.
- Identify internal and external factors that influence an individual's professional socialization.
- Describe developmental models of professional socialization and how they can be used.
- Differentiate between the elements of professional socialization that are the responsibility of nursing programs and those that are the individual's responsibility.
- Discuss Kramer's model for minimizing reality shock.
- Describe practical steps to ease the transition from student to professional nurse.
- Discuss employer expectations.

VOCABULARY

biculturalism	informal socialization	mutuality
cognitive rebellion	internal factors	preceptor
culture of nursing	internalize	professional socialization
dissonance	internship	reality shock
external factors	job hopping	resocialization
formal socialization	mentor	work ethic
inertia	modeling	

In Chapter 3, societal influences that have affected the development of nursing were discussed, and the media's impact on nursing's image was explored. It is clear that the image of nursing held by the public over the years has been influenced in large measure by books, television, and motion pictures. Nursing students, too, are affected by the images portrayed by these media as well as by contact with nurses they know. They bring an outsider's view of the nursing profession to school with them.

During formal schooling, the complex process of exchanging an outsider's perception for an insider's understanding of what nursing really is begins. This process requires that students **internalize,** or take in, the knowledge, skills, attitudes, beliefs, norms, culture, values, and ethical standards of nursing and make them a part of their own self-image and behavior (Jacox, 1973).

The process of internalization and development of an occupational identity is known as **professional socialization.** Put another way, "Socialization brings nurses into *existence*" (Colucciello, 1990, p. 17). Professional socialization in nursing is believed to occur largely, but not entirely, during the period students are in basic nursing programs. It continues after graduation when they enter nursing practice. In this chapter, the effects of both school and work settings on nurses' professional socialization are examined.

EDUCATION AND PROFESSIONAL SOCIALIZATION

What kinds of educational experiences are needed to make the transition from student to professional nurse? How does a student make the transition from novice to a person who thinks and feels like a nurse? Learning any new role is derived from a mixture of formal and informal socialization. Little boys, for example, learn how to assume the father role by what their own fathers purposely teach them (formal socialization) and by how they observe their own and other fathers behaving (informal socialization). In nursing, **formal socialization** includes lessons the faculty intend to teach—such as how to plan nursing care, how to perform a physical examination on a healthy child, or how to communicate with a psychiatric patient (Fig. 8–1). **Informal socialization** includes lessons that occur incidentally, such as overhearing a nurse teach a young mother how to care for her premature infant, participating in the student nurse association, or sitting in on a nursing ethics committee meeting. Part of professional socialization is simply absorbing the **culture of nursing,** that is, the rites, rituals, and valued behaviors of the profession. This requires that students spend enough time with nurses in work settings for adequate exposure to the nursing culture to occur. Most nurses agree that informal socialization is often more powerful and memorable than formal socialization.

Learning a new vocabulary is also part of professional socialization. Each profession has its own jargon, which is not generally understood by outsiders. Professional students usually enjoy acquiring the new vocabulary and practicing it among themselves.

Learning any new role creates some degree of anxiety (Wooley, 1978). Disappointment and frustration sometimes occur when students' learning expectations come into conflict with educational realities. Students' ideas of what they need to learn, when they need to learn it, and what might be the best way to learn it may differ from what actually occurs. They sometimes become disillusioned when they observe nurses behaving in ways that differ from their ideas about how nurses *should* behave. Knowing in advance that these things may happen can help students accurately assess the sources of their anxiety and manage it more effectively.

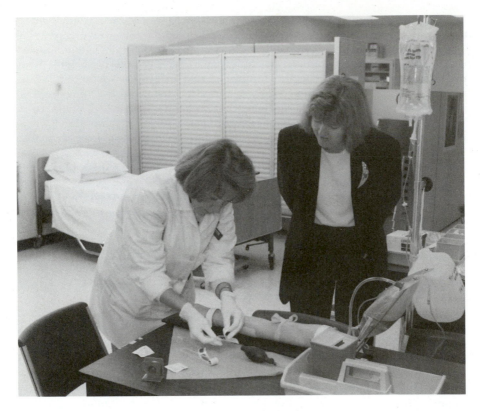

FIGURE   8 – 1
During formal schooling, students internalize the knowledge, skills, and beliefs of nursing. (Courtesy of University of Akron.)

Internal Influencing Factors

As students progress through nursing programs, a variety of internal and external factors challenge their customary ways of thinking. **Internal factors** include personal feelings and beliefs they bring with them. Some of these may conflict with professional values. For example, if they believe in a higher power, they may be uncomfortable working with patients who have no such belief. Yet nursing's code of ethics requires that nurses work with all patients regardless of their beliefs (American Nurses Association, 1976). Other areas that sometimes challenge students' thinking are substance abuse; self-destructive behaviors; abortion; and issues related to sexuality, such as sexual preference.

External Influencing Factors

External factors also influence professional development. Growing children are first influenced by the values, beliefs, and behaviors of the significant adults around them and later by peers. Ideas about health, health care, and nursing are also shaped through this process. If a nurse's family valued fitness, for example, it may be difficult for that nurse to empathize with an overweight patient who refuses to exercise. In this example, a family value (fitness) comes into conflict with a professional value (empathy toward all patients without judging them).

Nurses need to be aware of their biases and discuss them with peers, instructors, and professional role models. Failure to do so may adversely affect the nursing care provided to certain patients. Professional nurses make every effort to avoid imposing their beliefs on others. See Chapter 18 for further discussion of self-awareness and nonjudgmentalism as necessary attributes of professional nurses.

As seen from this brief discussion, socialization is much more than the transmission of knowledge and skills. It serves to develop a common nursing consciousness and is the key to keeping the profession vital and dynamic. It is not surprising, therefore, that a good deal of attention has been paid to this important process.

MODELS OF PROFESSIONAL SOCIALIZATION

In thinking about professional socialization, it is helpful to have theoretical models to consider. Cohen (1981) and Hinshaw (1976) described developmental models appropriate for beginning nursing students. Bandura (1977) described an informal type of socialization he called **modeling,** which is useful when learning any new behavior. Throwe and Fought (1987) described a developmental model of professional socialization specifically designed to meet the needs of registered nurse (RN) students. Each of these models is considered briefly.

Cohen's Model

Cohen (1981) proposed a model of professional socialization consisting of four stages. Basing her work on developmental theories and studies of students' attitudes toward nursing, she asserted, "Students must experience each stage in sequence to feel comfortable in the professional role" (p. 16). She believed that a positive outcome in all of the four stages is necessary for satisfactory socialization to occur.

Cohen called the first stage in her model *stage I, unilateral dependence.* Owing to inexperience and lack of knowledge, students at this stage rely on external limits and controls established by authority figures such as teachers. During stage I, students are unlikely to question or analyze critically the concepts teachers present because they lack the necessary background to do so.

In *stage II, negativity/independence,* students' critical thinking abilities and knowledge bases expand. They begin to question authority figures. Cohen called this **cognitive rebellion.** Much as a young child learns that he can say no, students at this level begin to free themselves from external controls and to rely more on their own judgment. They think critically about what they are being taught.

In *stage III, dependence/mutuality,* Cohen described students' more reasoned

TABLE 8–1	
Cohen's Stages of Professional Socialization	
Stage	**Key Behaviors**
Stage I: unilateral dependence	Reliant on external authority; limited questioning or critical analysis
Stage II: negativity/independence	Cognitive rebellion; diminished reliance on external authority
Stage III: dependence/mutuality	Reasoned appraisal; begins integration of facts and opinions following objective testing
Stage IV: interdependence	Collaborative decision making; commitment to professional role; self-concept now includes professional role identity

Reprinted with permission of Cohen, H. A. (1981). *The nurse's quest for professional identity*. Menlo Park, CA: Addison-Wesley.

evaluation of other's ideas. They develop an increasingly realistic appraisal process and learn to test concepts, facts, ideas, and models objectively. Students at this stage are more impartial; they accept some ideas and reject others.

In *stage IV, interdependence*, students' needs for both independence and **mutuality** (sharing jointly with others) come together. They develop the capacity to make decisions in collaboration with others. The successfully socialized student completes stage IV with a self-concept that includes a professional role identity that is personally and professionally acceptable and compatible with other life roles (Cohen, 1981). Table 8–1 summarizes the key behaviors associated with each stage.

Readers may wish to compare themselves and nursing classmates to these four stages. A word of caution, however: Although it is interesting and useful, this is a model that has not been scientifically tested and validated (confirmed). At least one researcher, McCain (1985), concluded that her study "did not support the Cohen model . . ." because students in McCain's sample of 422 BSN (bachelor of science in nursing) student volunteers in a large southern state university did not show evidence of progression through Cohen's developmental stages (p. 185). McCain recommended further testing of Cohen's model.

Hinshaw's Model

Another potentially useful model describing the educational aspect of professional socialization was proposed by Hinshaw in a 1976 publication for the National League for Nursing.

In this model, stage I, *initial innocence*, is characterized by idealized images and expectations of nursing. Students have gained these images from the media and from their own experiences with nurses. For example, they may expect that as nursing students they will immediately begin to work with sick patients, or that nurses are always treated with the utmost respect by other health care workers, or that they will always be able to make things better for their patients.

In stage II, *incongruities*, students realize that their innocent images of nursing differ from reality. For example, they discover that they must complete anatomy, physiology, nutrition, and a host of other courses before working with patients, or they discover that students are expected to defer to more experienced nurses and physicians, or they encounter patients with chronic, intractable pain. This **dissonance** (lack of harmony) between their expectations and reality produces tension and frustration. During the dissonant stage, differences are sufficiently well formulated to discuss with others. Students at this stage may overtly question whether or not they should continue in the program and may choose not to do so (Hinshaw, 1976).

In stage III, *identification*, students select and carefully observe role models. Role models may be particularly admired instructors or nurses seen in clinical settings. This stage is closely followed by stage IV, *role simulation*, in which they practice the role behaviors they observed. At first, the new behaviors may feel strange or phony, which sometimes causes confusion and self-doubt (Hinshaw, 1976). Students learning therapeutic communication techniques, for example, often feel awkward and obvious when they first try out these techniques in conversation.

In stage V, *vacillation*, there is a desire to cling to the old ideas and images about nursing while recognizing that new ideas and images are based on reality (Hinshaw, 1976). Evidence of this stage can be seen in new graduates who feel guilty when they are unable to provide intense, individualized care for every patient because of patient load and time constraints.

The last stage, *internalization*, occurs when there is stable and reliable use of the internalized professional model (Hinshaw, 1976). This can be seen in nurses who, after practicing for some time, have developed a balance between their expectations of themselves as professionals, employers' expectations, and their other life role expectations. Table 8–2 contains the stages of socialization described in the Hinshaw model.

TABLE 8–2
Hinshaw's Stages of Professional Socialization

Stage	Key Behaviors
Stage I: Initial innocence	Initial image of nursing unaffected by reality
Stage II: Incongruities	Initial expectations and reality collide; questions career choice; may drop out
Stage II: Identification	Observes behaviors of experienced nurses
Stage IV: Role simulation	Practices observed behaviors; may feel unnatural in role
Stage V: Vacillation	Old images emerge and conflict with new professional image
Stage VI: Internalization	Acceptance and comfort with new role

Adapted with permission of Hinshaw, A. S. (1976). *Socialization and resocialization of nurses for professional nursing practice*. New York: National League for Nursing.

TABLE 8–3
Bandura's Concept of Modeling

Role Model(s)	Student
Are competent practitioners	Consciously identifies and selects role model(s)
Manifest values, attitudes, and behaviors appreciated by student	Takes opportunities to practice desired behaviors

Reprinted with permission of Bandura, A. (1977). *Social learning theory.* Englewood Cliffs, NJ: Prentice-Hall.

Bandura's Concept of Modeling

Another method of professional socialization is modeling, discussed by Bandura (1977). In modeling, students learn by observing role models. Bandura believed that there are two requirements for successful modeling: Models must be seen as competent, and students must have an opportunity to practice the behaviors they see modeled. This is different from the informal socialization process described earlier because modeling involves a conscious decision on the part of learners to model themselves after the selected role model.

Students who wish to try modeling should identify nurses or instructors who share their values and attitudes and observe them closely. The next step is to "try out" the behaviors they most admire. Because people are not equally talented in all areas, students may choose to observe several models, each of whom excels in a different area. The basis of modeling as a method of professional socialization is careful observation and intentional simulation of the admired behaviors or characteristics. This is a legitimate method of acquiring desirable professional behaviors that can be useful to students interested in being more active in their own socialization. Table 8–3 summarizes Bandura's concept of modeling.

Throwe and Fought's Model for Socialization of Registered Nurse Students

When RNs return to school to work on their baccalaureate degrees, their needs are different from those of basic nursing students. They may experience feelings of frustration and anger caused by returning to the student role. Often, these nurses have practiced for years and wonder what anyone can teach them about nursing. It may seem almost insulting when they are placed in classes with students who are just beginning in nursing education. These RNs are not being socialized into nursing; if anything, they are in the process of **resocialization,** a process that often creates uncomfortable tension.

Throwe and Fought (1987) believed that the stages RNs must master during resocialization could be assessed using Erikson's theory. Erikson's (1950) theory described eight developmental stages individuals master as they progress from infancy to old age. Throwe and Fought designed a framework for RNs in BSN programs to assess their own growth as they progress through school. The framework can also be used by faculty and non-RN students to help them appreciate RNs' experiences. Table 8–4 contains Throwe and Fought's assessment tool.

TABLE 8–4
Assessment Tool for Socialization to the Professional Nurse Role

Developmental Task	Role-Resisting Behaviors Observed	Role-Accepting Behaviors Observed
Trust/mistrust: Learns to trust the worlds of education and work through consistency and repetitive experiences	Physically isolated from peers both in class, clinical Does not initiate interactions with others Responds only if called on	Involved with classmates Readily and quickly forms/joins groups when directed Initiates discussions with others Asks for clarification
Autonomy/doubt: Begins to develop independence while under supervision	Delays joining groups for unstructured activities Does not contribute equally Forgets or suppresses assignment dates Does not meet target dates Self-conscious about being evaluated by others	Joins groups for unstructured activities (study groups) Shares information with group; prepares for activities Meets target dates Able to interact in the teaching/learning environment Begins to develop independence with guidance
Initiative/guilt: Can independently identify, plan, and implement skills/assignments	Perceives objectives and assignments as not worthwhile Stress-related symptoms increase Has difficulty setting priorities Waits for instructor to initiate priority setting Lacks initiative to deal with conflicts Unaware of available resources	Objectives and assignments take on meaning Applies new skills, content to other work settings Effective in time management Renegotiates deadline extensions when appropriate Takes initiative in resolving conflict situations Aware of and uses available resources
Industry/inferiority: Behavior is dominated by performance of tasks and curiosity—individuals need encouragement to attempt and master skills	Elicits performance rewards and feedback from others Needs direct encouragement, especially when performing affective and cognitive skills Last to volunteer to demonstrate new behaviors Seeks rewards by performing old familiar skills rather than those in new dimensions Demonstrates disengaging behaviors (late, uninterested, resistive to learning opportunities)	Able to reward self Confidence thrives Eager to try out new skills; takes risks Volunteers to demonstrate new behaviors Profits from guidance and direction of others Applies self beyond family/work settings Curiosity channeled through educational system

(continued)

TABLE 8–4 *(Continued)*

Developmental Task	Role-Resisting Behaviors Observed	Role-Accepting Behaviors Observed
Generativity/stagnation: Efforts are made to guide and direct incoming students; assists others	Avoids social interaction and information sharing with incoming students Provides minimal care; unconcerned about continuity of patient care Selects patients with common, familiar clinical disorders No increased ease of learning or improved test-taking abilities Does not elect to test out of course requirements Stagnates in same job setting	Guides and directs incoming students Provides quality nursing care to patient, family, and community Takes calculated risks (questions level of care, seeks multiple learning opportunities, shares level of expertise, elects to test out of required/ elective courses) Demonstrates critical problem-solving skills Attains mastery of test-taking skills Self-directed learner Demonstrates clinical problem solving in own work setting Uses holistic approach to delivery of health care
Ego integrity/despair: Acceptance of one's own progress, achievement, and goals through realistic self-appraisal	Frustrated with progress and achievement; stagnated in developing new goals Crisis prone when changing roles Self-appraisal unrealistic Does not participate in structured educational opportunities Returns to old job and does not modify role performance Sees no reward in risk taking High risk for dissatisfaction with profession	Accepts progress, achievement, and goal attainment Realistic in self-appraisal Resets professional goals (graduate school, participation in continuing education, certification) Joins new perspectives on old job by use of critical thinking Takes risks (new jobs, different clinical setting, and leadership roles)

(continued)

TABLE 8–4   *(Continued)*

Developmental Task	Role-Resisting Behaviors Observed	Role-Accepting Behaviors Observed
Identity/role confusion: The individual searches for continuity and structure; is concerned with how he or she is accepted by others; is concerned how he or she is accepted by self; each individual struggles to shape or formulate own identity	Needs a structured clinical setting to develop ego identity further Sees old job as ideal and denies need for change Serious about learning (content and clinical practice) Frustrated with nursing as a career choice Too ideological or overly critical of others	Searches for continuity and structure but can adapt to unstructured clinical settings Identifies role models in clinical setting Articulates need for change or for modification of job-related roles and procedures Appears to enjoy learning and performing in clinical settings Realistic about own achievements and progress in educational system
Intimacy/isolation: Seeks to combine his or her identity with other self-selected individuals	Participates as a member, but resists group leader role Does not participate in professional meetings Unsupportive of others' educational advancement Feels no increased esteem in performing new role behaviors Meets minimal requirements and sees instructor only in evaluative role Resists using newly developed skills; more comfortable with previous level of performance Avoids giving feedback to agency personnel	Volunteers to lead work/study groups Participates in professional organizations Recruits others and represents school Demonstrates pride in new role behaviors and shares with others in work settings Seeks out instructor for additional learning, information, and professional growth opportunities Values symbols of profession (using assessment tools, RN name tags) Evaluates ability of clinical agencies to facilitate meeting learner objectives Provides feedback to agency personnel

Reprinted with permission of Throwe, A. N., and Fought, S. G. (1987). Landmarks in the socialization process from RN to BSN. *Nurse Educator*, 12(6), 15–18.

ACTIVELY PARTICIPATING IN ONE'S OWN PROFESSIONAL SOCIALIZATION

So far in this discussion, professional socialization has sounded like something that happens to students. Although much is out of their control, students do not have to be passive recipients of socialization. As active participants, they can influence the socialization process. For some ideas about how to become an active participant in the socialization process, use the checklist in Box 8–1.

B O X   8 – 1
A Do-It-Yourself Guide to Professional Socialization

Listed are 20 possible behaviors demonstrated by students who take responsibility for their own professional socialization. Place a check next to the behaviors you regularly exhibit. Be honest with yourself.

1. I interact with other students in and out of class.
2. I participate in class by asking intelligent questions and initiating discussion occasionally.
3. I have formed or joined a study group.
4. I use the library, labs, and teachers as resources.
5. I organize my work so I can meet deadlines.
6. If I have a conflict with another student or a teacher, I take the initiative to resolve it.
7. I don't let minor personality problems distract me from my goals.
8. I seek out new learning experiences and sometimes volunteer to demonstrate new skills to others.
9. I have chosen professional role models.
10. I am realistic about my performance.
11. I try to accept constructive criticism undefensively.
12. I recognize that *trying* to do good work is not the same as *doing* good work.
13. I recognize that each teacher has different expectations, and it is my responsibility to learn what is expected by each.
14. I demonstrate respect for my teachers' time by making appointments whenever possible.
15. I demonstrate respect for my classmates and patients by never coming to class or clinical workshops unprepared.
16. I recognize my responsibility to help create a dynamic learning environment and am not satisfied to be merely an academic spectator.
17. I participate in the student nurse association and encourage others to do the same.
18. I represent my school with pride.
19. I project a professional appearance.
20. One of my goals is to become a self-directed, lifelong learner.

Scoring: 1 to 10 checks: You need to examine your behavior and think about taking more responsibility for your own socialization.

11 to 15 checks: You are active in your own behalf. See if you can begin using some of the remaining behaviors on the list or come up with your own.

More than 15 checks: You are a role model of positive action in your own professional socialization process.

As consumers of educational services, students need to know what to expect of their nursing programs in terms of professional socialization. Schools are responsible for some activities, whereas the individual is responsible for others. The checklist in Box 8–2 provides ideas about what takes place in nursing programs around the United States to enhance students' professional socialization. Students can compare their experiences with those in this guide. The Research Note in this chapter describes the findings of a study of the socialization of students in nursing education programs.

BOX 8–2
A Consumer's Guide to Professional Socialization

The following statements indicate some positive socialization attitudes and behaviors students should expect in their nursing programs. Check the ones that apply to your program.

1. My teachers are interested in students' learning.
2. My teachers can tolerate ideas that are different from their own.
3. My program offers me the opportunity to explore differing values.
4. Considering the size of the community, my program offers me rich clinical opportunities.
5. My program emphasizes knowledge and techniques as well as values, ethics, and social behaviors of the profession.
6. My teachers provide regular, direct, constructive feedback on my performance.
7. The program's philosophy and curriculum have been explained to me.
8. The faculty members take pride in the school and actively work to improve it.
9. Faculty members model healthy personal behaviors.
10. Faculty members model professional behavior and project a positive nursing image on campus and in the community.
11. My teachers model respect for each other and for nurses in agencies where we have clinical labs.
12. Faculty members respect students and avoid authoritarianism (BIG ME/little you).
13. My program makes every effort to accept students who have the potential to succeed.
14. My teachers maintain school standards.
15. My teachers help students cope with anxiety.
16. My program encourages students to participate in extracurricular activities available in the larger institution.
17. My teachers avoid favoritism.
18. My teachers keep on top of new developments in nursing and health care and are clinically competent.
19. My teachers value teaching as much as they value their other academic interests.
20. My teachers view me as a consumer of educational services.

Scoring: Compare your responses to other students' and identify commonly agreed-on areas of strength and weakness. Discuss both strengths and weaknesses in class. With your teacher as a resource, decide how to use the information in a positive way.

RESEARCH NOTE

Because she believed that "the primary purpose of socialization is to transmit and transform our culture" (p. 17), Margaret L. Colucciello designed a study to examine the degree of professional socialization of 216 Midwestern university nursing students at sophomore, senior, and graduate levels. The student volunteers each completed a 25-item inventory developed by Richard Hall that measures degree of professionalism on five attitudinal dimensions: the use of professional organization(s) as a major reference; a belief in service to the public; a belief in self-regulation; a sense of calling to the field; and autonomy.

The study findings were surprising and dismaying: The degree of professionalism for each attribute was actually *lower* as the students progressed academically. According to Colucciello, this finding "is antithetical to nursing education's curriculum goals. It appears that socialization into the profession of nursing creates nurses who exhibit average or minimal commitment to the field" (p. 24). She cited other studies that showed that as nurses become "more socialized they begin to face the realities of their role expectations and responsibilities. The idealistic view of nursing is replaced by an awareness of the actuality" (p. 25).

Colucciello called for curriculum changes in nursing education to improve role socialization, a rethinking of the role of the nurse educator, use of nontraditional scheduling and adult learning strategies to promote autonomy, and fostering students' identification and internalization of nursing's role by increasing clinical practicum experiences to learn the work culture of nursing. She encouraged the use of debates, simulations, role reversals, and realistic, autonomous clinical experiences and research with instructor guidance and collaboration with nursing administration in clinical settings to make students feel more a part of the system.

Adapted with permission of Colucciello, M. L. (1990). Socialization into nursing: A developmental approach. *NursingConnections*, 3(2), 17–27.

Socialization to the Work Setting

When nurses graduate, is their professional socialization over? Most authorities believe that socialization, similar to learning, is a lifelong activity. The transition from student to professional is just another of life's challenges and, similar to most transitions, is one that helps people grow. Most new nursing graduates feel somewhat unprepared and overwhelmed with the responsibilities of their first positions. Although agencies that employ new graduates realize that the orientation period will take time, graduates may have unrealistic expectations of themselves and others.

During the early days of practice, most graduate nurses quickly realize that the ideals taught in school are not always possible to achieve in everyday practice. This is largely due to time constraints and produces feelings of conflict and even guilt. In school, students are taught to spend time with patients and to consider their emotional as well as their physical needs. In practice, the emphasis seems to be on getting things done, and talking with patients, engaging in patient teaching, or counseling with family members may be viewed as unproductive.

Comprehensive, individualized nursing care planning, such a staple of life for nursing students, may become an unrealistic luxury.

New nurses also must adapt to depending on other nursing care personnel, such as nursing assistants, patient technicians, and other unlicensed assistive personnel to assist them in caring for patients. This is a difficult adjustment for some nurses who are unaccustomed to delegating, are unsure of the abilities of others, or believe only they can provide quality care.

REALITY SHOCK

Kramer (1974) termed the feelings of powerlessness and ineffectiveness experienced by new graduates **reality shock.** Psychological stresses generated by reality shock decrease the ability of individuals to cope effectively with the demands of the new role. Unfortunately, some new nurses drop out at this point before they take steps to resolve reality shock.

Kramer identified several ways to drop out: dropping out mentally and becoming part of the problem; driving self and others to the breaking point trying to do it all; dropping out by **"job hopping"** (looking for the perfect, nonstressful job that is perfectly compatible with professional values); or dropping out by prematurely returning to school. Sadly, both for themselves and the nursing profession, some even sacrifice all the years of education they have invested in nursing and decide not to work in nursing at all. This is a loss neither nursing nor society can afford.

Being aware that there are stages most new graduates go through before settling comfortably into their professional roles can help reduce anxiety and increase coping. Kramer identified a model for resolving reality shock that consists of four stages.

1. *Mastery of skills and routines.* In busy acute care settings, which most new nurses choose for their first jobs, certain activities must be accomplished each day, and specific behaviors are required to accomplish them. During this stage, nurses focus on the mastery of essential skills and routines. They may temporarily lose sight of the bigger picture and may have to be reminded not to get so focused on the technical aspects of care that they fail to see patients' emotional needs.
2. *Social integration.* In this stage, which overlaps with stage 1, new nurses face the challenge of fitting into the work group. Issues of getting along and being accepted surface. Most people have a desire for peer recognition and approval. It is sometimes a challenge to retain the goodwill of co-workers while keeping high ideals and standards. Learning that they may have to sacrifice the esteem of some workers to maintain their professional values can be a painful, but necessary, lesson for nurses in this stage.
3. *Moral outrage.* Once they realize that they cannot do it all because their commitments to the needs of the organization (hospital), to the profession, and to patients often conflict, frustration and anger result. Is it more important to attend a staff meeting or to talk to Mr. Jameson's daughter, who needs to discuss home care versus nursing home placement for her father?

Managing these sorts of priorities is a challenge even for experienced nurses.
4. *Conflict resolution.* Kramer identified several possible resolutions of these problems:
   a. Change behavior while retaining values. For example, find a new work setting that is more compatible with beliefs or, if that is impossible, leave nursing altogether.
   b. Give up professional values (attending to patients' emotional needs) and accept bureaucracy's values (get work done quickly); just try to fit into the system.
   c. Give up both sets of values; for example, adopt a "go-with-the-flow" attitude; survival becomes the goal.
   d. Become a "bicultural nurse" (p. 162), who learns to use the values of both profession and bureaucracy to influence positive change in the system.

According to Kramer, adopting **biculturalism** is the most effective of these options.

BICULTURALISM

Biculturalism is a term Kramer used to describe nurses who learn to balance both cultures—the ideal nursing culture they learned about in school and the real one they experience in practice—and use the best of both.

How do bicultural nurses behave? First, they are realists. They recognize that there is no perfect work situation. They also recognize that if they are able to establish credibility and gain respect, they can later be leaders in making improvements.

Next, they accept the fact that newcomers have to demonstrate competence before they can become leaders. They know that people follow only those whom they respect. So they invest time in proving themselves before they start trying to make changes in the system. During that time, they demonstrate, through their own work, the approach to nursing care they value. They do this quietly and without fanfare, however, seeking support from like-minded peers.

Bicultural nurses observe the political system around them. Who are the real opinion makers? Who are the formal and informal leaders? Are they the same? When changes are made, who is involved, and how is it done? Who can be counted on to react to new ideas positively, and who is always negative and complaining? Is there anything that "turns on" the complainers? Are there some people who are so chronically underfunctioning that they just cannot or will not change? Answering these questions provides an appraisal of some of the political realities in the system.

Bicultural nurses willingly serve on committees to demonstrate their ability to address institutionwide issues and to meet others within the system who may share their values. They limit their committee service, however, to those that they believe are useful and constructive.

Bicultural nurses work at having rewarding personal lives. They realize that when people get most of their emotional needs met at work, they are vulnerable.

They want to fit in so badly that they tend to sacrifice their professional values if they conflict with the system or the values of others.

Bicultural nurses take care of themselves. They negotiate for a position, not just accept what is offered. They expect reasonable compensation and expect reasonable work hours most of the time, although they work their fair share of undesirable shifts. They do not routinely allow the system to take advantage of them and set them up for physical and emotional exhaustion, or burnout. They are cooperative. They demonstrate commitment and loyalty to the organization and show that nursing is more than just a job to them.

Bicultural nurses demonstrate many of the behaviors discussed in Chapter 6. In the final analysis, biculturalism and professionalism have many of the same attributes.

Minimizing Reality Shock

Much can be done to reduce reality shock in the transition from student to professional. Students must recognize that schools cannot provide enough clinical experience to make graduates comfortable on their first day as new nurses. They can take responsibility for obtaining as much practical experience as possible outside of school. Working in a health care setting during summers, on school breaks, and on weekends is helpful. They should avoid work during the school week, if at all possible, or keep it to an absolute minimum because academic responsibilities take priority during that time, and exhausted students make poor learners.

Some schools offer programs in which students are paired with practicing nurses (**preceptors**) and work closely with them to experience life as RNs do. If your school offers such a program, take advantage of it. If not, seek out information about similar programs at areas hospitals. Many hospitals are now providing excellent opportunities for students nearing graduation to function in expanded roles.

KNOWING EMPLOYERS' EXPECTATIONS

New nurses approaching graduation should realistically appraise their strengths, weaknesses, and preferences. To reduce reality shock, it is important to ensure that there is a good "match" between one's abilities and employers' expectations. Ellis and Hartley (1988, pp. 346–349) suggest that nurses examine themselves in seven areas in which employers of new graduates have expectations.

1. *Theoretical knowledge* should be adequate to provide basic patient care and make clinical judgments. Employers expect new nurses to be able to recognize the early signs and symptoms of patient problems, such as an allergic reaction to a blood transfusion, and take the appropriate nursing action, that is, turn off the transfusion. They are expected to know potential problems related to various patient conditions, such as postoperative status, and what nursing actions to take to prevent complications.

2. The ability to *use the nursing process* systematically as a means of planning nursing care is important. Employers evaluate nurses' understanding of the phases of the process: assessment, analysis, nursing diagnosis, planning, intervention, and evaluation. They expect nurses to ensure that all elements of a nursing care plan are used in delivering nursing care and that there is documentation in the patient's record to that effect.

3. *Self-awareness* is critically important. Employers ask prospective employees to identify their own strengths and weaknesses. They need to know that new nurses are willing to ask for help and recognize their limitations. New graduates who are unable or unwilling to request help pose a risk to patients that employers are unwilling to accept.

4. *Record-keeping ability* is an increasingly important skill that employers value. Although patient documentation systems differ from facility to facility, employers expect new graduates to know what patient data should be charted and that all nursing care should be entered in patient documents. Accuracy, legibility, spelling, and use of correct grammar and approved abbreviations are all minimal expectations.

5. *Work ethic* is another area in which employers are vitally interested. **Work ethic** means that prospective employees understand what is expected of them and are committed to providing it. Nursing is not, and never has been, a nine-to-five profession. Although work schedules are more flexible today than ever before, patient care still goes on around the clock, on weekends, and on holidays. Employers expect new graduates to recognize that the most desirable positions and work hours do not usually go to entry-level workers in any field. Nursing is no different in this respect from accounting, broadcasting, or investment banking. In nursing, others cannot leave work until they turn patient care responsibilities over to a qualified replacement; therefore, being late to work or "calling in sick" when not genuinely incapacitated are luxuries professional nurses cannot afford. Tardy nurses quickly lose credibility with their peers. Employers expect new nurses to recognize and accept that employment means some sacrifices in personal convenience—as in every other profession.

6. *Skill proficiency* of new graduates varies widely, and employers are aware of this. Most large facilities now provide fairly lengthy orientation periods when each nurse's skills are appraised and opportunities are provided to practice new procedures. In general, smaller and rural facilities have less formalized orientation programs, and earlier independent functioning is expected. It is useful to keep a log of nursing procedures learned during school. Many schools provide a skills checklist that is helpful in identifying areas in which students need more practice. Students can then be assertive in seeking specific types of patient assignments.

7. *Speed of functioning* is another area in which new nurses vary widely. By the end of the orientation period, the new graduate should be able to care for the average patient load without too much difficulty. Time management is a skill that is closely related to speed of functioning. Managing time well means managing yourself well and requires self-discipline. The ability to organize and prioritize nursing care for a group of patients requires time management skills. See Box 8–3 to determine what can be done to keep poor time management from being a problem.

B O X 8 – 3
Time Management Self-Assessment

Good time management is a skill that can be developed. Listed are principles reflecting good time management. *Circle* the answer most characteristic of how you manage your time.

1. I spend some time each day planning how to accomplish my school and other responsibilities.
   0. Rarely
   1. Sometimes
   2. Frequently
2. I set specific goals and dates for accomplishing them.
   0. Rarely
   1. Sometimes
   2. Frequently
3. Each day I make a "to do" list and prioritize it. I complete the most important tasks first.
   0. Rarely
   1. Sometimes
   2. Frequently
4. I plan time in my schedule for unexpected problems and unanticipated delays.
   0. Rarely
   1. Sometimes
   2. Frequently
5. I ask others for help when possible.
   0. Rarely
   1. Sometimes
   2. Frequently
6. I take advantage of short but regular breaks to refresh myself and stay alert.
   0. Rarely
   1. Sometimes
   2. Frequently

7. When I really need to concentrate, I work in a specific area that is free from distractions and interruptions.
   0. Rarely
   1. Sometimes
   2. Frequently
8. When working, I turn down other people's requests when they would interfere with my completing my priority tasks.
   0. Rarely
   1. Sometimes
   2. Frequently
9. I avoid unproductive and prolonged socializing with fellow students or employees during my workday.
   0. Rarely
   1. Sometimes
   2. Frequently
10. I keep a calendar of important meetings, dates, and deadlines and carry it with me.
    0. Rarely
    1. Sometimes
    2. Frequently

Scoring: Give yourself 2 points for each "Frequently."
  1 point for each "Sometimes."
  0 points for each "Rarely."
  If your score is:
  0–10: You need to improve your time management skills.
  11–15: You are doing fine and can still improve.
  16–18: You have very good time management skills.
  19–20: Your time management skills are too good to be true!

OTHER MEASURES TO REDUCE REALITY SHOCK

Other measures to reduce reality shock include seeking an employment situation with an **internship** or long orientation period. Inquire about preceptor opportunities, that is, working alongside an experienced nurse, and assess the level of professional development activities offered in each facility under consideration.

Recognize that all large systems have a certain amount of **inertia** (disinclination to change), and as good as a new nurse's ideas are, they may not be welcomed. Learning how change is accomplished in the institution is an important first step in becoming a positive influence on the system. Identifying which battles to fight and which to ignore is a learning process for all new professionals.

Talking with other new graduates about feelings is one of the best ways to combat reality shock. Take the initiative to form a group for mutual support—others need it too!

Another interpersonal strategy is to seek a professional mentor. A **mentor** is an experienced nurse who is committed to nursing and to sharing knowledge with less experienced nurses to help advance their careers. A mentor can be a great source of all types of knowledge as well as another source of support. Mentoring involves forming a relationship through which ideas, experiences, and successful behavior patterns are transmitted.

Ask an admired nurse to be a mentor and identify what he or she can offer. Some inexperienced nurses are fearful of approaching potential mentors with this request. They should remember that this process is not a one-way street; it has benefits to both parties because it complements and validates the mentor's self-esteem as well as providing important information and support to the nurse being mentored.

In preparing for a relationship with a mentor, you must first (Hagenow and McCrea, 1994):

1. Complete a self-assessment to identify your professional and personal needs and skills.
2. Select a mentor who seems to share your nursing values and beliefs.
3. Ask for an appointment to share your needs and values and determine mutual interest in the mentoring process.
4. Be prepared to communicate openly with your mentor. Be aware that you must be willing to identify your vulnerabilities to grow.

SUMMARY

Professional socialization is a critical process that turns novices into fully functioning professionals. The two major components of socialization to professional nursing are socialization through education and socialization in the workplace. There are several models of professional socialization that identify stages in the process and key behaviors occurring at each stage. Individuals have significant responsibility for active participation in their own professional socialization. They can identify needed learning experiences and seek opportunities that provide them. Reality shock has been identified as a stressful period new nurses may experience on entering nursing practice. Understanding the stages and how to resolve them can assist new graduates through this transition. In addition, knowing what employers expect can help students plan more effectively and help them be more assertive in seeking experiences they need.

REVIEW AND DISCUSSION QUESTIONS

1. Describe how both formal and informal socialization experiences in school have modified the image of nursing you brought with you.
2. Select one model of socialization discussed in this chapter and place yourself in one of the stages. Give your rationale for that placement. If none of the models fit your experience, design one and share it with the class.
3. List five things you can do to take active responsibility for your own professional socialization.
4. Interview a new nurse and assess his or her reality shock experience. How is this individual handling the transition from student to practicing nurse? What can you learn from his or her experience?
5. Identify several personal and professional areas in which a mentor might be helpful to you.

REFERENCES

American Nurses Association (1976). *Code for nurses with interpretive statements.* Kansas City, MO: Author.

Bandura, A. (1977). *Social learning theory.* Englewood Cliffs, NJ: Prentice-Hall.

Cohen, H. A. (1981). *The nurse's quest for professional identity.* Menlo Park, CA: Addison-Wesley.

Colucciello, M. L. (1990). Socialization into nursing: A developmental approach. *NursingConnections*, 3(2), 17–27.

Ellis, J. R., and Hartley, C. L. (1988). *Nursing in today's world: Challenges, issues, trends* (3rd ed.). Philadelphia: J.B. Lippincott.

Erikson, E. (1950). *Childhood and society.* New York: W.W. Norton.

Hagenow, N. R., and McCrea, M. A. (1994). A mentoring relationship: Two viewpoints. *Nursing Management*, 25(12), 42–43.

Hinshaw, A. S. (1976). *Socialization and resocialization of nurses for professional nursing practice.* New York: National League for Nursing.

Jacox, A. (1973). Professional socialization of nurses. *Journal of the New York State Nurses' Association*, 4(4), 6–15.

Kramer, M. (1974). *Reality shock: Why nurses leave nursing.* St. Louis, MO: C.V. Mosby.

McCain, N. L. (1985). A test of Cohen's developmental model for professional socialization with baccalaureate nursing students. *Journal of Nursing Education*, 24(5), 180–186.

Throwe, A. N., and Fought, S. G. (1987). Landmarks in the socialization process from RN to BSN. *Nurse Educator*, 12(6), 15–18.

Wooley, A. S. (1978). From RN to BSN: Faculty perceptions. *Nursing Outlook*, 26(2), 104–106.

CHAPTER 9

Kay K. Chitty*

Philosophies of Nursing

OBJECTIVES
- Define and give an example of a belief.
- Define and give an example of a value.
- Cite examples of nursing philosophies.
- Discuss the impact of beliefs and values on nurses' professional behaviors.
- Explain why nurses need a philosophy of nursing.
- Begin to identify personal beliefs, values, and philosophies as they relate to nursing.

VOCABULARY

aesthetics	ethics	philosophy
belief	logic	politics
bioethics	metaphysics	values
epistemology	nonjudgmental	

Up to now, this book has focused on describing and defining nursing from the outside. The historical milestones of the profession, how its practitioners are educated, the social context in which nursing has evolved, the organizations nurses belong to, how nursing measures up as a profession, how nurses define their profession, and how new nurses are socialized have all been examined. Now the book begins to examine what nurses themselves think, believe, and value and how their care of patients is influenced by these thoughts, beliefs, and values. In other words, nursing is explored from the inside.

Certain beliefs about what nursing is have evolved during the development of professional nursing. Specific statements of beliefs were generated by the members of the American Nurses Association (ANA) and published in the *Code for Nurses with Interpretive Statements* (see Box 4–1). Statements such as the code

*The author wishes to acknowledge the contributions of Marilynn K. Bodie to the preparation of this chapter.

174

exist to affirm the beliefs of the profession as a whole and to guide the practice of nursing.

This chapter examines the relationship of beliefs, values, and philosophies to the practice of nursing; reviews several philosophies of nursing that were developed by an individual, two hospitals, and a school of nursing; and assists readers in beginning to develop their own philosophies of nursing.

BELIEFS

A **belief** represents the intellectual acceptance of something as true or correct. Beliefs can also be described as convictions or creeds. Beliefs are opinions that may be, in reality, true or false. They are based on attitudes that have been acquired and verified by experience. Beliefs are generally transmitted from generation to generation.

Although all people have beliefs, few have spent much time examining their beliefs. In nursing, it is important to know and understand one's beliefs because the practice of nursing frequently challenges nurses' beliefs. Although this may create temporary discomfort, it is ultimately good because it forces nurses to consider their beliefs carefully. They have to answer the question: "Is this something I really believe, or have I accepted it because some influential person [such as a parent or teacher] said it?" Abortion, living wills, the right to die, the right to refuse treatment, alternative lifestyles, and similar issues confront all members of contemporary society. Professional nurses must develop and refine their beliefs about these and many other issues. This is often difficult to do but is nevertheless a worthy goal.

Beliefs are exhibited through attitudes and behaviors. Simply observing how nurses relate to patients, their families, and nursing peers reveals something about those nurses' beliefs. Every day nurses meet people whose beliefs are different from, or even diametrically opposed to, their own. Effective nurses recognize that they need to adopt **nonjudgmental** attitudes toward patients' beliefs. A nurse with a nonjudgmental attitude makes every effort to convey neither approval nor disapproval of patients' beliefs and respects each person's right to his or her beliefs (Fig. 9–1).

An example of differences in beliefs that directly affect nursing is the position taken by some religious groups that all healing should be left to a divine power. Seeking medical treatment, even lifesaving ones such as blood transfusions or chemotherapy for cancer, is not condoned. From time to time, there have been news reports of parents who are charged with criminal acts because they did not take a sick child to a physician. One such incident was reported in Pennsylvania when a 2-year-old boy developed a form of kidney cancer. His parents never took him to a physician because they believed that ". . . life rests in God's hands and that trust in medicine harms one's spiritual and eternal interests, which are more important than physical well-being . . ." (Levine, 1989, p. 220). These parents were ultimately convicted of involuntary manslaughter and endangering the welfare of a child. Think about how your health care beliefs differ from or concur with those of this family. What feelings might you have if assigned to work with a family with these beliefs? From this brief exercise, it can

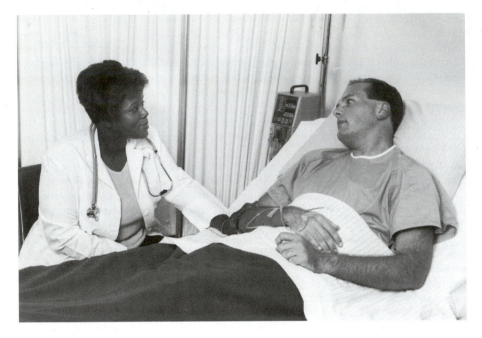

Professional nurses make every effort to maintain a nonjudgmental attitude toward patients. (Photo by Fielding Freed.)

be seen how difficult maintaining a nonjudgmental attitude toward the beliefs of patients can be.

Three Categories of Beliefs

People often use the terms *beliefs* and *values* interchangeably. Even experts disagree about whether they differ or are the same. Although they are related, beliefs and values are differentiated in this chapter and discussed separately.

Rokeach (1973, pp. 6–7) identified three main categories of beliefs:

1. *Descriptive* or *existential beliefs* are those that can be shown to be true or false. An example of a descriptive belief is: "The sun will come up each morning."
2. *Evaluative beliefs* are those in which there is a judgment about good or bad. The belief "Dancing is immoral" is an example of an evaluative belief.
3. *Prescriptive* (encouraged) and *proscriptive* (prohibited) *beliefs* are those in which certain actions are judged to be desirable or undesirable. The belief "Every citizen of voting age should vote in every election" is a prescriptive belief, whereas the belief "People should not engage in sexual intercourse outside of marriage" is a proscriptive belief. Prescriptive and proscriptive beliefs are closely related to values.

VALUES

Values are the social principles, ideals, or standards held by an individual, class, or group that give meaning and direction to life. A value is an abstract representation of what is right, worthwhile, or desirable. Values reflect what people consider desirable and consist of the subjective assignment of worth to behavior. Although many people are unaware of it, values help them make both small, day-to-day choices and important life decisions. Just as beliefs influence nursing practice, values also influence how nurses practice their profession, often without their conscious awareness. Diann Uustal (1985), a contemporary nurse who has written and spoken extensively about values, said, "Everything we do, every decision we make and course of action we take is based on our consciously and unconsciously chosen beliefs, attitudes and values" (p. 100). Uustal asserts that "Nursing is a behavioral manifestation of the nurse's value system. It is not merely a career, a job, an assignment; it is *a ministry*" (1993, p. 10). She believes that nurses must give "caring attentiveness and presence" to their patients and to do otherwise "is equivalent to psychological and spiritual abandonment" (Uustal, 1993).

Nature of Human Values

Values evolve as people mature. An individual's values today are undoubtedly different from those of ten, or even five, years ago. Rokeach (1973, p. 3) made several assertions about the nature of human values:

1. Each person has a relatively small number of values.
2. All human beings, regardless of location or culture, possess basically the same values to differing degrees.
3. People organize their values into value systems.
4. People develop values in response to culture, society, and even individual personality traits.
5. Most observable human behaviors are manifestations or consequences of human values.

Authorities agree that values influence behavior and that people with unclear values lack direction, persistence, and decision-making skill (Raths, Harmin, and Simon, 1978). Because much of nursing involves having a clear sense of direction, the ability to persevere, and the ability to make sound decisions quickly and frequently, effective nurses must have a strong set of professional nursing values. Uustal (1985) identified a number of professional nursing values; the complete list is found in Box 9–1.

Process of Valuing

Valuing is the process by which values are determined. Raths and colleagues (1978) identified steps in the process of valuing. They divided the process into three main components: choosing, prizing, and acting.

> **BOX 9-1**
> **Professional Nursing Values**
>
> - Nonjudgmental attitude
> - Honesty with patients
> - Involvement with families
> - Listening
> - Patient advocacy
> - Cooperative work relationships among staff
> - Dignity of the patient
> - Sharing self through nursing interventions
> - Integrity of profession through each nurse's example
> - Promotion of health
> - Providing care regardless of patient's ability to pay
> - Patient education
> - Emotional involvement with patients
> - Quality care (physical, emotional, spiritual, social, intellectual)
>
> - Individualized patient care
> - Knowledge
> - Competence
> - Empathy
> - Flexibility
> - Openness to learning
> - Trust
> - Teamwork
> - Promotion of patient self-determination
> - Collaboration between patient and nurse
> - Dependability
> - Support of fellow nurses
> - Accountability
>
> Adapted with permission of Uustal, D. B. (1985). *Values and ethics in nursing: From theory to practice.* East Greenwich, R.I.: Educational Resources in Nursing and Wholistic Health.

Choosing is the cognitive (intellectual) aspect of valuing. Ideally, people choose their values freely from all alternatives after considering the possible consequences of their choices.

Prizing is the affective (emotional) aspect of valuing. People usually feel good about their values and cherish the choices they make.

Acting is the behavioral aspect of valuing. When people affirm their values publicly by acting on their choices, they make their values part of their behavior. A real value is repeated consistently in behavior.

All three steps must be taken, or the process of valuing is incomplete. For example, a professional nurse might believe that learning is a lifelong process and that nurses have an obligation to keep up with new developments in the profession. This nurse would choose continued learning and appreciate the consequences of the choice. He or she might even publicly affirm this choice and feel good about it. If the nurse follows through consistently with behaviors such as reading journals, attending conferences, and seeking out other learning opportunities, continued learning can be seen as a true value in his or her life.

Values Clarification

Nurses as well as people in other helping professions need to understand their values. This is the first step in self-awareness, which is important in maintaining a nonjudgmental approach to patients.

A variety of values clarification exercises have been developed to help people understand their values. Considering your reactions to these statements can help in the beginning identification of some nursing values:

1. Patients should always be told the truth about their diagnoses.
2. Nurses, if asked, should assist terminally ill patients to die.
3. Severely impaired infants should be kept alive, regardless of their future quality of life.
4. Nurses should never accept gifts from patients.
5. A college professor should receive a heart transplant before a homeless person does.
6. Nurses should be role models of healthy behavior.

As you react both emotionally and intellectually to these statements, something about your personal and professional values is revealed. Determining where you stand on these and other nursing issues is an important step in clarifying your values. Box 9–2 contains a values clarification exercise you may want to complete to assist you further in understanding the valuing process.

Values Undergirding Nursing's Social Policy Statement

Groups, such as nursing, "have collective identities that are evidenced by their actions. These actions stem from a set of values and choices . . . [and] by examining the actions of groups, . . . their basic values can be logically inferred" (Mohr, 1995, p. 30).

Organized nursing, through the ANA, sets forth the values that undergird the profession. This is done in a document published from time to time that is designed to explain "nursing's relationship with society and nursing's obligation to those who receive nursing care" (American Nurses Association, 1995, p. 1). The most recent version, entitled *Nursing's Social Policy Statement*, was published in 1995. It set forth several underlying values and assumptions on which the *Statement* is based (American Nurses Association, 1995, pp. 3–4):

- Humans manifest an essential unity of mind/body/spirit.
- Human experience is contextually and culturally defined.
- Health and illness are human experiences.
- The presence of illness does not preclude health nor does optimal health preclude illness.

Another value inherent in this document is that "the relationship between a nurse and patient involves full and active participation of the patient and the nurse in the plan of care and occurs within the context of the values and beliefs of the patient and the nurse" (American Nurses Association, 1995, p. 4). Chapter 19 contains more about values and their relationship to nursing practice.

PHILOSOPHIES

Philosophy is defined as the study of the truths and principles of being, knowledge, or conduct (Flexner, 1994). A more literal translation, based on the Greek

---

BOX 9–2
Clarifying Your Values

Once you have identified a value, it is important to assess its significance to you and to clarify your willingness to act on the value. The following clarifying questions are organized based on the steps of the valuing process and can help you answer questions about what you value. Identify a value (or values) that is (are) important to you. Write your value(s) in the space provided.

_____

_____

_____

Next, use these questions to assess the importance of a belief or attitude and to determine if it is a value. Rephrase the questions to suit your own style of conversation.

Choosing freely
1. Am I sure I've thought about this value and chosen to believe it myself?
2. Who first taught me this value?
3. How do I know I'm "right"?

Choosing from among alternatives
4. What other alternatives are possible?
5. Which alternative has the most appeal for me and why?
6. Have I thought much about this value/alternative?

Choosing after considering the consequences
7. What consequences do I think might occur as a result of my holding this value?
8. What "price" will I pay for my position?

9. Is this value worth the "price" I might pay?

Complement to other values
10. Does this value "fit" with my other values, and is it consistent with them?
11. Am I sure this value doesn't conflict with other values I deem important to me?

Prize and cherish
12. Am I proud of my position and value? Is this something I feel good about?
13. How important is this value to me?
14. If this were not my value, how different would my life be?

Public affirmation
15. Am I willing to speak out for this value?

Action
16. Am I willing to put this value into action?
17. Do I act on this value? When? How consistently?
18. Is this a value that can guide me in other situations?
19. Would I want others who are important to me to follow this value?
20. Do I think I'll always believe this? How committed to this value am I?
21. Am I willing to do anything about this value?
22. How do I know this value is "right"? Are my values ethical?

Reprinted with permission of Uustal, D. B. (1993). *Clinical ethics and values: Issues and insights in a changing healthcare environment.* East Greenwich, R.I.: Educational Resources in Healthcare, pp. 36–37.

---

root words, means "the love of exercising one's curiosity and intelligence" (Edwards, 1967, p. 216). Nursing students often learn about philosophers such as Plato, Socrates, Aristotle, Bacon, Kant, Descartes, and others in nonnursing classes. These philosophers were searching for the underlying principles of reality and truth.

Philosophy begins when someone contemplates, or wonders, about something. If a group of friends sometimes sit and discuss the relationship between men and women and ponder the differences in men's and women's natures and approaches to life, one might say that they were developing a philosophy about male and female ways of being. It is important to remember that philosophy is not the exclusive domain of a few erudite individuals; everyone has a personal philosophy of life which is unique from all others'.

People develop personal philosophies as they mature. These philosophies serve as blueprints or guides and incorporate each individual's value and belief systems. Nurses' personal philosophies interact directly with their philosophies of nursing and influence professional behaviors.

Branches of Philosophy

Before examining professional philosophies, we briefly explore the discipline of philosophy itself. Philosophy has been divided into specific areas of study. This section reviews six branches: epistemology, logic, aesthetics, ethics, politics, and metaphysics.

1. **Epistemology** is the branch of philosophy dealing with the theory of knowledge. The epistemologist attempts to answer such questions as: "What can be known?" Epistemology attempts to determine how we can know whether our beliefs about the world are true.
2. **Logic** is the study of correct and incorrect reasoning. In logic, the nature of reasoning itself is the subject. It is logical behavior, for example, for fair-skinned individuals to stay out of the midday sun unless wearing protective clothing. Chapter 15 presents the method of logical thinking that nurses use to plan and implement effective patient care, called the *nursing process*.
3. **Aesthetics** is the study of what is beautiful. Painting, sculpture, music, dance, and literature are all associated with beauty. Judgments about what is beautiful, however, differ from individual to individual and culture to culture. For example, Eastern music may sound discordant to the Western ear and vice versa.
4. **Ethics** is the branch of philosophy that studies the propriety of certain courses of action. Moral principles and values make up a system of ethics. Behavior depends on moral principles and values. Ethics, therefore, underlie the standards of behavior that govern us as individuals and as nurses. **Bioethics** is a term describing the branch of ethics that deals with biological issues. Bioethics and nursing ethics are complex areas of study that are explored in Chapter 19.
5. **Politics,** in the context of a discussion of philosophy, means the area of philosophy that deals with the regulation and control of people living in society. Political philosophers study the conditions of society and suggest recommendations for improving them.
6. **Metaphysics** is the consideration of the ultimate nature of existence, reality, and experience. Metaphysicians believe that we can gain a more complete understanding of reality than even science can provide.

This brief review of the branches of philosophy is presented as a backdrop for the discussion of philosophies of nursing.

Philosophies of Nursing

Philosophies of nursing are statements of beliefs about nursing and expressions of values in nursing that are used as bases for thinking and acting. Most philosophies of nursing are built on a foundation of beliefs about people, environment, health, and nursing. Each of these four foundational concepts of nursing is discussed in Chapter 10.

INDIVIDUAL PHILOSOPHIES

If asked, most nurses could list their beliefs about nursing, but it is doubtful that many have written a formal philosophy of nursing. They are influenced on a day-to-day basis, however, by their unwritten, informal philosophies. It is useful to go through the process of writing down one's own professional philosophy and revising it from time to time. Comparing recent and earlier versions can reveal professional and personal growth over time. It is also helpful to read one's philosophy of nursing from time to time to make sure daily behaviors are consistent with deeply held beliefs. Box 9–3 contains one nurse's philosophy of nursing.

COLLECTIVE PHILOSOPHIES

Although few individuals write down their nursing philosophies, it is common for hospitals and schools of nursing to express their collective beliefs about nursing in written philosophies. In fact, both hospitals and schools of nursing are required by their accrediting bodies to develop statements of philosophy. Philosophical statements should be relevant to the setting. They are intended to guide the practice of nurses employed in that setting. Examining some of these statements clarifies what constitutes a collective philosophy of nursing.

Philosophies of Nursing in Two Hospital Settings.   First look at the philosophy of the Division of Nursing at Beth Israel Hospital in Boston (Box 9–4). Notice that this philosophy includes statements of belief about nursing services, recipients of nursing care, and professional nurses themselves.

Box 9–5 contains the philosophy of nursing of Memorial Hospital in Chattanooga, Tennessee. It describes a commitment to excellence in nursing service, practice, and leadership.

Notice differences and similarities in the two philosophies as well as statements with which one might agree or disagree. Remember that these are both philosophies of departments of nursing in hospital settings. Before taking a position in a hospital or health care agency, it is a good idea to ask for a copy of the philosophy of nursing in that institution. Read it carefully, and make sure you accept the beliefs and values it contains.

BOX 9–3
One Nurse's Philosophy

I believe that the essence of nursing is caring about and caring for human beings who are unable to care for themselves. I believe that the central core of nursing is the nurse-patient relationship and that through that relationship I can make a difference in the lives of others at a time when they are most vulnerable.

Human beings generally do the best they can. When they are uncooperative, critical, or otherwise unpleasant, it is usually because they are frightened; therefore, I will remain pleasant and nondefensive and try to understand the patient's perception of the situation. I pledge to be trustworthy and an advocate for my patients.

I realize that my cultural background affects how I deliver nursing care and that my patients' cultural backgrounds affect how they receive my care. I try to learn as much as I can about each individual's cultural beliefs and individualize care accordingly.

My vision for myself as a nurse is that I will provide the best care I can to all patients, regardless of their financial situation, social status, lifestyle choices, or spiritual beliefs. I will form partnerships with my patients, their families, and my health care colleagues and work cooperatively with them, valuing and respecting what each brings to the situation.

I am individually accountable for the care I provide, for what I fail to do and to know. Therefore, I pledge to remain a learner all my life and actively seek opportunities to learn how to be a more effective nurse.

I will strive for a balance of personal and professional responsibilities. This means I will take care of myself physically, emotionally, socially, and spiritually so I can continue to be a productive caregiver.

Philosophy of a School of Nursing. Now examine a philosophical statement of a school of nursing. The philosophy of the faculty in the School of Nursing at the University of Tennessee, Chattanooga, is printed in Box 9–6. After reading it, identify the differences between the philosophies of nursing in hospitals and the one in this school of nursing.

An important point about philosophies of nursing is that they are dynamic and change over time. When a collective philosophy is written, it reflects the existing values and beliefs of the particular group of people who wrote it. When the group members change, the philosophy may change. Therefore, once a collective philosophy is written, it should be "revisited" regularly and modified to reflect accurately the group's current beliefs about nursing practice (Cody, 1990).

DEVELOPING A PERSONAL PHILOSOPHY OF NURSING

Developing a philosophy of nursing is not merely an academic exercise required by accrediting bodies. Having a written philosophy can help guide nurses in the daily decisions they must make in nursing practice. Because many nurses have ill-defined, uneasy feelings about committing their philosophies of nursing to paper, few have done so.

BOX 9-4
Beth Israel Hospital Philosophy of Nursing

Introduction

This revised statement of philosophy and purpose has drawn on the seminal thinking of Benner, Henderson, Orlando, and Wiedenbach and on multiple documents developed by the Beth Israel Hospital nursing services and programs over a twenty-year period, including the Statement of Philosophy first issued in 1974.

Statements such as this are meaningless unless they are translated into action. Our philosophy and purpose are perhaps most succinctly expressed in the words of one of our patients: "My primary nurse was truly a gem in the profession of nursing. She combines not only the highest level of professionalism in nursing, but also the many personal qualities which go beyond that in assisting patients to make a full recovery. She had a knack for getting me to motivate myself. Her concern was genuine, her advice sound, and her willingness to assist in my long-range rehabilitation goals ever present."

Purpose

The purpose of the Beth Israel's nursing services and programs is to ensure that each patient receives professional nursing care that is patient-centered and goal-directed, and to support healthcare education and research in nursing and other disciplines. Beth Israel nurses and their associates in the division of nursing carry out their activities with one focus in mind—assisting the patient to achieve optimal health outcomes.

Philosophy

Nursing as a Professional Service

We agree with Virginia Henderson that professional nursing is a complex service that assists ". . . people (sick or well) in the performance of those activities contributing to health, or its recovery (or to a peaceful death) that they would perform unaided if they had the necessary strength, will, or knowledge. It is likewise the unique contribution of nursing to help people to be independent of such assistance as soon as possible." The activities that nurses help patients carry out (or those that nurses carry out for patients) include the therapeutic plans prescribed by physicians, by other health care providers, and by nurses themselves. In carrying out these activities, nurses practice an art through which technical, observational, analytical, and communication skills as well as scientific knowledge and clinical judgement are systematically applied to the health needs of others in a caring manner. Caring means being connected and having things matter. Thus by caring, the nurse creates possibilities for coping in the face of risk and vulnerability.

We believe that physical and emotional comfort is a universal health need, the provision of which is a historical and fundamental nursing responsibility. Nursing is further distinguished from other direct healthcare services by its tradition of continuity. For hospitalized patients, this includes 24-hour accountability for observing, recording, and reporting of the patient's condition, and for direct provision of care and comfort. For patients residing in the community, care is generally provided on an intermittent basis, incorporating the family and/or significant other in the plan to insure continuity. The nursing care in this setting includes identifying and facilitating access to community resources and supports, and encouraging patients to achieve their optimal level of functioning. Continuity of care across the spectrum of health and illness is valued and provided by all Beth Israel nurses whatever their area of practice.

We believe that for each patient, continuity, personalization, and excellence of care is best achieved when it is planned and evaluated by a collaborative patient

(continued)

BOX 9-4   *(Continued)*

care team whose individual members have continuous accountability for that care. We further believe that nursing care for each patient should be planned, coordinated, and delivered by a professional registered nurse, and that direct care should be provided by a primary nurse and any designated associates. The desired endpoint of all nursing activity is to maintain or improve the patient's health status and comfort.

The art and science of professional nursing is acquired through formal high-

er education. It becomes refined through continuing education and training, experience, self-evaluation, evaluation by a manager, and peer review.

. . .

The Beth Israel Nursing Services philosophy also contains statements about patients, families, professional nursing, and the environment for nursing care.

Reprinted with permission of Beth Israel Corporation, Boston. Copyright the Beth Israel Corporation 1996. All rights reserved.

Writing a philosophy is not a complex, time-consuming task. It simply involves writing down one's beliefs and values about nursing. It answers the question: Why do you practice nursing the way you do? A philosophy should provide direction and promote effectiveness. If it does not, it is a time-wasting collection of words.

Box 9–7 is designed to help you get started in developing your own personal philosophy of nursing. After you develop a beginning philosophy, save it. As you progress through your educational program, take it out and revise it regularly, saving each version. After you graduate, look back at all the different versions and see how your values and beliefs about nursing have changed over time.

SUMMARY

People develop beliefs and values that affect their attitudes and behaviors. Beliefs and values influence how nurses practice their profession. Nurses need to be aware of their beliefs and values to prevent the unintentional intrusion of personal values into the nurse-patient relationship. A statement of beliefs can be called a philosophy. There are numerous philosophical statements about nursing. Examples in this chapter demonstrate that philosophies rest on a basis of beliefs and values. As nurses progress professionally, they collect ideas about the practice of nursing that they agree with and support. From these, they develop their own personal philosophies of nursing. The purpose of developing a philosophy of nursing is to shape and guide nursing practice. As nurses mature in the profession, they may find that their philosophies about nursing also change, even though underlying values may not.

REVIEW AND DISCUSSION QUESTIONS

1. Name two of your health-related values. How did these become your values? Describe how you expect these values to influence your nursing practice.

Memorial Hospital Philosophy of Nursing

Philosophy of Nursing

The Department of Nursing at Memorial Hospital is committed to upholding the corporate values of the Sisters of Charity of Nazareth Health System and promoting the mission of Memorial Hospital. We affirm that the corporate values of

JUSTICE
QUALITY
COMPASSION
STEWARDSHIP
COLLABORATION

are in congruence with our professional values.

Therefore, we believe that the following principles must characterize the Department of Nursing.

Excellence in Service

We believe . . .

That each of our patients, regardless of circumstances, possess intrinsic value from God and should be treated with dignity and respect.

That each encounter with patients and families should portray compassion and concern.

That each patient should receive quality care that is cost-effective, competitive, and based on the latest technology.

That patient confidentiality and privacy should be preserved.

That meeting the needs of patients and other customers should always be our number one priority.

Excellence in Practice

We believe . . .

That our profession is a science and an art, the essence of which is nurturing and caring.

That our primary duty is to restore and maintain the health of our patients in a spirit of compassion and concern.

That the nursing process is an integral part of our practice as professional nurses.

That nurses should collaborate with other health care team members to meet the holistic needs of our patients, which include physical, psychosocial, and spiritual aspects of care.

That we should aggressively promote patient and family education to allow each individual the opportunity to prevent illness and/or achieve optimal health.

That we are accountable to our patients, patients' families and to each other for our professional practice.

That monitoring and evaluating nursing practice is our responsibility and is necessary to continuously improve care.

That we should pursue professional growth and development through education, participation in professional organizations, and support of research.

Excellence in Leadership

We believe . . .

That we should provide a progressive environment, utilizing current technology, guided by responsible stewardship to promote the highest quality patient care and employee satisfaction.

That we should encourage and support collaborative decision-making by those who are closest to the situation, even at the risk of failure.

That compassion should be characterized in our day to day personal interactions as well as being a motivating factor in management decisions.

That we should be sensitive to individual needs and give support, praise, and recognition to encourage professional and personal development.

That we should possess an energy level and personal style that empowers and inspires enthusiasm in others.

That we should consider suggestions and criticisms as challenges for improvement and innovation.

That justice should be applied equitably in all employment practices and personnel policies.

Reprinted by permission of the Department of Nursing, Memorial Hospital, a division of the Sisters of Charity of Nazareth Health System. (1995). (*Philosophy of nursing.* Chattanooga, TN: Author.

Philosophy of the School of Nursing, University of Tennessee at Chattanooga

The faculty believe that:

Human beings are holistic and live in an ever-changing environment. Through the life span, people function as individuals within a variety of systems including the family, other groups, and the community. Individuals have a life-long capacity for growth and strive for self-actualization. While attempting to meet their own needs, individuals have a personal responsibility to maintain a balance within the ecosystem (a community of living things and their environment in interaction with each other). Imbalance in the ecosystem alters the health care requirements of the individual and the larger society.

Society is composed of individuals, families and communities sharing a variety of common goals and values which change as interests and priorities of the members change. Social change evolves through the mutuality of relationships and the interaction of political and social forces which affect the individual's rights, responsibilities and obligations.

Health is an ever-changing state varying from high level wellness through illness to death. The potential for wellness is influenced by adaptation to inborn and developed capabilities, internal and external stresses, state of development, values and beliefs, and by interaction with the environment.

Nursing is one of the major sectors of the health care system. It is a part of an interdisciplinary effort to promote and maintain health, to prevent disease and disability, and to care for, cure and rehabilitate the sick. This effort also includes helping clients and families cope with suffering and death. The faculty believe that the uniqueness of nursing resides in its humanistic, holistic, and collaborative approach to the health care of people throughout the life span.

Professional nursing is a practice discipline with an academic foundation that focuses on health. Building on the study of the biological, physical, and behavioral sciences and the humanities, nursing develops theories and conducts research to improve practice.

The practice of nursing is a blend of knowledge, skills, caring, and nurturing. The practice is designed to assist individuals, groups, or larger systems to achieve self-determined health goals, to reach a state of adaptation to their unique environments, and to maintain adequate or improved patterns of functioning.

The practice of nursing affects and is affected by societal changes and health care delivery systems. The nurse fulfills present and emerging roles, some of which are the practitioner, teacher, collaborator, counselor, manager, nurturer, advocate, and researcher. Nursing practice is based upon the nursing process. Nursing practice requires that knowledge be updated in an ongoing manner.

Learning is a dynamic process involving the acquisition of cognitive, affective, and psychomotor skills. Learning is sequential and is achieved by active, direct participation in didactic and experiential situations. Learning at its best fosters autonomy and a sense of responsibility. Learning for professional practice is a life-long endeavor. Learners have varied backgrounds and different styles of learning. They should be responsible for self-direction and their own learning. Educators are responsible for providing an environment conducive to learning, identifying the needs of the learner, encouraging independence, fostering the spirit of inquiry, and guiding the learning experiences. The faculty view the expansion of knowledge as a social process. Knowledge is developed as students and faculty, individually and collectively, engage in various forms of purposeful activity; close continuous interpersonal contact is therefore essential between students and faculty among students.

Reprinted by permission of School of Nursing, University of Tennessee at Chattanooga. (1995). *Philosophy of the School of Nursing.* Chattanooga, TN: Author.

BOX 9-7
Philosophy of Nursing Work Sheet

Purpose: To write a beginning philosophy of nursing that reflects the beliefs and values of _____. [Your Name].
Today's date is: _____.
I chose nursing as my profession because nursing is _____.
I believe that the core of nursing is _____.
I believe that the focus of nursing is _____.

My vision for myself as a nurse is that I will _____.
To live out my philosophy of nursing, every day I must remember this about:
a.   My patients _____.
b.   My patients' families _____.
c.   My fellow health care professionals _____.
d.   My own health _____.

---

2. Compare the nursing philosophies of Beth Israel and Memorial hospitals. What are three common elements and three differences?: If you or a family member needed to be hospitalized, which hospital would you choose, based on these philosophies? Why?
3. Obtain the philosophy statement of the faculty of your school of nursing. What concepts are included? Which beliefs do you agree with and disagree with? Why?
4. Using the work sheet in Box 9–7, write a beginning philosophy of nursing. Share your philosophy with one other person.
5. Discuss how having or not having a philosophy of nursing influences a nurse's practice.
6. Discuss how the current focus on the business aspects of health care and cost savings impact your own and nursing's professional values.

REFERENCES

American Nurses Association (1995). *Nursing's social policy statement*. Washington, D.C.: Author.

Beth Israel Hospital Division of Nursing (1996). Statement of philosophy and purpose. Boston: Author.

Cody, B. (1990). Shaping the future through a philosophy of nursing. *Journal of Nursing Administration*, 20(10), 16–22.

Edwards, P. (Ed.). (1967). *Encyclopedia of philosophy*. New York: Macmillan.

Flexner, S. B. (Ed.). (1994). *The Random House dictionary*. New York: Random House.

Levine, C. (1989). God's will versus doc-

tor's orders. *Parents' Magazine*, 64(3), 220, 222, 226–227.

Memorial Hospital Department of Nursing. (1995). Memorial Hospital philosophy of nursing. Chattanooga, TN: Author.

Mohr, W. K. (1995). Values, ideologies, and dilemmas: Professional and occupational contradictions. *Journal of Psychosocial Nursing*, 33(1), 29–34.

Raths, L., Harmin, M., and Simon, S. (1978). *Values and teaching* (2nd ed.). Columbus, OH: Charles Merrill.

Rokeach, M. (1973). *The nature of human values*. New York: Free Press.

School of Nursing, The University of Tennessee at Chattanooga (1995). Philosophy of the School of Nursing. Chattanooga, TN: Author.

Uustal, D. B. (1993). *Clinical ethics and values: Issues and insights in a changing healthcare environment*. East Greenwich, R.I.: Educational Resources in Healthcare.

Uustal, D. B. (1985). *Values and ethics in nursing: From theory to practice*. East Greenwich, RI: Educational Resources in Nursing and Wholistic Health.

10

Kay K. Chitty*

Major Concepts in Nursing

O B J E C T I V E S

- Summarize the concepts basic to professional nursing.
- Describe the components and processes of general systems theory.
- Explain human needs theory.
- Recognize how environmental factors such as family, culture, social support, and community influence health.
- Explain the significance of a holistic approach to nursing care.
- Apply Rosenstock's model of health beliefs and Bandura's theory of perceived self-efficacy to personal health adoption behaviors and the behaviors of others.
- Devise a personal plan for achieving high-level wellness.

V O C A B U L A R Y

adaptation	health beliefs	output
closed system	high-level wellness	person
culture	holism	self-actualization
environment	homeostasis	self-efficacy
evaluation	input	subsystems
extended family	Abraham Maslow	suprasystem
feedback	nuclear families	system
general systems theory	nursing	theory of human
health	open system	motivation
health behaviors		

There are certain basic concepts, or ideas, that are essential to an understanding of professional nursing practice; they are the building blocks of nursing. These concepts are person, environment, and health. Everything professional nurses do is in some way related to one of these basic concepts. These concepts are interrelated, as seen in Figure 10–1. Before addressing each of the concepts,

*The author wishes to acknowledge the contributions of Marilynn K. Bodie to the preparation of this chapter.

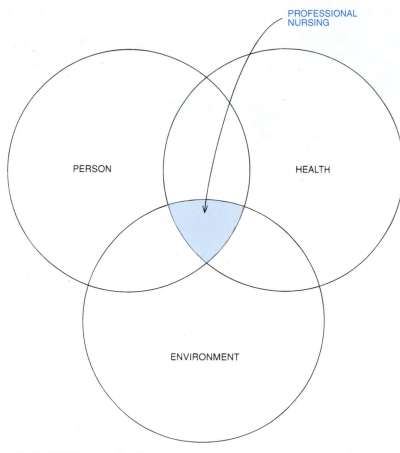

Relationship of concepts basic to professional nursing.

it is important to have an understanding of general systems theory (von Berta-lanffy, 1968), which helps explain how the concepts relate to each other.

GENERAL SYSTEMS THEORY

von Bertalanffy described **general systems theory** in the late 1930s. **A system** is a set of interrelated parts that come together to form a whole. Each part is a necessary or integral component required to make a complete, meaningful whole. These parts are input, output, evaluation, and feedback.

The first component of a system is **input,** which is the information, energy, or matter that enters a system. For a system to work well, input should contribute to achieving the purpose of the system.

A second component of a system is **output,** the end result or product of the system. Outputs vary widely, depending on the type and purpose of the system.

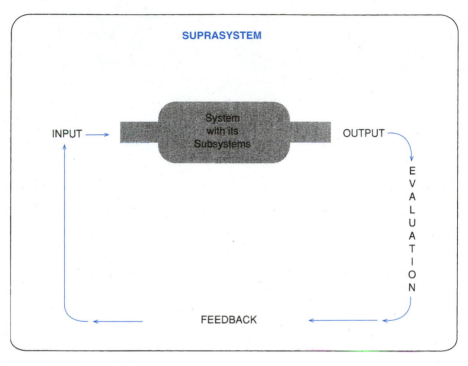

F I G U R E   1 0 – 2
General systems model.

Evaluation is the third component of a system. Evaluation means measuring the success or failure of the output and consequently the effectiveness of the system. For evaluation to be meaningful in any system, outcome criteria, against which performance or product quality is measured, must be identified.

The process of communicating what is found in evaluation of the system is called **feedback,** the final component of a system. Feedback is the information given back into the system to determine whether or not the purpose, or end result, of the system has been achieved. Figure 10–2 is a pictorial explanation of general systems theory.

It may be helpful to use a simple example to clarify the components of systems. In a college system, *input* consists of students, faculty, ideas, the desire to learn, and knowledge. Because the purpose of the system is to educate, the students need to be ready to learn, the faculty should be prepared to teach, and the ideas and knowledge transmitted must be clear and understandable. The *output*, or product, of the system is educated graduates. For *evaluation* of the output, a standardized examination of reading comprehension, mathematics, and analytical skills may be used. Student scores on the comprehensive examination provide *feedback* to the faculty and administrators. If they score well, the system has achieved its purpose. If not, changes need to be made in the input or in the system itself, for example, to admit brighter students, hire more talented faculty, or design more rigorous courses and curricula.

Systems are usually complex and consist of several parts called **subsystems.**

Let us examine a hospital as a system. Technically, it is a system for providing health care, but the success of the system depends on the functioning of many subsystems. The subsystems include the laboratory, radiology, housekeeping, laundry, central supply, medical records, dietetics, nursing, pharmacy, and medical staff. All these subsystems function collaboratively to make the health care provider system—the hospital—work.

The hospital and all its subsystems are **open systems.** An open system promotes the exchange of matter, energy, and information with other systems and the environment. The larger environment outside the hospital is called the **suprasystem.** A **closed system** does not interact with other systems or with the surrounding environment. Matter, energy, and information do not flow into or out of a closed system. There are few totally closed systems. A completely balanced aquarium comes close to being a closed system.

Two more points are essential to a beginning understanding of systems theory. First, the whole is different from and greater than the sum of its parts. Stated another way, the system is different from and greater than the sum of its subsystems. Anyone who has ever been in a hospital, for example, knows that what happens there is different from and more than the sum of the following equation: Laundry + pharmacy + nurses + physicians = hospital. Something additional occurs when all the various subsystems and the people who make them up join forces to work with patients and their families.

The final point to be made about systems is that change in one part of the system creates change in other parts. If the hospital admissions office, for example, decides to admit patients only between the hours of 8:00 A.M. and 10:00 A.M., that decision creates change on the nursing units, in housekeeping, the business office, surgery, the laboratory, and other hospital subsystems. If that change were implemented without prior communication to the other subsystems and coordinated planning, it could create chaos in the system.

The exchange of energy and information *within* open systems and *between* open systems and their suprasystems is continuous. The dynamic balance within and between the subsystems, the system, and the suprasystems helps create and maintain **homeostasis,** or internal stability.

All living systems are open systems. The internal environment is in constant interaction with a changing environment external to the organism. As change occurs in one, the other is affected. For example, walking into a cold room (change in the external environment) affects a variety of physiological and psychological subsystems of the person's internal environment. These, in turn, change a person's blood flow, ability to concentrate, feeling of comfort, and so on (changes in internal environment).

The openness of human systems makes nursing intervention possible. Understanding systems theory helps nurses assess relationships among all the factors that affect patients, including the influence of nurses themselves. Nurses who understand systems theory view patients holistically, including the subsystems (respiratory system, gastrointestinal system, and so on) and suprasystem (family and community). These nurses appreciate the influence of change in any part of the system. For instance, when a diabetic patient has pneumonia (change in subsystem), the infection increases the blood sugar and may result in hospitalization. Hospitalization may adversely affect the patient's role in the family and community (change in suprasystem). Key concepts of general systems theory are

---

BOX 10–1

Key Concepts in General Systems Theory

- A system is a set of interrelated parts.
- The parts form a meaningful whole.
- The whole is different from and greater than the sum of its parts.

- Systems may be open or closed.
- All living systems are open systems.
- Systems strive for homeostasis (internal stability).

---

summarized in Box 10–1. With this beginning understanding of general systems theory as a foundation, the three basic concepts that are fundamental to the practice of professional nursing can now be examined.

PERSON

The term **person** is used to describe each individual man, woman, or child. There are a number of different approaches to the study of person. This chapter briefly examines the concept of person according to general systems theory and human needs theory.

As mentioned previously, each individual has numerous subsystems that make up the whole person. There are circulatory, musculoskeletal, respiratory, and neurological subsystems that compose the physiological subsystem. There are also psychological, social, and spiritual subsystems that combine with the physiological subsystem to make the whole person. Each person is unique and different from all others. This uniqueness is determined both genetically and environmentally.

Certain personal characteristics are determined before birth by the genes received from parents. Genetically determined characteristics include eye, skin, and hair color; height; gender; and a variety of other features. Other characteristics about persons are determined by the environment. Such environmental factors as the presence or absence of loving parents or parent substitutes, the presence or absence of sufficient nutritious foods, educational opportunities or lack of them, adequate or inadequate housing, the quality and quantity of parental supervision, and safety are all environmental factors that influence how a person develops.

Human Needs Theory

In addition to having personal characteristics, people have needs. A human *need* is something that is a requirement for the person's well-being. In 1954, psychologist **Abraham Maslow** published *Motivation and Personality*. In this book, Maslow discussed his **theory of human motivation** and the relationship of motivation and needs. He suggested that human behavior is motivated by needs. He identified five levels of needs and organized them into a hierarchical order, as shown in Figure 10–3.

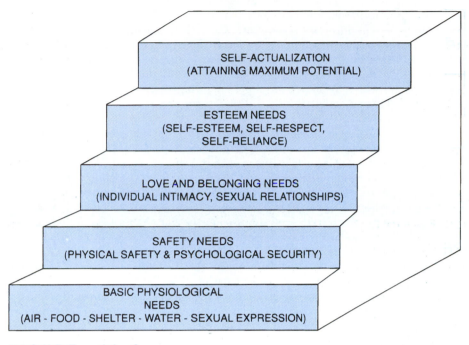

F I G U R E   1 0 – 3
Maslow's hierarchy of needs.

   The most basic level of needs consists of those necessary for physiological survival: food, oxygen, rest, activity, shelter, and sexual expression. These are
needs all human beings, regardless of location or culture, have in common.
Maslow identified the second level of needs as safety and security needs. These
include both physical safety and security needs and psychological safety and security needs. Psychological safety and security include having a fairly predictable environment with which one has some familiarity. The third level of
needs consists of love and belonging needs. Each person needs close, intimate
relationships, social relationships, and group affiliations. Next in Maslow's hierarchy is the need for self-esteem. This includes the need to feel self-worth, self-
respect, and self-reliance. The highest level of needs was termed **self-actualization.** Self-actualized people have realized their maximum potential and use their
capabilities to the fullest extent possible. People do not stay in a state of self-
actualization but may have "peak experiences" during which they realize self-
actualization for some period of time. Maslow believed that many people strive
for self-actualization, but few reach that level.
   Maslow's hierarchy rests on several basic assumptions about human needs.
One assumption is that the more basic needs must be at least partially satisfied
before higher-order needs can become relevant to the individual. For example,
a starving person can hardly be concerned with self-esteem needs until a life-
sustaining level of nutrition is established.
   A second assumption about human needs is that individuals meet their needs
in different ways. One person may need eight or nine hours of sleep to feel rest-

ed, whereas another may require only five or six hours. Each individual's sleep needs may vary at different stages of life. Older people usually require less sleep than younger people. Individuals also eat different diets in differing quantities and at differing intervals. Some prefer to eat only twice a day, whereas others may snack six or eight times a day to meet their nutritional needs. Sexual energy also varies widely from person to person. The frequency with which normal adults desire sexual activity is difficult to determine owing to the broad range of individual interests.

Even though sleep, food, and sex are considered basic human needs, the manner in which these needs are met as well as the extent to which any one of them is considered a need varies according to each individual. It is therefore extremely important to determine what a person's needs are to provide appropriate, individualized nursing care. If a patient is uncomfortable eating three large meals such as those served in most hospitals, nurses can help that person by saving parts of the large meals in the refrigerator on the nursing unit and serving them to the patient between regularly scheduled meals. This is a simple example of what is meant by the term *individualized nursing care*. Individualized nursing care recognizes each individual's unique needs and tailors the plan of nursing care to take that uniqueness into consideration.

Another aspect of human needs that must be considered is that people change, grow, and develop. Carl Rogers (1961), a well-known psychologist, built a theory of personhood based on the idea that people are constantly adapting and discovering themselves. His book *On Becoming a Person* is considered a classic in psychological literature. Rogers's idea that a person's needs change as the person changes is important for nurses to remember. Nurses can tap into the human potential to grow and develop to assist patients to change unhealthy behaviors and to reach the highest level of wellness possible. The concept of **adaptation** is also helpful in understanding that people admitted to hospitals and removed from their customary, familiar environments frequently become anxious. Even the most confident person can become fearful when in an uncertain, perhaps threatening, situation. Under these circumstances, nurses have learned to expect people to regress slightly and to become more concerned with basic needs and less focused on the higher needs in Maslow's hierarchy. A "take-charge" professional person, for example, may become somewhat demanding and self-absorbed when hospitalized.

Homeostasis

When a person's needs are not met, homeostasis is threatened. Remember that homeostasis is a dynamic balance achieved by effectively functioning open systems. It is a state of equilibrium, a tendency to maintain internal stability. In humans, homeostasis is attained by coordinated responses of organ systems that automatically compensate for environmental changes. When someone goes for a brisk walk, for example, heartbeat and respiratory rates automatically increase to keep vital organs supplied with oxygen. When the individual comes home and sits down to read the newspaper, heart rate and breathing slow down. No conscious decision to speed up or slow down these physiological functions has to be made. Adjustments occur automatically to maintain homeostasis.

Individuals, as open systems, also endeavor to maintain balance between external and internal forces. When that balance is achieved, the person is healthy, or at least is resistant to disease. When environmental factors affect the homeostasis of a person, the person attempts to adapt to the change. If adaptation is unsuccessful, disequilibrium may occur, setting the stage for the development of illness or disease. How individuals respond to *stress* is a major factor in the development of illness. Stress is discussed more fully in Chapter 17.

ENVIRONMENT

The second concept basic to professional nursing practice is **environment.** Environment includes all the circumstances, influences, and conditions that surround and affect individuals. The environment can be as small as a premature infant's incubator or as large as the universe. Included in environment are the social and cultural attitudes that profoundly shape human experience.

The environment can either promote or interfere with homeostasis and well-being of individuals. As seen in Maslow's hierarchy of needs, there is a dynamic interaction between a person's needs, which are internal, and the satisfaction of those needs, which is often environmentally determined.

Nurses have always been aware of the influence of environment on people, beginning with Florence Nightingale, who "believed in creating an environment for the patient in which restoration and preservation of health and prevention of disease and injury were possible" (Spellbring, 1991, p. 805). Concerns about the health of the public have led governmental entities at local, state, and national levels to promulgate standards and regulations that assure citizens of the safety of their food, water, air, cosmetics, medications, workplaces, and other potential health hazards. Environmental factors to be discussed in this section are family, culture, social support, and community.

Family Influences

The most direct environmental influence on people is the family. The quality and amount of parenting provided to infants and growing children constitute a major determinant of health. Children who are nurtured when young and vulnerable, who are allowed to grow in independence and self-determination, and who are taught the skills they need for social living are likely to grow into strong, productive, autonomous adults.

For most of the history of humankind, immediate and **extended families** were relatively intact units that lived together or lived within close proximity to each other. Children were nurtured by a variety of relatives as well as by their own parents. This closeness was profoundly affected by industrialization, which fostered urbanization. When families ceased farming, which was a family endeavor, and moved to cities where fathers worked in factories, the first dilution of family influence on children began. Former sources of nurturing such as grandparents, aunts, uncles, and other extended family members often stayed in rural areas, whereas the **nuclear family** (mother, father, and their children) moved away.

During World War II, more women began to work, taking them out of the home and away from young children for hours each day. The increased geographic mobility of families since World War II also had a destructive effect on the role of extended family in the lives of children, as nuclear families often live half a continent or more away from grandparents and other family members. The intense attention children traditionally received from adult relatives diminished, sometimes to the detriment of the child's well-being.

Today, there are more single-parent families in the United States than ever before, most of which are headed by women. The 1990 U.S. census revealed that there are more than 10 million women with a total of 16 million children under age 21 and no father present (U.S. Bureau of the Census, 1990, p. 20). This represents a 39 percent increase in such families in a decade. Only half of the single and divorced mothers are receiving child support due from absent fathers, according to the U.S. Census Bureau. Louis Sullivan, former secretary of the Department of Health and Human Services, stated, "Many of this country's societal problems can be traced back to parents not supporting their children" ("Half of single moms . . . ," 1991). Lack of money often means adequate nutrition and health care are not attainable, adversely affecting the health status of all the family members.

In addition to single mothers, there are nearly 3 million single fathers in the United States (U.S. Bureau of the Census, 1990, p. 20). Life is challenging for single parents of both sexes who must perform traditional breadwinner roles as well as traditional nurturing roles in the family. The combination of bearing multiple roles over long periods of time can be extremely stressful, even exhausting, to single parents. Long-term stress affects the mental and physical health of these adults, which, in turn, affects their parenting abilities. Although many single parents manage stress well and are able to provide excellent parenting, some children's needs are neglected. The impact of this neglect can be seen in the behavior and school performance of children who have not learned the skills they need to be successful.

The examples given are only a few of the ways families influence the well-being of individuals. There are many others. Understanding a patient's family and home environment is part of a complete nursing assessment. Modification of the home environment may be needed, particularly when a person is returning home with a physical disability, in cases of child neglect, and in abuse cases. Nurses, social workers, and discharge planners often collaborate to ensure that needed changes occur before patients are discharged to homes and families.

Cultural Influences

Culture is another important environmental influence affecting individuals. Culture consists of the attitudes, beliefs, and behaviors of social and ethnic groups that have been perpetuated through generations. Patterns of dress; eating habits; activities of daily living; attitudes toward those outside the culture; health beliefs and values; spiritual beliefs or religious orientation; and attitudes toward children, women, men, work, and recreation all are influenced by culture.

Nearly 20 million Americans were born in other countries, and approximately 32 million speak non-English languages at home. As mentioned in Chapter 3, the United States is fast becoming the "first truly multicultural society" (Gross-man, 1994, p. 58). Because a person's basic beliefs about health and illness vary widely from culture to culture, nurses need to develop *cultural competence* to meet the needs of culturally diverse patients. For example, "Among some South-ern African-Americans . . . health is considered a gift from God and illness ret-ribution for sin" (Grossman, 1994, p. 58). These beliefs may cause delays in seek-ing treatments. "A traditional Vietnamese folk remedy, *ventouse*, . . . involves placing a heated cup on the skin. It's believed that as the cup cools, it draws away excess energy or 'wind' causing the illness" (Grossman, 1994, p. 58). This prac-tice can cause bruising, which in a child can be mistaken for a sign of abuse. Giv-en these examples, it is easy to see that cultural beliefs of patients have great rel-evance to nurses.

Effective nurses learn to be aware of and to respect cultural influences on pa-tients. Whenever possible, they pay attention to patients' cultural preferences. As in the previous example, they recognize that some cultural groups attribute illness to bad fortune. Individuals from these cultures do not see themselves as active participants in their own health status. This attitude is a challenge for nurses who value the collaboration of patients in their own health care planning.

These are only a few examples of the influence of cultural beliefs on the nurse-patient interaction. Wise nurses realize that integration of a patient's cultural health beliefs into the individualized treatment plan can make a strong impact on that patient's desire and ability to get well.

Understanding the relationship between culture and health is the basis for "transcultural nursing," a field of nursing practice initiated by nurse-sociologist Madeline Leininger. Additional discussion of the influence of culture is included in Chapters 3 and 17.

Influence of the Social Environment

In addition to families and cultural groups, individuals are also influenced by the social environment in which they live. Social institutions such as families, neighborhoods, schools, churches, professional associations, civic groups, and recreational groups all may constitute a form of social support. Social support also includes such factors as presence in the home of a spouse; proximity to neigh-bors, children, and other supportive individuals; access to medical care; coping abilities; educational level; and so on.

Holmes and Rahe (1967) published a study of the relationship of social change to the subsequent development of illness. People with many social changes that disrupt social support, such as death of a loved one, divorce, job changes, mov-ing, or unemployment, were much more likely to experience illness in the fol-lowing 12 months than were people with few social changes. Both positive and negative changes created the need for social readjustment. Box 10–2 lists the 43 life events studied by Holmes and Rahe.

Broadhead and colleagues, in a 1983 review of the literature, found additional evidence that social support has a direct relationship to health. They reviewed a number of studies that indicated that poor social support preceded declining health in the subjects studied. They concluded that further research is needed to determine more precisely the type(s) of social support people most need.

BOX 10-2
Holmes and Rahe's Social Readjustment Rating Scale

Each of the 43 life events is ranked in order of the average length of time following the event it is believed to take people to readjust. Notice that life events include both positive and negative changes.

1. Death of spouse
2. Divorce
3. Marital separation
4. Jail term
5. Death of close family member
6. Personal injury or illness
7. Marriage
8. Fired at work
9. Marital reconciliation
10. Retirement
11. Change in health of family member
12. Pregnancy
13. Sex difficulties
14. Gain of new family member
15. Business readjustment
16. Change in financial state
17. Death of close friend
18. Change to different line of work
19. Change in number of arguments with spouse
20. Mortgage over $10,000 (in 1967 dollars)
21. Foreclosure of mortgage or loan
22. Change in responsibilities at work
23. Son or daughter leaving home
24. Trouble with in-laws
25. Outstanding personal achievement
26. Wife begin or stop work
27. Begin or end school
28. Change in living conditions
29. Revision of personal habits
30. Trouble with boss
31. Change in work hours or conditions
32. Change in residence
33. Change in schools
34. Change in recreation
35. Change in church activities
36. Change in social activities
37. Mortgage or loan less than $10,000 (in 1967 dollars)
38. Change in sleeping habits
39. Change in number of family get-togethers
40. Change in eating habits
41. Vacation
42. Christmas
43. Minor violations of the law

(Reprinted with permission of Holmes, T. H., and Rahe, R. H. (1967). The social readjustment rating scale. *Journal of Psychosomatic Research*, 11(2), 213–218.)

In assessing patients, nurses need to remember that the adequacy of social support is determined by the patient, not the nurse. Individuals vary in their need and desire for social support. When it is determined that strengthening social support is desirable, nurses can encourage patients to use interest groups, parenting classes, marriage enrichment groups, religious groups, formal and informal educational groups, and self-help groups to develop stronger support from the social environment.

Community, National, and World Influences

Community environment also influences the health status of people. The types and availability of jobs, housing, schools, and health care as well as the overall economic well-being of a community all profoundly affect its citizens. Although it may not seem an obvious nursing role, nurses can be instrumental in improving community environment. Identifying health needs and bringing these to the attention of community planners, offering screening programs, serving on health-related committees and advisory boards, and lobbying political leaders all can bring about positive community change. Nurses also have become politically active by running for elected offices at local, state, and national levels. They can actively support political candidates who have sound environmental platforms. More about political activism in nursing is found in Chapter 21.

On a broader perspective, environment also includes the nation, the world, and the universe. An isolated incident such as a volcano eruption in the Philippines may have worldwide environmental repercussions. Although nothing can be done to prevent natural disasters, nurses can contribute to a healthier world environment by promoting or participating in humanitarian responses to international disasters. Individual nurses, in the interest of world health, may choose to engage in a variety of environmentally sound practices and encourage others to do the same. These include recycling, using pump rather than aerosol sprayers, avoiding insecticides and unnecessary use of gardening chemicals, buying energy-efficient appliances and automobiles, walking when possible instead of driving, and boycotting companies that engage in environmentally unsound practices such as polluting air and water.

Hospitals are among the highest producers of waste. In an effort to reduce environmental pollution, some hospitals have committees dedicated to identifying and recommending environmentally sound products. Nurses may wish to consider reducing the amount of solid waste generated by hospitals by recommending the purchase of fewer disposable products and avoiding products with wasteful packaging.

HEALTH

Health is the third concept fundamental to the practice of professional nursing. Health can be viewed as a continuum, or series of events, rather than as an absolute state. Each individual's health status varies from day to day, depending on a variety of factors, such as rest, nutrition, and stressors (Fig. 10–4). Illness is also not an absolute state. People can have chronic illnesses such as diabetes or seizure disorders and still work, take part in recreational activities, and maintain acceptably healthy lives.

Defining Health

There are numerous definitions of health. The World Health Organization (WHO) defined health as "a state of complete physical, mental and social well-being and not merely the absence of disease or infirmity" (1947, p. 29). This definition was the first modern recognition of health as multidimensional. The WHO definition presented a holistic view of health that reflected the interplay between the psychological, social, spiritual, and physical aspects of human life.

A holistic view of health focuses on the interrelationship of all the parts that make up a whole person. Jan Christian Smuts (1926) first introduced the concept of **holism** in modern Western thought by emphasizing the harmony between

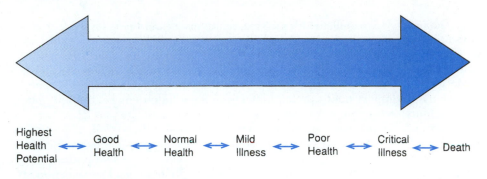

| Highest Health Potential | ⟷ | Good Health | ⟷ | Normal Health | ⟷ | Mild Illness | ⟷ | Poor Health | ⟷ | Critical Illness | ⟷ | Death |

F I G U R E   1 0 – 4

The health-illness continuum—a holistic health model. (Adapted with permission of Flynn, J., and Heffron, P. (1984). *Nursing: From concept to practice*. East Norwalk, CT: Appleton & Lange.)

people and nature. When viewing health holistically, individual health practices must be taken into account. Health practices are culturally determined and include nutritional habits, type and amount of exercise and rest, how one copes with stress, quality of interpersonal relationships, and other lifestyle factors. As a profession, nurses value a holistic view of health.

Parsons (1959) defined health as "the state of optimum capacity of an individual for the effective performance of his roles and tasks." This definition focused on the roles individuals assume in life and the impact health or illness has on the fulfillment of those roles. A few examples of roles that are familiar may include the student role, the parent role, the breadwinner role, and the friend role. Given the activities inherent in each of these roles, it is easily seen that the state of health profoundly influences how people carry out their roles in life.

Yet another description of health is the opposite of illness (Dunn, 1959). Dunn, in his classic text, *High Level Wellness* (1961), described health as a continuum with high-level wellness at one end and death at the other. He described **high-level wellness** as functioning at maximum potential in an integrated way within the environment. A prisoner of war kept in solitary confinement and given a diet of rice for many months certainly would have difficulty maintaining health. If he keeps active, both physically and mentally, and retains a positive outlook, however, he is likely to be healthier than the prisoner who does none of these things. Using Dunn's definition and taking his environment into consideration, the prisoner may even be said to have attained high-level wellness.

Nurse-theorist Nola Pender (1987) described health promotion as "approach behavior," whereas prevention is "avoidance behavior" (p. 5). This may be a useful concept for nurses to keep in mind when seeking to help patients expand their positive potential for health.

A National Health Initiative: Healthy People 2000

On September 6, 1990, then U.S. Secretary of Health and Human Services, Louis W. Sullivan, released a report to the United States entitled *Healthy Peo-*

ple 2000. Heralded as an unprecedented cooperative effort, the preparation of the report involved government, private businesses, voluntary and professional associations, and concerned individual citizens. *Healthy People 2000* was designed to stimulate initiatives to improve significantly the health of all Americans in the last decade of the century. Three broad goals for health of the public in the 1990s were identified (U.S. Department of Health and Human Services, 1990, p. 1):

1. "Increase the span of healthy life for Americans."
2. "Reduce health disparities among Americans."
3. "Achieve access to preventive services for all Americans."

To meet these goals, 300 measurable objectives were identified in 22 different priority areas under the broad categories of health promotion, health protection, and preventive services. The report challenged American citizens, organizations, and communities to change behaviors and environments to support good health for all. U.S. public health agencies were charged with the responsibility for overseeing the initiatives in each of the 22 priority areas. Box 10–3 lists the *Health People 2000* priority areas.

It was the hope of those involved in preparing the plan that it would stimulate sustained support from a diverse base of individuals, groups, communities, associations, and governmental agencies to improve health outcomes. Particular emphasis was placed on improving access to health care by the poor, minorities, and rural populations, all of whom have borne "a disproportionate burden of suffering compared to the total population" (p. 1).

Although the Healthy People 2000 initiative stimulated much discussion and activity among those concerned about health, as of 1995, progress with respect to the health of U.S. citizens was mixed. According to McGinnis and Lee (1995),

---

BOX 10–3
Healthy People 2000 **Priority Areas**

- Physical activity and fitness
- Nutrition
- Tobacco
- Alcohol and other drugs
- Family planning
- Mental health and mental disorders
- Violent and abusive behavior
- Educational and community-based programs
- Unintentional injuries
- Occupational safety and health
- Environmental health
- Food and drug safety
- Oral health
- Maternal and infant health

- Heart disease and stroke
- Cancer
- Diabetes and chronic disabling conditions
- HIV* infection
- Sexually transmitted diseases
- Immunization and infectious diseases
- Clinical preventive services
- Surveillance and data systems

*HIV, Human immunodeficiency virus. (Reprinted with permission of U.S. Department of Health and Human Services. (1990). *Healthy people 2000:* Fact sheet. Washington, D.C.: Author.)

a preliminary examination of trends shows mixed results. In the area of health promotion, 10 of the 17 priority areas were

> proceeding in the right direction, four are proceeding in the wrong direction, one is without change, and two have no data available on which to make comments. Particularly good progress continued for reductions in adult use of tobacco products and in alcohol-related automobile deaths. Positive but less striking gains are recorded for the proportion of adults exercising regularly, eating less fatty diets, and reporting stress-related problems (pp. 1124–1125).

They attribute some of the gains to the fact that more workplaces have health promotion programs for their workers. On the downside, the number of people with sedentary lifestyles was unchanged and a higher proportion of the population was overweight in 1995 than in 1990. The trends for youth were also mixed with improvements in tobacco, alcohol, and marijuana use but alarming increases in the areas of homocides, other violence, and pregnancies.

Reporting on the 10 *Healthy People 2000* priorities in the area of health protection, McGinnis and Lee reported that 8 of the 10 were "proceeding in the right direction while one is progressing in the wrong direction and one has insufficient data available on which to base a conclusion" (p. 1125). There were fewer motor vehicle deaths, owing to reductions in drunk driving, increased use of child safety devices, increased seat belt use, speed limit enforcement, and the introduction of air bags in new cars. Air quality had improved, and reductions were noted in blood lead levels in children. Indoor air quality remained a challenge as did the incidence of work-related injuries. Food safety had improved. Fewer old people had complete tooth loss, although children's oral health was not documented.

The mid-decade report also pointed out progress in reducing cholesterol levels and controlling hypertension, reductions in coronary heart disease deaths and stroke deaths, and increasing use of recommended cancer screening services. Prenatal care during the first trimester had also improved, as had the number of children receiving childhood immunizations. They pointed out that problems remained for vulnerable populations, such as ethnic minorities and the chronically ill. As a result of the mixed progress, a number of midcourse corrections have been recommended and will be implemented (McGinnis and Lee, 1995).

Health Beliefs and Health Behaviors

Health is affected by **health beliefs** and **health behaviors.** Health behaviors include those choices and habitual actions that promote or diminish health, such as eating habits, frequency of exercise, use of tobacco products and alcohol, sexual practices, and adequacy of rest and sleep (Fig. 10–5).

Rosenstock (1966) was interested in determining why some people change their health behaviors, whereas others do not. For example, when the surgeon general's report on smoking first came out in 1960, some people immediately quit smoking. Over the years, condemning evidence against smoking has accumulated and been widely communicated, yet many intelligent people still smoke.

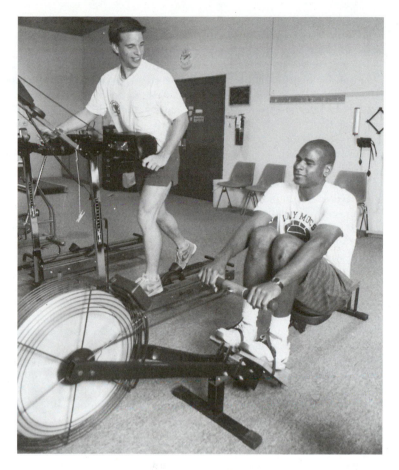

FIGURE   10-5
More Americans are engaging in health behaviors such as regular exercise. (Photo by
Fielding Freed.)

Rosenstock wondered why. He formulated a model of health beliefs that illustrates how people behave in relationship to health maintenance activities. His
model included three components:

1. An evaluation of one's vulnerability to a condition and the seriousness of
   that condition.
2. An evaluation of how effective the health maintenance behavior might be.
3. The presence of a trigger event that precipitates the health maintenance behavior.

Using Rosenstock's model, a man chooses to participate in a stop-smoking
program depending on his perception of smoking-related heart disease and his
personal susceptibility to it. If because of family history he believes he is sus-

ceptible to heart disease and that it may cause his early death, and if he believes that not smoking will substantially reduce his risk, he is likely to participate in the program. If, however, the stop-smoking program is in an inconvenient location, scheduled at an inconvenient time, or not affordable, he is less likely to participate. If his older brother, who smokes, has a massive heart attack, he may be motivated to attend the stop-smoking program despite the inconvenience and cost. The illness of his brother is what Rosenstock termed "a cue to action," or trigger event. A trigger event propels a previously unmotivated individual into changing health behaviors.

Albert Bandura (1992), a cognitive psychologist, developed an approach designed to assist people to exercise influence over their own health-related behaviors. He observed that whether people considered altering detrimental health habits depended upon their belief in themselves as having the ability to modify their own behavior. He called this belief in their own abilities perceived **self-efficacy.** High belief in one's self-efficacy leads to efforts to change, whereas low perceived self-efficacy leads to a fatalistic lack of change.

Bandura identified four components needed for an effective program of lifestyle change: information, skill development, skill enhancement through guided practice and feedback, and creating social supports for change (Bandura, 1992).

Using Bandura's model, a man wishing to stop smoking needs knowledge of the potential dangers of smoking, guidance on how to translate concern into action, extensive practice and opportunities to perfect skills, and strong involvement in a social network supportive of nonsmoking.

According to nurse-writer Patricia Butterfield, most health belief models place "the burden of action exclusively on the client and assume that only clients who have distorted or negative perceptions will fail to act" (1995, p. 74). She suggested that nurses familiarize themselves with the work of Nancy Milio (1976) and focus their attention "upstream" at the causes of poor health of the entire population. Milio recommended intervening at the population level rather than attempting to change individual behaviors. She advocated making health-promoting choices more readily available and cheaper than health-damaging options and using national-level policy-making to impact society's health.

Using the Milio/Butterfield model of health behaviors, a man wishing to stop smoking would be supported by population-based interventions such as "mobilizing comprehensive smoking cessation programs in schools and workplaces and encouraging politicians to end federal subsidization of the tobacco industry" (Butterfield, 1995, p. 76).

No one definition or theory of behavior can fully explain the complex state called health. It is important for nurses to recognize that health is relative, ever changing, and affected by both genetics and environment. It affects the entire person physically, socially, psychologically, and spiritually.

Devising a Personal Plan for High-Level Wellness

Each individual nurse has a personal definition of health, certain health beliefs, and individual health behaviors. How nurses view health behaviors in their own lives has both direct and indirect impact on nursing practice. Sedentary nurses, for example, are less likely to encourage patients to become fit. This has a direct

impact on their effectiveness as nurses. Because not exercising is a health behavior that most agree disqualifies people as healthy role models, being unfit also
has an indirect effect by portraying a poor image of nursing.

Nurses have a professional responsibility to model positive health behaviors
in their own lives, but nurses are people, too. Being or becoming a healthy role
model may require some effort. Box 10–4 will help you get started.

BOX 10–4
Self-Assessment: Developing a Personal Plan for High-Level Wellness

Nurses' personal health behaviors send a powerful message to consumers of nursing care. Are you in a position to demonstrate that you practice what you preach? In answering the following questions, you can assess how well you are meeting your responsibilities in this area of nursing.

1. I weigh no more than 10 pounds over or under my ideal weight.

   T   F

2. I eat a balanced diet including breakfast each day.

   T   F

3. Of the total calories in my diet, less than 30 percent come from fat.

   T   F

4. I exercise aerobically at least three times each week.

   T   F

5. I get at least seven hours of sleep each night.

   T   F

6. I do not smoke or use any other form of tobacco.

   T   F

7. I use alcohol in moderation and take mood-altering medication only when prescribed by my physician.

   T   F

8. I identify and control the sources of stress in my life.

   T   F

9. I have a balanced lifestyle, with work and diversional activities both playing an important role.

   T   F

10. I have friends, neighbors, or family members who are sources of social support for me.

   T   F

11. I practice safe sex.

   T   F

Directions for scoring: If you could not honestly answer "True" to all 11 questions, you need to set goals for yourself to enable you to do so.

1. On a piece of paper, begin your personal plan for high-level wellness. Write down at least two things you can do to address each "False" answer you gave to the self-assessment questions.
2. Share your health goals with one other person in your class. Make a contract with that person to serve as your "health coach."
3. Review your progress with your health coach at least once per week for the remainder of the term.
4. Begin your quest for high-level wellness today!

PUTTING IT ALL TOGETHER: NURSING

Nursing integrates concepts from person, environment, and health to form a meaningful whole. Nursing is an example of an open system that freely interacts with, influences, and is influenced by external and internal forces. Nursing is the provision of health care services that focus on maintaining, promoting, and restoring health. Nursing involves collaborating with patients and their families to help them cope and adapt to situations of disequilibrium in an effort to regain homeostasis. Nursing is also health and wellness promotion, including patient teaching to maximize rehabilitation and restoration of high-level wellness.

Nursing is integrally involved with people at points along the health-illness continuum. The purpose of nursing is to assist people in maintaining health, avoiding or minimizing disease and disability, restoring them to wellness, or assisting them to achieve a peaceful death. Nursing care is provided regardless of diagnosis, individual differences, age, beliefs, gender, sexual preference, or other factors. As a profession, nursing supports the value, dignity, and uniqueness of every person.

Nurses require advanced knowledge and skills; they also must care about their patients. Nursing requires concern, compassion, respect, and warmth as well as comprehensive, individualized planning of care to facilitate patients' growth toward wellness. Nursing links theory and research in an effort to answer difficult questions generated during nursing practice. Nursing's role is to assist patients to achieve health at the highest possible level.

S U M M A R Y

Nursing integrates three basic components—person, environment, and health—to form its focus. General systems theory and needs theory can be used to understand these components. Persons are viewed as unique open systems who are motivated by needs. Maslow organized human needs into a hierarchy consisting of five levels that range from basic physiological needs, which are common to all people, to self-actualization, which is attained by few. Environment consists of all the circumstances, influences, and conditions that affect an individual. The physical environment and family, cultural, social, and community environments all have impact.

Health is dynamic and viewed as a continuum. There are numerous definitions of health. Nurses view health holistically, including its effect on an individual's physical, emotional, social, and spiritual functioning as well as the impact on the family. Health is affected by health beliefs and health behaviors.

Nursing integrates person, environment, and health into a meaningful whole. Nursing assists people to achieve health at the highest possible level, given their environmental and genetic constraints.

R E V I E W A N D D I S C U S S I O N Q U E S T I O N S

1. Discuss general systems theory in relation to your family. What are the family equivalents of inputs, subsystems, suprasystems, outputs, evaluation, and feedback? Is your family an open or closed system?

2. Describe Maslow's hierarchy of needs and place yourself on the hierarchy today; one week ago; and when you were a senior in high school.

3. Write your own personal definition of health and share it with one other person. Evaluate your definition in terms of holism.

4. What are factors that influence an individual's personal health behaviors? Make a list of your health behaviors, including those that promote health and those that diminish health. Analyze why you continue both the healthy and the nonhealthy behaviors. Identify population-based initiatives that could influence you to make more health generating choices.

5. Conduct an assessment of your community in terms of one of the following: availability of jobs, quality of public education, availability of health services, environmental hazards, and quality of air and water. What is the impact of the factor you selected on the health of the community's citizens? What can you do to strengthen the environmental health of your community?

6. Look through the yellow pages of your local telephone book under "social services" and "organizations." What types of social support do you find that might be useful to patients?

REFERENCES

Bandura, A. (1992). A social cognitive approach to the exercise of control over AIDS infection. In R. J. DiClemente (Ed.), *Adolescents and AIDS: A generation in jeopardy*. Newbury Park, CA: Sage Publications.

Broadhead, W. E., et al. (1983). The epidemiologic evidence for a relationship between social support and health. *American Journal of Epidemiology*, 117(5), 521–531.

Butterfield, P. G. (1995). Thinking upstream: Conceptualizing health from a population perspective. In J. M. Swanson and M. Albrecht (Eds.), *Community health nursing*. Philadelphia: W. B. Saunders.

Dunn, H. L. (1961). *High level wellness*. Thorofare, NJ: Slack, Inc.

Dunn, H. L. (1959). High-level wellness for man and society. *American Journal of Public Health*, 49(6), 786–792.

Flynn, J., and Heffron, P. (1984). *Nursing: From concept to practice*. East Norwalk, CT: Appleton & Lange.

Grossman, D. (1994). Enhancing your cultural competence. *American Journal of Nursing*, 94(7), 58–62.

Half of single moms get support. (1991). *Citizen-News* (Dalton, GA), October 14, 1991, p. 4A.

Holmes, T. H., and Rahe, R. H. (1967). The social readjustment rating scale. *Journal of Psychosomatic Research*, 11(2), 213–218.

Maslow, A. (1954). *Motivation and personality*. New York: Harper & Row.

McGinnis, J. M., and Lee, P. R. (1995). *Healthy People 2000* at mid decade. JAMA, 273(14), 1123–1129.

Milio, N. (1976). A framework for prevention: Changing health-damaging to health-generating life patterns. *American Journal of Public Health*, 66, 435–439.

Parsons, T. (1959). Definitions of health and illness in light of American values and social structure. In E. G. Jaco (Ed.), *Patients, physicians and illness* (pp. 165–187). New York: Free Press.

Pender, N. J. (1987). *Health promotion in nursing practice*, 2nd ed. Norwalk, CT: Appleton & Lange.

Rogers, C. (1961). *On becoming a person*. Boston: Houghton Mifflin.

Rosenstock, I. M. (1966). Why people use health services, part II. *Milbank Memorial Fund Quarterly*, 44(3), 94–124.

Smuts, J. C. (1926). *Holism and evolution*. New York: Macmillan.

Spellbring, A. M. (1991). Nursing's role in health promotion: An overview. *Nursing Clinics of North America*, 26(4), 805–814.

U.S. Bureau of the Census. (1990). *Statistical abstract of the United States: 1990.* Washington, D.C.: Author.

U.S. Department of Health and Human Services. (1990). *Healthy people 2000: Fact sheet.* Washington, D.C.: Author.

von Bertalanffy, L. (1968). *General systems theory: Foundations, development, applications.* New York: George Braziller.

World Health Organization. (1947). *Constitution.* Geneva: Author.

Pamela J. Holder
Kay K. Chitty

Theory as a Basis for Professional Nursing

OBJECTIVES

- Differentiate among conceptual frameworks, models, and theories.
- Describe selected nonnursing theories including implications for nursing practice.
- Compare and contrast selected models of nursing theory.
- Explore the relationship of theory to nursing research and practice.
- Describe how nurses can participate in theory development.
- Explain the importance of theory-based nursing practice.

VOCABULARY

adaptation model	Madeleine Leininger	Sister Callista Roy
adaptation theory	model	self-care model
concept	Betty Neuman	set
conceptual framework	Dorothea Orem	stage theory
coping mechanisms	peer review process	stressors
cultural care, theory of	Nola Pender	systems model
developmental theory	phenomenon,	theory
growth	phenomena	unitary human beings,
health promotion model	proposition	science of
Virginia Henderson	Martha Rogers	Jean Watson
human caring, theory of		

As a science, nursing is in its infancy. Professional nurses are aware of this and conscious of the need for both nursing theory development and theory-based practice. As nursing comes of age, not only as a practice discipline, but also as a scholarly discipline, there will be increasing interest in delineating the theory base for nursing. Some believe that theory development is the most crucial task facing nursing.

There are three reasons for this interest in theory. First, as seen in Chapter 6, one criterion for professions is a distinct body of knowledge upon which practice is based. There has long been interest in identifying a body of nursing knowledge that is essential to professional nursing practice. Theory development contributes to knowledge building and is seen as a means of establishing nursing as a profession.

Second, commitment to practice based on sound, reliable knowledge is intrinsically valuable to nursing. That is to say, by its nature, knowledge is desirable. The growth and enrichment of theory in and of itself is an important goal for nursing, as a scholarly discipline, to pursue.

Third, theory is useful. Nursing practice settings are complex, and the amount of data available to nurses is virtually endless. Nurses must analyze a tremendous amount of information about each patient and decide what to do. If a theory helps practicing nurses categorize and understand what is going on in nursing practice, if it helps them predict patients' responses to nursing care, and if it is helpful in clinical decision making, it is useful as a guide to practice.

This chapter defines and differentiates among various terms used in discussing theory, examines several theories that have implications for nursing practice, and briefly reviews several theoretical nursing models.

WHAT IS THEORY?

Theories are general explanations used to explain, predict, control, and understand commonly occurring events. Theories provide a method of classifying and organizing data in a logical, meaningful manner.

Perhaps the best-known theory is Einstein's theory of relativity, which states that "matter and energy are equivalent and form the basis for nuclear energy and that space and time are relative rather than absolute concepts" (Flexner, 1980, p. 743). Although this theory may not be especially meaningful to non-physicists, it is clear that it is a logically connected group of general statements used as principles of explanation for a class of events. That is a good working definition of theory.

It is important to remember that a theory is an explanation that has not yet been disproved. Until disproved, it may be useful. When more knowledge becomes available, theories that are no longer useful are discarded, and new ones are generated.

Theories are best understood as preliminary explanations that reflect the current understanding of events. For the purposes of this chapter, **theory** is defined as a set of propositions or concepts used to describe, explain, predict, and control phenomena.

Useful Definitions

Several other terms and descriptions are useful in discussing our definition of theory:

- **Set.** A group of circumstances, situations, and so on, joined and treated as a whole. In mathematics, for example, negative numbers are treated as a set.
- **Propositions.** Statements about how two or more concepts are related. For example, "Heart rate increases as anxiety increases" is a proposition.

- **Concepts.** Abstract classification of data. For example, "temperature" is a concept.
- **Describe.** To tell about in detail.
- **Explain.** To offer reasons for.
- **Predict.** To foretell.
- **Control.** To exercise a regulating influence over.
- **Phenomena.** Occurrences or incidents; events. (Singular form is **phenomenon.**)

Four Functions of Theory

Each of the four functions of theory—description, explanation, prediction, and control—represents a different phase of theory development. The perfect theory would do all four things well. No perfect theories, however, exist in any discipline. Because science is evolving and because humans are fallible, that is, liable to make mistakes, theories are always changing. At any given point in time in a given area of study, theories in all stages of development can be found. This is certainly true in nursing, as seen later in this chapter.

Some theories are specifically designed as explanations, without having any intention of predicting. An example is the theory of evolution. Other theories are designed to predict but do not provide control. For example, plate tectonic theory may someday contribute to the ability of geologists to predict earthquakes, but it is doubtful that humans can ever control them. The world of theory building is an imperfect but dynamic one, always in a state of evolution to higher levels of scientific thought.

Conceptual Frameworks and Models

People often use the terms *theory* and *conceptual framework* interchangeably. The term *model* may be used in the same discussion. This imprecise usage of terms results in a state of confusion in which terms have little meaning. Nurses need a clear understanding of these terms to participate effectively in theory building.

CONCEPTUAL FRAMEWORKS

Conceptual frameworks and theories overlap somewhat because both use concepts as major developmental components (Polit and Hungler, 1991). Fawcett (1984) defined a conceptual framework as "a set of concepts and those assumptions that integrate them into a meaningful configuration" (p. 2). A conceptual framework is not a theory. A conceptual framework is a less formal and somewhat more abstract explanatory framework than a theory. It is the degree of formality and abstractness that differentiates between theories and conceptual frameworks (Fawcett, 1984).

MODELS

Model is a third term that frequently appears in nursing literature. A key idea in understanding models is that they are not the real thing but attempt to make concrete the concepts they represent. A model replicates reality with various degrees of precision. The symbolic form of a model may consist of words, mathematical notations, or physical material, as in a model airplane. Models use a minimal amount of language. They are useful in understanding concepts that cannot be directly observed or visualized. A visit to a planetarium, for example, allows one to gain an understanding of the universe, a phenomenon so vast that it is otherwise difficult to grasp. In theory building, theories are often graphically represented by means of models.

NONNURSING THEORIES USEFUL IN NURSING PRACTICE

The contributions of many theorists outside of nursing formed the knowledge base for nursing practice for many years. New disciplines are often slow to develop their own theories, and nursing was no exception. Even now, theories from the physical, biological, social, and behavioral sciences, in addition to more recent nursing models and theories, are used extensively in nursing practice.

Nurses use theories developed outside of nursing to understand, explain, and intervene in relationships between people. They also use these theories to understand, explain, and predict changes in health and the environment. Adaptation, systems, stress, developmental, role, human motivation, and communication theories are all heavily used in nursing.

Several nonnursing theories used by nurses are covered elsewhere in this textbook: Systems theory is discussed in some detail in Chapter 10; Selye's (1976) stress theory is covered in Chapter 17; communication theory is discussed in Chapter 18; and theories of moral development are explored in Chapter 19. Even though they are not nursing theories, these theories are all relevant and useful in nursing practice. Additional nonnursing theories that nurses use extensively are adaptation theories and developmental theories. These are discussed to show how nonnursing theories enhance nursing practice.

Adaptation Theories

Adaptation theories are based on systems theory and view change in terms of cause and effect. People have to adjust to changes every day. Adaptation theories provide ways to understand how balance is maintained in the face of change and the possible effects of disturbed equilibrium. Adaptation theories have been widely used to explain, predict, and control biological responses of people.

In adaptation theory, the human body is seen as functioning as a whole. All body cells are affected by the activities of other cells. This communication is made possible because all cells are surrounded by the same fluids (e.g., blood, lymph, and interstitial fluid), which form an internal environment for the entire body. The internal environment provides a medium for the exchange of nutrients and wastes, and it provides a stable physiochemical environment for cell function.

Normal cells require that constancy of the body's internal environment be maintained within relatively narrow limits. These limits must be maintained even though the body is constantly responding to interactions between internal and external environments. Stability of the internal environment is maintained through feedback mechanisms. As changes occur in the internal environment, regulatory systems, such as the nervous system and the endocrine system, respond to keep the change within limits the body can tolerate. The word *homeostasis* was originally used by Cannon (1929) to describe a state of relative constancy of the body's internal environment because of the action of regulatory mechanisms. Constancy does not imply that the internal environment is static. It is constantly changing, but *relative* equilibrium is maintained. For example, when blood sugar drops, the endocrine system responds by secreting cortisone, which both decreases the rate at which cells use glucose and stimulates the conversion of amino acids into glucose. These compensatory actions cause blood sugar to rise. If blood sugar rises above acceptable limits, the endocrine system again responds by increasing insulin secretion, which increases the rate of glucose uptake by cells. These compensatory actions cause the blood glucose level to fall. In both situations, homeostasis is maintained.

STRESSORS

In adaptation theories, stimuli that tend to disturb equilibrium are called **stressors.** Stressors are factors that create change in the external or internal environments, thus placing demands on the body to compensate. Potential external stressors include such things as environmental temperature and noise level. Internal stressors include such factors as hunger, joy, and infection. Stressors may be beneficial or harmful, but they all require the body to respond. The response of the body is called adaptation. As mentioned in Chapter 10, the ability to adapt effectively to changes in life events is believed to be a major factor in determining a person's potential for health or disease (Holmes and Rahe, 1967).

COPING

One way that a person adapts is by means of **coping mechanisms.** Coping mechanisms are psychological devices a person uses when threat is perceived. A person's reaction to stress, therefore, occurs on two levels: (1) the cognitive level, at which appraisal of the stress occurs and resulting psychological coping methods are begun, and (2) the physiological level, at which compensatory reactions occur.

USING ADAPTATION THEORIES IN NURSING PRACTICE

Adaptation theories are useful in nursing practice because they allow nurses to assess patients' stressors and abilities to cope. Illness is stressful, as is being hospitalized or otherwise unable to meet one's usual responsibilities. Not all people react the same way to these stressors. Nurses familiar with adaptation theories can help patients realistically appraise their stressors, examine their usual coping responses, and, if necessary, learn new ones. If a patient is newly diagnosed with a chronic health problem, such as diabetes, nurses using adaptation theories help patients learn to anticipate and cope with the stress of life changes created by the disease.

Adaptation theories are also useful to nurses working in the area of health promotion. Predicting and eliminating stressors and strengthening coping abilities are valuable steps in promoting health.

Developmental Theories

Developmental theories, sometimes called theories of growth and development, assume that human growth is linear, has predictable irreversible direction, occurs in degrees (stages), and progresses toward maximum potential (Chin, 1980). Nurses use developmental theories in planning future-oriented nursing interventions because knowing developmental theories makes it possible for nurses to describe and predict patient behavior.

GROWTH

In developmental theory, **growth** is defined as an increase in physical size and shape to a point of optimal maturity (Billingham, 1982, p. 4). Because no change occurs in isolation, each modifies the individual as a whole. Thus, assessment of maturation requires data about all aspects of the individual—physical, intellectual, psychological, spiritual, and social.

Growth is continuous and orderly, with regular trends in direction. For example, the direction of motor growth proceeds from the head to the extremities and from the central part of the body toward the periphery. As a result, a child sits before standing and can control shoulder movements before those of the fingers. Although growth is patterned and continuous, it is not always smooth and gradual. Different aspects of a person develop at different rates. Adolescents, for example, sometimes experience pain in the long bones of their legs when growth spurts occur. This results when leg muscles do not develop as rapidly as the bones grow.

DEVELOPMENT

Although growth is quantitative, development is related to functional changes that are usually qualitative. As with growth, multiple factors influence development, and authorities have differing opinions about the relative importance of maturational versus environmental influences on development. All aspects of human development are interrelated and integrated. Because development proceeds in a sequential pattern, realistic expectations for behavior can be predicted for various stages of development.

There are a number of theories about how development occurs. The classic approach is called **stage theory.** This theory proposes that all people pass through a number of levels (stages). The stages differ in quality and duration, but the order is fixed, and a person cannot skip a stage or reorder the stages. Mastering the tasks of one stage forms the basis for mastering the tasks of the next. Individuals differ in the speed with which they move through these stages and in the level of development that they finally reach.

Various developmental or stage theorists, such as Erikson, Kohlberg, and Piaget, have described particular aspects of human development. Erikson described the stages of human development from birth to death, including the developmental "tasks" that must be accomplished at each stage. Kohlberg explored the stages of moral development. Piaget (1969) delineated the cognitive (intellectual) stages of development.

USING DEVELOPMENTAL THEORIES IN NURSING PRACTICE

The value of developmental theories in nursing practice is undeniable. They are particularly useful in assessing whether a child's growth pattern and developmental stage are keeping pace with his or her chronological age. There are broad ranges of "normal" growth and development, but when children fall outside of these ranges, medical and nursing interventions are often required.

Growth and development theories are also useful to nurses teaching parents about what to expect from their children at certain ages and stages. Sometimes parents expect young children to have abilities beyond their level of maturation; for example, they may become frustrated when their 9-month-old is not toilet trained. Using developmental theories, nurses can explain that children do not have sufficient control of the muscles involved in toilet training until 2 years or even older. If the mother of a 5-year-old child is concerned that the child tells "lies," it is helpful for the nurse to explain that a child of this age often has difficulty separating fact from fantasy and is not simply being "bad."

When studying developmental theories, nurses should remember that although knowing characteristic traits, developmental tasks, and stages is useful, each individual is unique in style and behavior.

MODELS OF NURSING THEORY

Until the 1950s, nursing knowledge was principally derived from social, biological, and medical theories. With recognition of the importance that theory plays in developing a scientific discipline, and awareness that theories in other disciplines were insufficient to describe nursing, nurses began to develop their own theories. With the exception of the work of Florence Nightingale (1859), who was ahead of her time, nursing theory began with the publication of Hildegarde Peplau's *Interpersonal Relations in Nursing* (1952). Peplau was the first to describe the phases of the nurse-patient relationship and the factors that influence that relationship.

As the number of doctorally prepared nurses increased, interest in developing nursing knowledge flourished. In addition to developing nursing philosophies

TABLE 11–1
Historical Development of Nursing Theory

Year	Theorist	Name of Model or Theory
1859	Florence Nightingale	Sometimes referred to as Environmental Model; writings explored the nature of nursing
1966	Virginia Henderson	Need-Based Model; defined nursing; identified 14 basic patient needs
1970	Martha Rogers	The Science of Unitary Human Beings
1971	Dorothea Orem	Self-Care Deficit Theory of Nursing
1972	Betty Neuman	Systems Model of Nursing
1976	Sr. Callista Roy	Adaptation Model of Nursing
1978	Madeleine Leininger	Cultural Care Theory
1979	Jean Watson	Theory of Caring
1982	Nola Pender	Health Promotion Model

Data from Marriner-Tomey, A. (1994). *Nursing theorists and their work* (3rd ed.). St. Louis: Mosby.

and conceptual models and applying theories of other disciplines, nurse theorists have created two types of theories: those that broadly define nursing and those that are grounded in nursing practice.

Descriptions of nursing and nursing models evolved from the personal, professional, and educational experiences of nurse theorists and reflect their perception of "ideal" nursing practice. Most theoretical models in nursing are based on the major concepts basic to nursing discussed in Chapter 10. They describe the nature of nursing, the individual recipient of care (patient), the context of nurse-patient interactions (environment), and health (Fawcett, 1984). As can be seen in Table 11–1, a number of nursing scholars have been thinking and writing about nursing knowledge in the second half of the twentieth century. This section presents an overview of selected nursing models.

Nightingale's Environmental Model

Nightingale conceptualized disease as a reparative process and described the nurse's role as manipulating the environment to facilitate this process. Her ideas about ventilation, warmth, light, diet, cleanliness, variety, and noise are presented in her classic nursing textbook *Notes on Nursing* (1859). Nightingale's intent was to describe nursing and provide guidelines for nursing practice and education. She defined nursing as a service to people and viewed a healthful environment as critically important.

MAJOR CONCEPTS AS DEFINED BY NIGHTINGALE

- Patient. Individuals; responsible, creative, in control of their lives and health, and desiring good health.
- Health. A state of being well; using one's powers to the fullest.

- Illness. The reaction of nature against the conditions in which we have placed ourselves. Disease is a reparative mechanism, an effort of nature to remedy a process of decay.
- Environment. External to the person, but affecting the health of both sick and well persons. The environment, one of the chief sources of infection, must include fresh air, fresh water, efficient drainage, cleanliness, and light.
- Nursing. A service to people intended to relieve pain and suffering. The goal of nursing is to promote the reparative process by manipulating the environment.

Henderson's Need-Based Model

Virginia Henderson viewed nursing as an art and a discipline separate from medicine. As discussed in Chapter 7, she believed that the "unique function of the nurse . . . is to assist the individual, sick or well in the performance of those activities contributing to health or its recovery (or a peaceful death) that he would perform unaided if he had the necessary strength, will or knowledge" (Henderson, 1966, p. 15).

Henderson viewed the nurse's role as that of a substitute for the patient, a helper to the patient, and a partner with the patient. She listed 14 basic needs that nurses should assist patients with if patients are unable to perform them unaided. These basic needs compose Henderson's components of nursing care. Box 11–1 contains Henderson's 14 basic needs of patients.

BOX 11–1
Henderson's Fourteen Basic Needs of the Patient

1. Breathe normally.
2. Eat and drink adequately.
3. Eliminate body wastes.
4. Move and maintain desirable position.
5. Sleep and rest.
6. Select suitable clothes—dress and undress.
7. Maintain body temperature within normal range by adjusting clothing and modifying the environment.
8. Keep the body clean and well groomed and protect the integument (skin).
9. Avoid dangers in the environment and avoid injuring others.
10. Communicate with others in expressing emotions, needs, fears, or opinions.
11. Worship according to one's faith.
12. Work in such a way that there is a sense of accomplishment.
13. Play or participate in various forms of recreation.
14. Learn, discover, or satisfy the curiosity that leads to normal development and health and use the available health facilities.

(Reprinted with permission of Henderson, V. (1966). *The nature of nursing: A definition and its implications for practice, research, and education.* New York: Macmillan.)

MAJOR CONCEPTS AS DEFINED BY HENDERSON

- Patient. Individual; requires assistance to achieve health and independence or a peaceful death. Individuals achieve or maintain health if they have the necessary strength, will, or knowledge. The individual and family are viewed as a unit.
- Health. A quality of life basic to human functioning. Equated with independence.
- Illness. A lack of independence.
- Environment. All external conditions and influences that affect life and development.
- Nursing. A unique function of assisting sick or well individuals in a complementary role. The goal of nursing is to help the individual gain independence as rapidly as possible.

Orem's Self-Care Model

Dorothea Orem first published her concepts of nursing in 1959, refining them in 1980 and 1985 (Orem, 1980, 1985). Originally, she designed her model for nursing school curricula to help students differentiate among nursing actions. This model focuses on identifying the patient's self-care needs and nursing actions designed to meet the patient's needs.

Today, Orem's **self-care model** is widely used in nursing education and practice. It is useful for comprehensive assessment and analysis of individuals. The model is useful for nurses working with chronically ill patients in the hospital or in other settings. It can also be used in health maintenance and illness prevention: primary, secondary, and tertiary.

MAJOR CONCEPTS AS DEFINED BY OREM

- Patient. Individual unable to maintain self-care continuously in sustaining life and health, in recovering from disease or injury, or in coping with their effects.
- Health. Ability to meet self-care demands that contribute to the maintenance and promotion of structural integrity, functioning, and development.
- Illness. Occurs when an individual is incapable of maintaining self-care as a result of health-related limitations.
- Environment. Any setting in which a patient has unmet self-care needs.
- Nursing. A service of deliberately selected and performed actions to assist individuals to maintain self-care, including structural integrity, functioning, and development.

Roy's Adaptation Model

Sister Callista Roy has continuously expanded her model from its inception in 1970 to the present (Roy, 1970). Roy's **adaptation model** is based on general systems theory. She focused on the individual as a biopsychosocial adaptive system and described nursing as a humanistic discipline that "places emphasis on the person's own coping abilities" (Roy, 1984, p. 32). According to Roy, the individual and the environment are sources of stimuli that require modification to promote adaptation. When the demands of environmental stimuli are too great or the person's adaptive mechanisms are too low, the person's behavioral responses are ineffective for coping. Effective adaptive responses promote the integrity of the individual by conserving energy and promoting the survival, growth, reproduction, and mastery of the human system.

MAJOR CONCEPTS AS DEFINED BY ROY

- Patient. Person or family with unusual stressors or ineffective coping mechanisms.
- Health. State and process of being and becoming integrated and whole.
- Illness. A lack of integration.
- Environment. All conditions, circumstances, and influences surrounding and affecting the development and behavior of persons or families.
- Nursing. Promotion of the patient's effective coping and progress toward integration.

Rogers's Model: Science of Unitary Human Beings

Martha Rogers first described her **science of unitary human beings** in 1970 (Rogers, 1970). She sought to develop a science unique to nursing and a basis for nursing practice, believing that without this body of knowledge, there was no need for higher education in nursing (Rogers, 1991, personal communication). Rogers defined *nursing* as a noun—a body of knowledge necessary for practice. She called this organized body of abstract knowledge *nursing science* and considered the imaginative and creative use of knowledge in practice as *art*. As both science and art, nursing is described as a learned profession that focuses on the nature and direction of human development and human betterment. Rogers viewed the interaction between humans and their environments as the central focus of nursing. Box 11–2 provides observations of a Rogerian practitioner.

MAJOR CONCEPTS AS DEFINED BY ROGERS

- Patient. "Unitary human being"; human field; an irreducible, pan-dimensional energy field identified by pattern and manifesting characteristics that are specific to the whole and that cannot be predicted from knowledge of the parts.
- Health.* Occurs when patterns of living are in harmony with environmental change.
- Illness.* Occurs when patterns of living conflict with environmental change and are deemed unacceptable.

*Rogers viewed the terms *health* and *illness* as value-laden, arbitrarily defined, and culturally infused. She saw them not as opposites but as part of the same continuum.

BOX 11–2
Using Nursing Science in Practice:
Observations of a Rogerian Practitioner

In this abstract system [the Rogerian model], the key is always listening to clients and allowing exploration of whatever they bring. Modalities I use to assist people in the discovery process and in creating change include therapeutic touch, imagery, hypnosis, poetry, music, humor, bibliotherapy, and journaling.

Therapeutic touch is based on the therapeutic use of hands, a human function that goes back to depictions in cave paintings calculated to be more than 15,000 years old. The basic skill in therapeutic touch is centering, a process of finely focusing one's consciousness. The centered nurse is attuned to the client's patterning process and with the client can assist in identifying direction for creative change. The goal is to regain balance, or repatterning.

My practice includes working with undergraduate nursing students in the home health setting, directing the Therapeutic Touch and Centering Clinic at the Arizona State University College of Nursing, and private practice. Using Rogers's science of unitary human beings in practice is health promoting, fulfilling, and exciting—for the nurse as well as the client!

(Courtesy of Katherine E. Rapacz, Ph.D., R.N., Arizona State University, 1992.)

- Environment. Environmental field; an irreducible, pan-dimensional energy field identified by pattern and integral with the human field.
- Nursing. A learned profession; a science and an art. The science of nursing is an organized body of abstract knowledge; a synthesis of facts and ideas. The art of nursing refers to the use of this knowledge in the delivery of nursing care for human betterment.

Neuman's Health Care Systems Model

Betty Neuman developed a **systems model** in response to student requests. They expressed a need to focus on breadth rather than depth in understanding human variables in nursing problems. First published in 1972, this model was refined and published in its present form in *The Neuman Systems Model* in 1989 (Neuman, 1989). This is a complex systems model, with a focus on stress reactions and stress reduction. This comprehensive model depicts the patient as the core of a circle with several protective layers. The patient is continuously exposed to internal and external stressors, which require lines of defense and reactions. Nursing interventions can occur before or after stressors and at three levels of prevention.

Neuman's model is applicable to all phases of the nursing process. It can be applied across all clinical areas and is especially useful for individuals and families. It is a holistic approach because each system or subsystem cannot be isolated; rather, the influence of each system on the whole must be considered. The three levels of prevention are useful guides for planning nursing interventions.

MAJOR CONCEPTS AS DEFINED BY NEUMAN

- Patient. Open system seeking balance and harmony. Composite of physiological, psychological, sociocultural, and developmental variables and viewed as a whole. Individuals, families, and communities.
- Health. Dynamic equilibrium of the normal line of defense.
- Illness. Caused by reaction to stressors with lines of resistance.
- Environment. Internal and external stressors and resistance factors.
- Nursing. Reduction of stressors through prevention activities at three levels.

Leininger's Cultural Care Theory

Madeleine Leininger's interest in cultural aspects of nursing grew out of her professional experiences in a child guidance home in the mid-1950s, where she observed that children of different cultures had widely varying behaviors and needs (Marriner-Tomey, 1994). She discussed the parallels between nursing and anthropology with the famed anthropologist Margaret Mead and decided to pursue doctoral study in cultural and psychological anthropology. Through her doctoral work, she became convinced that cultural differences were directly related to health beliefs and health practices, which led her to begin work on her **theory of cultural care** in nursing.

Transcultural nursing's goal involves more than simply being aware of different cultures. It involves planning nursing care that is "culturally defined, classified, and tested as a guide to provide nursing care" (Leininger, 1978, p. 12). Because of the increasingly diverse and multicultural world in which we live, many people believe that transcultural nursing knowledge is essential to guide nurses as they care for people of various cultures.

Leininger sees theory as a "systematic and creative way of discovering knowledge about something, or to account for some phenomenon that is understood in a limited way" (Marriner-Tomey, 1994, p. 427). She encourages nurses to discover creatively the cultural aspects of human needs and use them to make culturally congruent therapeutic decisions. Her theory is broadly holistic, taking into account all aspects of human life.

MAJOR CONCEPTS AS DEFINED BY LEININGER

- Patient. Individuals, families, groups, communities, and institutions in diverse health systems. They possess culturally determined world views (Leininger, 1991).
- Health. Culturally defined; varies from culture to culture. By studying care, beliefs, values, and practices, nurses can discover health in patients.
- Illness. Culturally defined; varies from culture to culture. Some cultures view illness as a personal experience (due to factors inside the person) and some view it as a cultural experience (due to factors outside the person).
- Environment. Political, religious, educational, technological, economic, kinship, values, beliefs, and lifeways of a given cultural group (Leininger, 1991).

- Nursing. Learned humanistic art and science that promotes and maintains health behaviors and recovery from illness taking into account physical, psychocultural, and social significance and meanings. The essence of nursing is caring.

Watson's Theory of Human Caring

Jean Watson has a background in psychiatric–mental health nursing. She began writing about her **theory of human caring** as she developed a graduate course at the University of Colorado Health Sciences Center, where she has been both a faculty member and administrator. She was instrumental in establishing the Center for Human Caring at the University of Colorado. It is the first interdisciplinary center in the United States with a goal of developing and using knowledge about human caring and healing as the basis of nursing practice and scholarship. The ultimate goal is to transform the health care system to one with a greater emphasis on human dignity and humanity (Marriner-Tomey, 1994).

Watson's theory is based on 10 factors she calls "carative" factors. She used the term *carative* as opposed to *curative* to help differentiate nursing from medicine. Watson's 10 carative factors are found in Box 11–3.

MAJOR CONCEPTS AS DEFINED BY WATSON

- Patient. Unique individuals with biophysical, psychophysical, psychosocial, and intrapersonal needs.

B O X　1 1 – 3
Watson's Ten Primary Carative Factors

1. The formation of a humanistic-altruistic system of values.
2. The instillation of faith-hope.
3. The cultivation of sensitivity to one's self and others.
4. The development of a helping-trust relationship.
5. The promotion and acceptance of the expression of positive and negative feelings.
6. The systematic use of the scientific problem-solving method for decision making.
7. The promotion of interpersonal teaching-learning.
8. The provision for a supportive, protective, and/or corrective mental, physical, sociocultural, and spiritual environment.
9. Assistance with the gratification of human needs.
10. The allowance for existential-phenomenological forces.

(Reprinted with permission of Marriner-Tomey, A. (1994). *Nursing theorists and their work* (pp. 151–153). St. Louis: Mosby.)

- Health. A "unity and harmony within the mind, body, and soul" that is associated with the "degree of congruence between the self as perceived and the self as experienced" (Watson, 1988, p. 48). Health is the responsibility of the client.
- Illness. Lack of harmony within the mind, body, and soul created by internal or external environments (or both).
- Environment. Internal environment includes mental and spiritual well-being and sociocultural beliefs. External environment includes epidemiological variables, comfort, privacy, safety, and clean, aesthetic surroundings (Watson, 1979).
- Nursing. A caring science based on human values and concern for the welfare of others. "Nursing is interested in understanding health, illness and the human experience . . . [and is] an interrelationship of quality of life, including death, as well as the prolongation of life" (Marriner-Tomey, 1994, p. 154). Nursing is concerned with health promotion, health restoration, and illness prevention.

Pender's Health Promotion Model

Nola Pender developed an interest in nursing as a child when her aunt was hospitalized. Later, during her doctoral study, she identified a gap between the capacity for prevention, early detection of illness, and use of available services and the rate at which people actually used these services. She began to explore what others had written about behavior and behavioral change and was influenced by the work of Bandura and Fishbein (Marriner-Tomey, 1994).

Pender's work is known as the **health promotion model** of nursing. She believes that such habits as smoking, substance abuse, overeating, and sedentary lifestyles produce chronic illnesses that can be prevented. Further, that improvement in the health status of people will come about only through aggressive prevention and health promotion efforts. In tandem with her economist husband, she also addresses the problems of shrinking finances in today's health care system.

Pender stresses the importance of appraising health risks of healthy people and instituting a protective plan of care. Her philosophy emphasizes personal control, freedom, and a feeling of well-being that are the rewards of good health (Pender, Barkauskas, Hayman, Rice, and Anderson, 1992).

MAJOR CONCEPTS AS DEFINED BY PENDER

- Patient. Individuals with personality traits and beliefs, culturally determined, that influence their choices of behavior and lifestyle. Each person has a basic drive toward health.
- Health. A positive, high-level state. Different with each patient and therefore must be carefully assessed. The absence of disease to some; illness prevention and a feeling of wellness to others.
- Illness. A state of feeling ill, influenced by each individual's patterns of cognitive-perceptual and modifying factors.

- Environment. Personal, interpersonal, and situational factors that influence health behavior, including patients' perceptions about the importance of health, assessment of their own vulnerability to disease, belief in the value of early detection, perception of the seriousness of a potential health problem, assessment of the efficacy of possible actions, and level of internal or external control (Pender, 1982).
- Nursing. A research-based discipline with the capacity to influence individuals' health-promoting behaviors through interaction, motivation, and education. Nursing has a role in delivering health-promotion services to people across the life span.

Ongoing Model Development

Each of these nurse theorists as well as a number of others has made significant contributions to the development of nursing's unique body of knowledge. Offering an assortment of perspectives, models of nursing theory vary in their level of abstraction and their conceptualization of the patient, health, illness, environment, and nursing. To describe any of the existing nursing models as a "theory" may be going too far. As in other disciplines, models of nursing theory are found at various stages of development, but no comprehensive theory is yet in existence. Some nurse theorists continue to develop and refine their models, whereas others are deceased or no longer actively work on theory development. Each theoretical model has followers who continue to expand, clarify, and refine the original work.

In the future, nursing models must clearly differentiate activities that are unique to nursing and different from other disciplines. Nursing must distinguish a separate body of knowledge or a distinct manner of applying shared knowledge. Future nursing theorists will strive to describe, explain, predict, and control patient outcomes. Theories facilitate the prevention of illness and the maintenance, promotion, and restoration of the patient's optimum health potential.

RELATIONSHIP OF THEORY TO NURSING PRACTICE AND RESEARCH

Nurses have traditionally based their practices on intuition, experience, or "the way I was taught." These methods lead to unimaginative, rote, and stereotypical practice. To move nursing practice forward and to improve the quality of nursing care, theory development and research were undertaken.

Theory-Based Practice

How is theory translated into practice? The answer to that question lies with theory-based practice. Theory-based practice enables nurses to challenge conventional views of patients, the health-illness continuum, and traditional nursing interventions. Theory-based practice encourages hypothesis formation, testing of hypotheses, drawing conclusions about nursing actions, and evaluating nursing actions.

Nurses who engage in theory-based practice must feed their findings back to nurse theorists and nurse researchers for theory, research, and practice to continue to energize each other and to advance the science of nursing.

Research

Nursing research is conducted to test and refine nursing's developing scientific base. Research is the best means to test and validate the usefulness of knowledge necessary for nursing practice. Ultimately, research will enable nurses to predict reliably how nursing actions influence patient outcomes. Research is the future

RESEARCH NOTE

Even though breast cancer is the leading cause of cancer mortality in African-American women, fewer than half of these women who are older than 50 years report ever having had mammograms and breast examinations. Two-thirds report not practicing regular breast self-examination. Puzzled by these findings, Brown and Williams used Leininger's Culture Care Theory and the Health Belief Model to explore factors that prevented these women from using screening services.

According to Leininger's work, African-Americans value extended family networks, religious values, interdependence with other African-Americans, daily survival, folk foods, and folk-healing modes. The five variables of the Health Belief Model are susceptibility, seriousness, benefits, barriers, and health motivation.

After an extensive literature review, they determined that some barriers to breast screening programs experienced by older African-American women were unique to their culture, whereas others were shared with all older women. Some barriers they identified that were unique to the African-American culture included heightened fear of cancer, underestimating its incidence, pessimism about cure, lack of awareness of screening tests, and use of a lay referral system that may delay treatment. In common with other older women, they attributed breast changes to age; were embarrassed; lacked knowledge about mammograms and breast self-examination; and believed that screening programs were too much trouble, inconvenient, or unnecessary. In addition, African-American individuals thought that health care providers were insensitive to their cultural and social needs.

Several practice implications were identified as a result of this literature review. Nurses can

- Encourage the use of screening methods daily in their interactions with older African-American women.
- Reduce costs by planning reduced-cost services.
- Increase the availability and accessibility of screening programs by using mobile units and community sites during evening and weekend hours.
- Plan and implement breast health educational programs using culturally sensitive materials.
- Work with African-American community leaders to promote breast cancer screening.

(Adapted with permission of Brown, L. W., and Williams, R. D. (1994). Culturally sensitive breast cancer screening programs for older Black women. Reproduced/adapted with permission from the March, 1994 issue of *The Nurse Practitioner*, © Springhouse Corporation.)

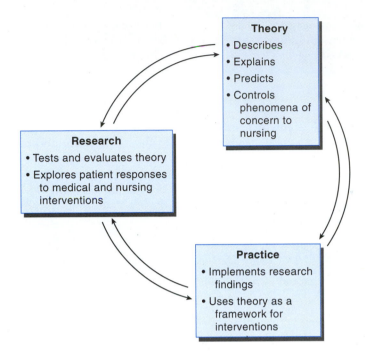

FIGURE 11–1
The interrelatedness of nursing theory, research, and practice.

of nursing. Chapter 12 is devoted to understanding the research process. For an example of how nurses use theory as a framework for research, refer to the accompanying Research Note.

It is important for nurses to understand that theory, nursing practice, and research are interrelated. Each stimulates, improves, and advances the others. Figure 11–1 illustrates the circularity of theory, research, and practice in nursing.

How Nurses Can Participate in Theory Development

Theory development is not a mysterious activity, and it is not restricted to a few nursing scholars. To the extent that nurses continue to think, read, study, and develop nursing practice, they are *all* scholars of nursing.

Many nurses have developed their ideas about nursing and continue to develop nursing assumptions based on experience, observation, and reading. Most nurses do not talk explicitly about their personal theories, although these theories probably influence the way these individuals practice nursing. Personal theories, however, tend to be incomplete or inconsistent. Therefore, using personal theory as a basis for practice is probably ineffective.

Public, systematic development of nursing theory is necessary to advance nursing. Nurses who devise theories of nursing must present them for public review by nursing colleagues, thus engaging in the **peer review process** essential to advancing theory development.

Theory building involves discovery and creativity. The aspiring theorist who approaches theory construction in a mechanical way through structured procedures has limited success. Although it is possible to teach specific theory-building techniques, how to facilitate creativity and originality is unknown. It has been said, "You can teach someone how to look, but not how to see; how to search, but not how to find" (Rosenberg, 1978, p. 2). A sense of imagination, playfulness, and participation is essential not only for theorists, but also for readers who seek to understand theories.

In addition to imagination, developing and presenting theories require personal discipline. Novel ideas tend to occur in a vague, disconnected, and tenuous form (Mills, 1959). Self-discipline is required to work with the idea, develop it, and express it in written form for others to review.

Astute observations and clinical interventions of nurses in practice settings can advance progress toward a distinct knowledge base for nursing. Nursing theorists rely on practicing nurses to test the usefulness of theories. Such clinical investigations cannot take place without the widespread support of practicing nurses who recognize the importance of theory-based practice. Professional nurses must participate in research investigations whenever possible. Their insights and observations about patients and nursing care provide invaluable contributions to nursing theory.

SUMMARY

Theory improves nursing practice by describing, explaining, predicting, and controlling phenomena of interest to nurses. Nurses who have and use theoretical knowledge are more likely to be reliably effective than those using trial and error, intuition, or ritual. Nurses who base their practices on theory can justify their decisions and explain them to others. This facilitates the transmission of nursing knowledge to students and neophytes in the profession as well as to those outside the profession.

Theory allows professional autonomy by guiding the practice, education, and research functions of the profession. The study of theory helps develop analytical skills, challenges thinking, and clarifies values and assumptions.

Building a sound nursing knowledge base requires that nurses test theory in practice. Contributions of practicing nurses through their active participation in research are of significant value to the development of nursing theory.

When nursing develops its own theory, validates research knowledge in the practice setting, and relies on this knowledge to direct nursing practice, it will be recognized as an independent, autonomous profession. At that point, nursing will no longer rely on knowledge from other disciplines but will use its own knowledge base, called nursing science, to guide nursing practice.

REVIEW AND DISCUSSION QUESTIONS

1. Why is theory development important to the profession of nursing?
2. From the brief summaries given, do any of the nursing theoretical models

described in this chapter appeal to you? Do any evoke a negative response from you? Identify the attractive and unattractive features of each.
3. Recognizing that your understanding of nursing theories is preliminary, make some predictions about how nurses using each model might behave.
4. Interview nurses to determine what nonnursing and nursing theories and theoretical models they use. Ask how theory is useful in their practices.

REFERENCES

Billingham, K. (1982). *Developmental psychology for the health care professions.* Boulder: Westview Press.

Brown, L. W., and Williams, R. D. (1994). Culturally sensitive breast cancer screening programs for older Black women. *Nurse Practitioner,* 19(3), 21, 25–26, 31, 35.

Cannon, W. (1929). The sympathetic division of the autonomic system in relation to homeostasis. *Archives of Neurological Psychology,* 22, 282–294.

Chin, R. (1980). The utility of systems models and developmental models for practitioners. In J. Riehl and C. Roy (Eds.), *Conceptual models for nursing practice* (2nd ed.) (pp. 21–37). New York: Appleton-Century-Crofts.

Chinn, P., and Kramer, M. (1995). *Theory and nursing: A systematic approach* (4th ed.). St. Louis: Mosby.

Fawcett, J. (1984). *Analysis and evaluation of conceptual models of nursing.* Philadelphia: F. A. Davis.

Flexner, S. B. (Ed.). (1980). *The Random House dictionary.* New York: Random House.

Henderson, V. (1966). *The nature of nursing: A definition and its implications for practice, research, and education.* New York: Macmillan.

Holmes, T., and Rahe, R. (1967). The social readjustment rating scale. *Journal of Psychosomatic Research,* 11(2), 213–218.

Leininger, M. (1991). *Culture care diversity and universality: A theory of nursing.* New York: National League for Nursing Press.

Leininger, M. (1978). *Transcultural nursing: Concepts, theories, and practices.* New York: John Wiley & Sons.

Marriner-Tomey, A. (1994). *Nursing theorists and their work* (3rd ed.). St. Louis: Mosby.

Mills, C. (1959). On intellectual craftsmanship. In L. Gross (Ed.). *Symposium on sociological theory.* Evanston, IL: Row, Peterson.

Neuman, B. (1989). *The Neuman systems model: Application to nursing theory and practice.* Norwalk: Appleton-Century-Crofts.

Nightingale, F. (1969 facsimile of 1859 edition). *Notes on nursing: What it is and what it is not.* New York: Dover Publications.

Orem, D. (1985). *Nursing: Concepts of practice* (3rd ed.). New York: McGraw-Hill.

Orem, D. (1980). *Nursing: Concepts of practice* (2nd ed.). New York: McGraw-Hill.

Pender, N. J. (1982). *Health promotion in nursing practice.* Norwalk: Appleton-Century-Crofts.

Pender, N. J., Barkauskas, V. H., Hayman, L., Rice, V. H., and Anderson, E. T. (1992). Health promotion and disease prevention: Towards excellence in nursing practice and education. *Nursing Outlook,* 40, 106–112.

Peplau, H. (1952). *Interpersonal relations in nursing.* New York: G. P. Putnam's Sons.

Piaget, J. (1969). *The psychology of the child.* New York: Basic Books.

Polit, D., and Hungler, B. (1991). *Nursing research: Principles and methods* (4th ed.). Philadelphia: J. B. Lippincott.

Rogers, M. (1970). *An introduction to the theoretical basis of nursing.* Philadelphia: F. A. Davis.

Rosenberg, J. (1978). *The practice of philosophy.* Englewood Cliffs, NJ: Prentice-Hall.

Roy, Sr. C. (1984). *Introduction to nurs-*

ing: An adaptation model (2nd ed.). Englewood Cliffs, NJ: Prentice-Hall.

Roy, Sr. C. (1970). Adaptation: A conceptual framework for nursing. *Nursing Outlook*, 18, 254–257.

Selye, H. (1976). *The stress of life*. New York: McGraw-Hill.

Watson, J. (1988). *Nursing: Human science and human care*. New York: National League for Nursing.

Watson, J. (1979). *Nursing: The philosophy and science of caring*. Boston: Little, Brown.

CHAPTER

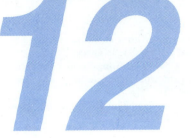

12

Carol T. Bush

Understanding the Scientific Method and Nursing Research

OBJECTIVES

- Differentiate between pure and applied science.
- Describe the historical development of the scientific method.
- Give examples of inductive and deductive reasoning.
- Discuss the limitations of the scientific method when applied to nursing.
- Differentiate between problem solving and research.
- List the steps in the research process.
- Discuss contributions nursing research has made to nursing practice and to health care.
- Describe the relationship of nursing research to nursing theory and practice.
- Identify sources of support for nursing research.
- Discuss the roles of nurses in research.

VOCABULARY

applied science	informed consent	pure science
conceptual framework	institutional review	qualitative research
confidentiality	board	quantitative research
data	Newton	reliable
deductive reasoning	nonexperimental design	replicate
disseminate	nursing research	research process
experimental design	peer review	research question
Galileo	phenomena	sample
generalizable	population	scientific method
hypothesis	problem solving	subjects
inductive reasoning	protocol	valid

In the 1960s, the nursing profession was poised on the threshold of a higher level of development. There was recognition that more mature professions had strong scientific bases, which were lacking in nursing. Nursing scholars realized that nursing could achieve its potential and desired professional status only to the extent that the discipline was based on a scientifically derived body of knowledge unique to nursing. As a result of that recognition, nursing researchers set about developing knowledge, and nursing theorists began developing theories and testing them.

About the same time, nurses realized that a similar professionalization of patient care practices was needed. Using traditional methods to deal with familiar patient problems and trial and error or intuition to deal with unfamiliar ones was no longer seen as an acceptable way to care for patients and move the profession toward science-based practice. Practitioners of nursing, therefore, also developed a more scientific approach to patient care that is an adaptation of the classic scientific method. This problem-solving approach is called the nursing process and is presented in more depth in Chapter 15. An understanding of the scientific method is helpful in appreciating both nursing research and the nursing process.

SCIENCE AND THE SCIENTIFIC METHOD

The study of any subject by using the scientific method or other methods of reasoning can be considered science. The **scientific method** is an orderly, systematic way of thinking about and solving problems. It has been used by scientists for centuries to discover and test facts and principles. When used under carefully planned and controlled conditions, the scientific method becomes research. The scientific method is the same, regardless of the discipline using it.

Pure and Applied Science and Research

Scientists divide scientific knowledge into two categories: pure and applied. **Pure science** or pure research, sometimes called basic science or basic research, summarizes and explains the universe without regard for whether the information is immediately useful. When Joseph Priestly discovered oxygen in 1774, he did not have an immediate use for that information. Therefore, that discovery could be classified as pure science, that is, information gathered solely for the sake of obtaining new knowledge. **Applied science** or applied research seeks to use scientific theory and laws in some practical way. The use of oxygen with premature infants is an example of applied science. The testing of this method to refine treatment guidelines is applied research. From this example, it can be seen that today's pure science can become tomorrow's applied science. Nursing makes use of applied scientific principles and is most effective in conducting applied research to improve nursing care.

History of the Scientific Method

Until the time of Hippocrates (ca. 460–377 B.C.), illness was believed to be caused by evil spirits. Gradually, over the years and through the efforts of many scientists, humankind has learned a great deal about the human body, health, and illness. Most of this knowledge was developed after the scientific method came into widespread use.

A period of great intellectual activity, known as the Age of Reason, began in the 1600s and lasted until the late 1700s. During that time, scientists made unparalleled advances in understanding the laws by which nature operates by using reason and experimentation. **Galileo** (1564–1642), the Italian physicist and astronomer, and Sir Isaac **Newton** (1642–1727), the English philosopher and mathematician, are usually credited with developing and refining the scientific method. A scientific revolution and technological explosion resulted from the use of the scientific method. In the area of health care alone, profound and far-reaching scientific discoveries have changed human life dramatically. Some important scientific discoveries related to health are listed in Box 12–1.

Inductive and Deductive Reasoning

The scientific method requires the use of two types of logic: inductive and deductive reasoning. In **inductive reasoning**, the process begins with a particular experience and proceeds to generalizations. Repeated observations of an experiment or event enable the observer to draw general conclusions. For example, the statement "All the St. Bernard dogs I have encountered are gentle; therefore, St. Bernards are gentle" is an example of inductive reasoning. It is obvious from this example that this type of logic leads to probabilities—not certainties—unless the world's entire population of St. Bernard dogs is observed.

Scientists also use **deductive reasoning,** a process through which conclusions are drawn by logical inference from given premises. It proceeds from the general case to the specific. For example, if the premises "All schoolchildren like chocolate" and "Missie is a schoolchild" are accepted, the conclusion, "Missie likes chocolate" can be drawn. It may be entirely possible, however, that Missie, although a schoolchild, does not like chocolate at all. In deductive reasoning, the premises used must be correct or the conclusions will not be. Conclusions drawn through deductive processes are called valid rather than true. **Valid** is a term meaning "soundly founded," whereas true means "in accordance with the fact or reality" (Flexner, Stein, and Su, 1980). It is possible for a conclusion to be solidly founded without its being true. There is a subtle but real difference in the two terms.

As seen by these examples, neither inductive nor deductive processes alone are adequate. If scientists used only deductive logic, experience would be ignored. If they used only inductive logic, relationships between facts and principles would be ignored. A combination of both types of reasoning processes in science unifies the theoretical and the practical, which is the basis for the scientific method and research.

Limitations of the Scientific Method in Nursing

Polit and Hungler (1995, p. 9) asserted that the scientific method is the "most sophisticated method of acquiring knowledge that humans have developed." Many authorities believe that using any other method is less than scientific and thus to be avoided. There are at least four reasons, however, why the scientific method has limitations when applied to nursing.

The first and most obvious drawback is that health care settings are not com-

BOX 12-1
Important Health-Related Events in the Evolution of Science

ca. 400 B.C.	Hippocrates taught that diseases have natural, not supernatural, causes.
A.D. 100	Galen laid the foundation for the study of anatomy and physiology.
ca. 1500	Leonardo da Vinci recognized the importance of observation and experimentation in learning.
1543	Andreas Vesalius published a book on human anatomy, based observation.
1628	William Harvey published his theory on the circulation of blood.
1774	Joseph Priestly discovered oxygen.
ca. 1796	Edward Jenner discovered a method of smallpox vaccination.
1839	Matthias Schleiden and Theodor Schwann developed the theory that all living things are composed of cells.
1866	Gregor Mendel demonstrated the laws of heredity.
ca. 1876	Louis Pasteur demonstrated that microorganisms cause fermentation and disease.
1882	Robert Koch isolated the bacterium that causes tuberculosis.
1895	Wilhelm K. Roentgen discovered x-rays.
1898	Marie and Pierre Curie isolated the element radium.
ca. 1900	Paul Ehrlich originated chemotherapy, the treatment of diseases with chemicals (drugs).
1928	Alexander Fleming discovered penicillin.
1953	Jonas Salk developed the first effective polio vaccine.
1957	Arthur Karnberg grew DNA (deoxyribonucleic acid), the basic chemical of genes, in a test tube.
1978	The world's first test tube baby was delivered.
1982	William DeVries implanted the world's first artificial heart.
1989	The first authorized use of genetic engineering involved injecting genetically altered cells into patients with malignant melanoma.
1992	A team of international scientists reported the discovery of the gene that causes fragile X syndrome, a common inherited form of mental retardation.

(Data from Kuhn, T. S. [1970]. The structure of scientific revolutions. In O. Neurath, [Ed.], *International encyclopedia of unified science* [2nd ed., vol 2]. Chicago: University of Chicago Press; and Ware, C. F., and Panikkar, K. M. [1966]. *The twentieth century: History of mankind, cultural and scientific development* [vol. 6]. New York: Harper & Row.

parable to laboratories. There are realities and priorities operating in health care settings that must take precedence over laboratory protocols. The safety and security of human patients are of the utmost importance and cannot be jeopardized.

Second, human beings are far more than collections of parts that can be dissected and subjected to examination or experimentation. A strength of nursing is that nurses view patients holistically, whereas the scientific method is based on dividing a problem into manageable problem statements, each of which can be tested. Because humans are complex organisms with interrelated parts and systems, the classic scientific method loses some of its usefulness.

A third limitation of the scientific method as the only approach to solving patient problems is the fact that it is so objective; it fails to take the meaning of patients' own experiences, that is, their subjective view of reality, into consideration. Nurses are keenly aware that patients' perceptions of their experiences, or subjective data, are just as important as objective data.

Finally, there are definite ethical implications involved in experimenting with humans that make reliance on the scientific method impractical. The rights of human subjects in research are paramount, as discussed elsewhere in this chapter.

NURSING RESEARCH BASED ON THE SCIENTIFIC METHOD

For many undergraduates their only exposure to research is in introductory psychology or sociology courses, in which they are subjects in a professor's research project. All they see of research are the boring forms they fill out or the nonsense syllables they memorize. This kind of orientation leads them to wonder what research could have to do with their ability to care for patients.

Before students of nursing write research off altogether, they should consider the value of a different kind of research—patient care research. Through patient care research, nurses "examine questions that nurses, patients, and families grapple with daily, attempting to find answers that make health care more efficient and effective, and that help patients cope with responses to illness and medical therapies" (Friends of the NINR 1995, pp. 7–8) (see News Note).

For example, nurses are often the key to life or death for low-birth-weight infants. What do nurses need to know to tip the balance in favor of life for those babies? A group of researchers at the University of Pennsylvania, led by nurse Barbara Medoff-Cooper (Medoff-Cooper and Ray, 1995), has considered this question. They are studying neonatal sucking behaviors. According to these researchers, "Effective sucking behaviors or feeding is not only a prerequisite for survival, but also implies that an infant has achieved the neurologic, behavioral, and physiologic maturity required for safe, effective oral feeding" (p. 195). Their finding that breast-feeding is easier and requires less energy expenditure by premature or sick infants than does bottle-feeding is important in their care. Then there is the question of pacifiers—are they useful or harmful? Known in the research literature as "nonnutritive sucking," pacifier usage for 5 minutes before feeding has been demonstrated to increase the time infants are awake. This knowledge provided the basis for nurses to experiment with giving pacifiers to infants who were being tube-fed. The use of the pacifier was found to help the tube-fed infants move more rapidly to normal oral feedings.

Another nurse researcher, Dr. Patricia Becker of the University of Wisconsin, has also studied low-birth-weight infants and the stress they experience during routine feeding, bathing, and intrusive procedures in neonatal intensive care units (NICUs). Her findings are expected to change NICU caregiving routines,

NEWS NOTE
"BEYOND TENDER LOVING CARE, NURSES ARE A FORCE IN RESEARCH"

The Florence Nightingales of the nation are busily adding a Louis Pasteur research component to their profession. And nursing's distinctly human, low-tech studies are bringing better and less costly medical care to millions of patients as well as helping relatives who care for them at home.

Since Congress established the National Center for Nursing Research over President Reagan's veto, federally financed studies by nurses have made important strides toward closing gaps in patient care that often lead to physical and emotional complications, prolonged hospital stays or failure to adapt to disease or its treatment.

. . . Nurse researchers at the University of Rochester found that when nurses or family members provided moral support for heart patients during their transfer out of the coronary care unit, fewer cardiovascular complications occurred and the patients stayed in the hospital an average of four days fewer than similar patients who weathered the transfer without added support.

A study by nurses at Ohio State University showed that several weeks of aerobic exercise before surgery and chemo-therapy for breast cancer speeded the patient's ability to return to normal activities.

. . . A recent analysis of 84 studies conducted by nurse researchers among a total of 4146 patients prompted Dr. Barbara S. Heater, associate professor of nursing at the University of Missouri in St. Louis, to conclude that "research-based nursing interventions can produce 28 percent better outcomes for 72 percent of patients" and save money by shortening hospital stays. . . .

. . . [N]urse researchers are carving out new territories in health promotion and disease prevention that have been all but ignored by physicians. Studies by nurses look, for example, at factors that help patients follow doctor's orders, to change their living habits after a heart attack, reasons many elderly patients fail to take influenza seriously, ways to help families cope with high cholesterol levels in children, and circumstances that keep women from following an exercise routine.

—Jane E. Brody. (Reprinted with permission of *The New York Times*, Tuesday, August 13, 1991. Copyright 1991 by the New York Times Company.)

thereby reducing complications and improving weight gain (Friends of the NINR, 1995). The sooner the infants gain weight, the sooner they can be discharged to their homes and families. From these examples, it is easily seen that studying newborn behavior yields a great deal of useful information that can improve nursing care and ultimately improve the health of infants.

Another example of nursing research that makes a difference is with geriatric patients. Some older persons lose strength in their lower extremities or lose their balance from time to time, leading to hip fractures and other injuries suffered during falls. Fractures can be set and hips surgically replaced, but it would be better if older people did not fall.

Elizabeth McNeely, a nurse who specializes in working with older persons, collaborated with researchers from other disciplines to study falls in elderly individuals. A group of older persons were taught "tai chi," a martial art form, to see if those who practiced tai chi would fall less often than others (McNeely, 1991, personal communication). The moves performed in tai chi exercises promote balance and strengthen muscles. When elderly people have better balance and are stronger, they are not as likely to fall, and they may avoid breaking bones. This study is expected to have an impact on the health of the elderly in the future.

Another example is provided by nurses who work with children. These nurse researchers use imagery to decrease the nausea and vomiting of children who are receiving cancer treatment. Imagery involves creating positive mental images that counteract unpleasant reality. It is sometimes used in stress reduction exercises. The nurse researchers design individual imagery programs for the children with whom they work. They make a tape with the child's favorite music in the background and talk the patient into relaxing while listening to the music. For children who have a favorite recording artist, the nurses play that artist's recordings and talk the children through a sequence of pleasant mental images. Children who have cancer respond in a positive way to music and images to which they can relate and thereby tolerate their treatments better.

This chapter describes some basic concepts of **nursing research.** The purpose is to introduce nursing research, demonstrate that nursing research has merit, and provide a beginning vocabulary for nursing research. The ultimate goal is for nurses to participate in the research process and apply research findings to clinical practice.

WHAT IS NURSING RESEARCH?

Nursing research is the systematic investigation of **phenomena** (events or circumstances) related to improving nursing care. When nurses have a question that they believe is necessary to answer to provide better care for patients, and they have the time, money, skill, and energy to study that question, they can do nursing research. Although it does not have to be a topic that others are interested in for it to be an appropriate research question, there is much to be gained from choosing research problems that are connected to work already done. This builds nursing knowledge in an orderly way.

Research problems should be pursued if they meet all three of the following tests:

1. There is a conceptual framework; that is, the researchers' ideas about the problem fit logically and dovetail with what is already known about the topic.
2. The proposed research project is based on related research findings published in professional journals or is networked with similar ongoing research in other settings.
3. The proposed research is carefully designed so that the results will be applicable in similar situations.

In addition to building nursing knowledge, studies that build on previous work are more likely to receive financial support. Research is expensive and often requires funding beyond what one nurse, hospital, or college can supply.

Nurses who want to do research usually find it necessary to obtain outside funding or compete with other aspiring researchers for limited internal (from within the agency) funding. Therefore, to receive funding, nurses must do research that interests others and that a funding agency is willing to support.

The agencies that fund nursing research look for ideas that build on and advance nursing knowledge. Thus, although nursing research may be broadly defined as anything that interests nurses and helps them provide better care, controversy exists as to what can legitimately be included. When choosing a topic, the wise nurse researcher considers the important issues of background and support.

Research is different from **problem solving.** Problem solving is specific to a given situation and is designed for immediate action, whereas research is **generalizable** (transferable) to other situations and deals with long-term solutions rather than immediate ones. For example, Mrs. Abney is an elderly patient who frequently was found wandering in the halls of the nursing home, unable to find her way back to her room. This was quite distressing to her and time-consuming for the nursing staff who helped her find her way "home." A nurse noticed that Mrs. Abney had no difficulty recognizing her daughter, so she taped a photograph of the daughter to Mrs. Abney's door. Now Mrs. Abney can find her room easily. She is less agitated, and the nursing staff time can be spent on other priorities.

This is an example of problem solving. It is effective in one set of circumstances and has immediate application. But the solution that worked for Mrs. Abney may not work for all confused patients. Table 12–1 compares problem solving and research.

Research Process

The nursing research process is the same as any other research process; it simply addresses a nursing-related problem. Research starts with a problem or stimulus. The stimulus for a research project may be the feeling that something needs to be addressed, that something is not right. It may be that there are insufficient data for resolving a problem, or the literature is unclear, or the data presented in the literature are conflicting. When there is a need for more information and no adequate information exists, research is in order.

TABLE 12–1
Comparison of Problem Solving and Research

Characteristic	Research	Problem Solving
Type of problems addressed	Widely experienced	Situation specific
Conceptual basis	Theoretical framework	Whatever works
Knowledge base needed	Review of literature	Practical knowledge, common sense, and experience
Scope of application	Generalizable to similar situations	Useful mainly in the immediate situation

There are two major categories of research: quantitative and qualitative. **Quantitative research** is generally considered objective and uses data-gathering techniques that can be repeated by others and verified. Data collected are quantifiable; that is, they can be counted, measured with standardized instruments, or observed with a high degree of agreement among observers.

Qualitative research is more subjective. Questions that cannot be answered by quantitative designs must be addressed by qualitative methods. Answering "why" questions requires the use of qualitative approaches. Why do persons with diabetes choose not to follow the diet prescribed for them? Why do chronically mentally ill individuals choose not to take the medications that would reduce psychotic symptoms? Qualitative research is useful in understanding the perceptions, feelings, and motivations of the research subjects.

Whether quantitative or qualitative, all research must be rigorously planned, carefully implemented, and scrupulously analyzed. Therefore, most research follows a formal process known as the **research process.** Students in baccalaureate nursing programs usually take a course in nursing research in which both qualitative and quantitative methods are described. This chapter looks at the steps in the quantitative research process.

There are several steps in the process:

1. Identification of a research problem.
2. Review of literature.
3. Formulation of the research question or hypothesis.
4. Design of the study.
5. Implementation.
6. Drawing conclusions based on findings.
7. Discussion of implications.
8. Dissemination of findings.

IDENTIFICATION OF A RESEARCH PROBLEM

Problems generally come from three sources: clinical situations, the literature, or theories. Clinical situations are rich sources for research problems. Nurses want to prevent elderly clients from wandering off the unit and getting lost. How can they do it? Asking this question can lead to a research problem. Or perhaps a nurse wonders if a time-honored method of providing care is, in fact, the best way of doing things. A research problem may result from her curiosity.

Sometimes researchers become interested in a problem because it has been written about in the literature. They may decide to **replicate** (repeat) the study or may design a similar one to test part of the original study in a new way.

The third source of research problems, theory, relates to testing theoretical models. Chapter 11 discussed several models of nursing theory that have been developed. If a theoretical model is designed to predict patients' responses to nursing actions, whether or not it actually does predict patients' responses can be tested through research. The researcher can create certain conditions and see if, in fact, the events happen as the theoretical model predicted. Most ideas for nursing research projects come from one of these three sources.

REVIEW OF LITERATURE

Once a problem is identified, the professional literature must be reviewed. A review of the literature is comprehensive and covers all relevant research and supporting documents in print. Doing a thorough review of the literature requires a lot of library time and detective work. Computer-generated searches of the literature can assist tremendously with this step but cannot totally replace the efforts of a dedicated researcher.

The literature review is essential to locate similar or related studies that have already been completed and upon which a new study can build. The review is helpful in creating a **conceptual framework,** or organization of supporting ideas, upon which to base the study. At this point, you may want to review the brief discussion of conceptual frameworks in Chapter 11.

FORMULATION OF THE RESEARCH QUESTION OR HYPOTHESIS

Once researchers have identified a research problem, are intimately acquainted with the relevant literature, and have chosen a conceptual framework that helps to focus the topic, they need to formulate the **research question.** The question may be stated in one of three forms: a statement, a question, or a hypothesis. If researchers are going to describe something, they may make a statement, such as: "The purpose of this study is to identify the five most frequently expressed needs of family members in intensive care unit waiting rooms." They could also ask a question, such as: "What are the characteristics of mothers who have difficulty bonding to their newborn babies?" If comparing the relationship of two variables, a question might be asked, such as: "What is the relationship of time spent studying and grade point averages?" If conducting an experiment, researchers must have a **hypothesis** (educated guess) as to what the outcome will be so that hypothesis-testing statistics may later be applied. For example, "First-time mothers who attend childbirth classes will demonstrate earlier bonding with their newborn babies than mothers who do not attend the classes" is a testable hypothesis. Whatever the form used, the research question must be expressed succinctly and clearly.

DESIGN OF THE STUDY

Once the research question is identified, the study must be designed. There are two broad categories of research designs: **experimental** and **nonexperimental.** If the researcher influences the **subjects** in any way, the research is experimental. If not, the research is nonexperimental. There are numerous types of research under each of these two categories, but the main difference between experimental and nonexperimental research is whether the researcher manipulates, or influences, the subjects.

True experimental designs provide evidence of a cause-and-effect relationship between actions. For example, testing the hypothesis "Patients who receive preoperative teaching need less pain medication in the first 72 hours postoperatively than those who do not" would provide evidence of a cause-and-effect relationship between teaching and pain. Sometimes it is impossible to conduct a true experimental study with human beings because to do so might endanger them in some way. In those instances, modified experimental studies are used.

Nonexperimental designs are frequently referred to as *descriptive designs* because the researcher describes what the situation is or was at some point in the past. There are many types of nonexperimental designs: surveys, descriptive comparisons, evaluation studies, exploratory studies, and historical-documentary research.

Whether the researcher chooses an experimental or nonexperimental design influences the data-collection process. The data-collection process includes selection of data collection instruments, design of the data collection protocol, the data analysis plan, subject selection, and informed consent and institutional review plans.

Data Collection Instruments. When designing a study, researchers must consider how the data will be collected. Data collection instruments, sometimes called data collection tools, range from simple survey forms to complex radiographic scanning devices. The instrument used must be **reliable,** or accurate. A reliable instrument is one that yields the same values dependably each time the instrument is used to measure the same thing. The tool must also be valid, which, when applied to a research instrument, means that it must measure what it is supposed to be measuring. If body temperature is being measured, a thermometer is an obvious data collection tool. When measuring an abstract factor, such as anxiety or depression, the best data collection tool is not as clear. To minimize measurement errors, beginning researchers usually choose instruments with published reliability and validity, rather than designing their own.

Data Collection Protocol. Another aspect of designing the study is deciding on the data collection **protocol** (procedure). The quality of the data depends on strict adherence to the plan. If, for example, the plan calls for administering a questionnaire to renal dialysis clients after their dialysis treatments, the data collectors must be sure that they give the questionnaires to all subjects only after their treatments. The data collection protocol answers the question: How will we go about gathering our data?

Data Analysis Plan. It may seem premature to decide how the data will be analyzed before it is even collected, but careful planning is important. The research design is developed with data analysis in mind. The analysis must be part of the planning process because what data are collected and the protocols for collecting the data depend on how the data will be analyzed. The data analysis plan answers the question: What will we do with the data once we gather it?

Subject Selection. Once the researcher knows what is to be done, the specifics of who is to be included are decided. The individual people or laboratory animals being studied are known as research subjects. If the researchers plan to study pain control in postoperative patients, for example, they have to decide the specific type of surgery and the age, sex, ethnicity, and geographic location of the patients as well as a variety of other factors in planning the subject

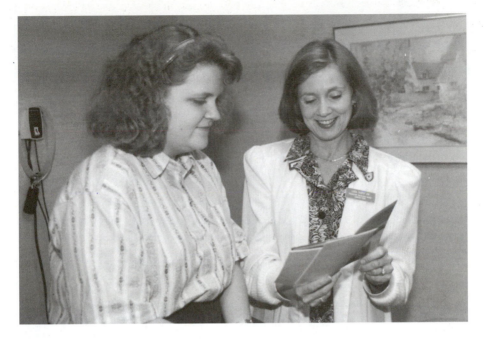

FIGURE 12-1

Research subjects are selected based on factors such as age, sex, condition, and location. (Courtesy of Memorial Hospital, Chattanooga, TN)

selection (Fig. 12–1). Subject selection answers the question: Who qualifies to be a participant in this study?

Rarely, all subjects in a particular group are studied. The term **population** refers to all subjects who meet the selection criteria. Usually, researchers have to use a **sample** (subgroup) of the entire population, however, and valid results can be obtained if the sample is properly selected.

Informed Consent and Institutional Review. Next, researchers who use human subjects must plan to protect the rights of those subjects. Research subjects must be asked to sign an **informed consent** form that describes the details of the study and what participation means for the subjects. Any risks involved in participating must be explained. No one should be pressured in any way to participate, and the **confidentiality** (privacy) of participants must be assured. (See Sidebar 12–1 for further information about including women in research.)

A related step when using human subjects is submitting the proposal to the institution, such as a hospital or clinic, where the research will take place. It must be approved by the **institutional review board.** Usually composed of individuals from different disciplines, these boards exist to ensure that research is well designed and ethical and does not violate the policies and procedures of their institutions. Only after the institutional review board approves the proposal can the study begin.

FYI

SIDEBAR 12–1
Including Women in Research

Nurses have a responsibility to apply appropriate ethical standards as they incorporate research findings into practice. Additionally, qualified nurses conducting research must do so in an ethical manner. Although these two statements may seem obvious, the practice is not as obvious or as easy as one might think.

For example, women have traditionally been excluded as subjects from research for seemingly appropriate reasons: (1) The drugs being tested in some experiments could be harmful to fetuses if women in the study were or became pregnant during the study, and (2) women might react differently to some experiments because of hormonal fluctuations.

There have been more serious problems with the misuse of women as subjects in research. An example was the use of gynecological patients in a pilot study to test antibody reaction to transplanted cancer cells without obtaining written permission from the subjects (although signed permission was obtained from male prison volunteers who were the healthy subjects). Another example was a study to determine the side effects of hormone contraceptives. Most of the women subjects were poor and from an ethnic or minority population who were seeking effective contraceptive measures after having had several pregnancies. More pregnan-

cies resulted in the placebo group. It was determined that the women were not informed about the risk of pregnancy in participating in the study.

Such examples provided the stimulus for the National Institutes of Health to publish guidelines for including women and minorities in research. The guidelines mandate:

- The inclusion of women and members of minorities in all human research.
- The inclusion of women and minorities in clinical trials to the degree that differences in intervention effect can be accomplished in the statistical analysis.
- The exclusion of cost as an acceptable reason to exclude groups.
- The initiation of programs and support for outreach efforts to recruit these groups into clinical studies.

The nurse's increased awareness of these potential dilemmas and subsequent action to prevent biased and discriminatory treatment can result in decreased vulnerability and oppression for women.

(Adapted with permission of Pinch, Winifred J. (1994). Women and research. *ANA Center for Ethics and Human Rights Communique*, 3(3), 4–5.)

IMPLEMENTATION

Up until this point, only planning has taken place. In the implementation phase, the actual study is conducted. The two main tasks during this phase are data collection and data analysis.

Data Collection. **Data** (research-generated information) should be collected only by those who understand the study. All research assistants should understand the purpose of the data and the importance of accuracy and careful record keeping. No matter who is collecting the data, however, the integrity of the project is ultimately the responsibility of the primary researcher.

Data Analysis. If all goes well, the data are analyzed exactly as proposed. In analyzing the data, most researchers use the same statistics consultants who assisted in planning the study. The researcher is well advised to work closely with the statistician in interpreting as well as analyzing the data. The nurse researcher is in charge, however, and he or she has the final word on what interpretations are made.

DRAWING CONCLUSIONS BASED ON FINDINGS

In writing the research report, the findings directly related to the research question are presented first. Findings are presented factually—without value judgments. The facts must speak for themselves. Simple presentation of the facts is all that is required. After findings related to the research question are reported, unexpected findings can be reported. Conclusions are then drawn. Conclusions answer the question: What do these findings mean? Here researchers can be more subjective and inject some of their own thinking but should stay within the boundaries of the study.

DISCUSSION OF IMPLICATIONS

Researchers are always on the lookout for the implications of their studies. Implications are suggestions of things that should be done in the future. Every good study raises more questions than it answers. In nursing studies, there may be indications for modifications in nursing education or nursing practice. Nearly every study has implications for further research, and if the findings are as expected, almost all studies should be carefully replicated. Replication can answer these and other questions: What needs to be known to develop more confidence in the findings? Will the research instrument produce similar results in a similar population in a different geographic location? Will the procedure be effective with patients having a slightly different type of surgery? Will age make a difference? Will cultural orientations make a difference? What else do we need to know to improve the care of patients?

DISSEMINATION OF FINDINGS

A study is not completed until the results are communicated to others who may find it useful. Most funding agencies want to know in advance how the researcher plans to **disseminate** the findings. The two major vehicles for knowledge dissemination are articles in professional journals and presentations at conferences. Examples of nursing research journals include *Clinical Nursing Research, Image, Nursing Research, Research in Nursing and Health Care,* and the *Western Journal of Nursing Research*. Because there are relatively few research journals in nursing, the competition for publishing might seem fierce, but editors say they have great difficulty getting well-written manuscripts on topics of interest to readers. A review process, called **peer review,** is the method most journals use to determine whether to publish a research report. During peer review, a manuscript is circulated to a review panel consisting of one or more experts in the area of study. They evaluate its appropriateness and accuracy and recommend that it be published, resubmitted with changes, or rejected. Most research that is carefully conceived, conducted, and presented can get published, although the researcher must be persistent and resilient in taking criticism and reworking manuscripts.

A somewhat easier, yet still discriminating, route to dissemination is presentation at one or more of the numerous nursing research conferences. Many research conferences also use the peer review process. In general, however, the proportion of abstracts (summaries of research) chosen for presentation at conferences is higher than the proportion of manuscripts chosen for publication.

Whether research is published or presented, it is important to disseminate research results to other nurses who may choose to use it to improve patient care practices.

INTERVIEWS WITH NURSE RESEARCHERS

The field of nursing research is growing, with many nurses actively involved in research. In this section, two nurse researchers tell about their work.

Research on Self-Esteem in Children

The first interview is with Maureen Killeen, an associate professor of nursing at the Medical College of Georgia (Fig. 12–2).

INTERVIEWER: Maureen, your research is with children and self-esteem; exactly what do you do?

RESEARCHER: I go into people's homes and ask children about themselves, and I ask the parents about the children. I ask the children, "What kinds of things are you good at?" And I ask them how important certain words are to them.

INTERVIEWER: What are some examples of the important words?

RESEARCHER: *Pretty, smart, honest, messy, lazy, active, careful, happy*— things like that. In another study, I am interested in the relationship between obesity and self-esteem. I go into a fifth-grade classroom and give everyone a self-concept scale and measure height and weight. I ask if they are heavier or thinner than others their age.

INTERVIEWER: How do you happen to be doing what you are doing?

RESEARCHER: I read about research on self-esteem in a "Social Psychology and the Self" course I took in graduate school. I read a lot of studies, and every study indicated that if you think of yourself in a certain way, this leads to certain behaviors. But there was nothing about how people come to think of themselves in certain ways. What are the characteristics or traits that get people thinking that way? I wanted to know the answer to that question.

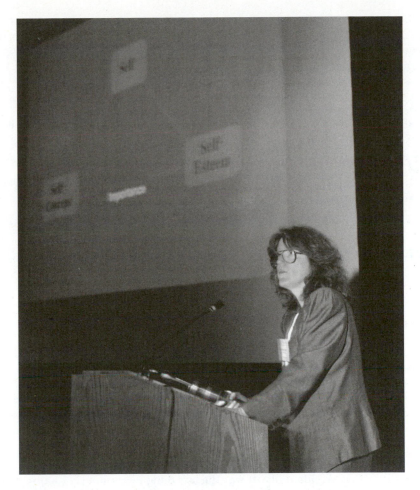

F I G U R E   1 2 – 2
Maureen Killeen presents her research at a psychiatric nursing conference.
(Courtesy of Maureen Killeen.)

INTERVIEWER: What impact do you hope your research will have on the care of children?

RESEARCHER: If we can figure out how other people affect children's ideas about themselves, how talk about children and talk to children affects them, then we can teach parents how to talk more effectively with their children. We can increase the relevance of treatment and therapy. We will know how to change how people feel about themselves. That is the treatment implication of this research.

INTERVIEWER: What has been most helpful to you in the process of becoming a nurse researcher?

RESEARCHER: Mentoring by more experienced researchers. I have benefited from the kindness of senior researchers who shared ideas. Experience is the best teacher, and I have been fortunate to have had good mentoring. Also, getting a funded grant to pay the bills while I do research has helped a lot!

INTERVIEWER: With regard to your professional life, what is the most fun for you?

RESEARCHER: Some aspects of research are the most fun, but teaching is close behind. If I can use my research in teaching—that's a *lot* of fun!

INTERVIEWER: What do you like the least of the things you have to do?

RESEARCHER: Writing. Writing is hard. There are constant revisions. I'm not sure it ever gets done.

INTERVIEWER: What would you like to say about research to nursing students?

RESEARCHER: Research can be a lot of fun. Hook up with someone who believes it's fun and asks interesting questions. It's very exciting!

Research on Decreasing Falls in the Elderly

The second nurse researcher interviewed was Elizabeth McNeely, who did the tai chi research with older people mentioned earlier. McNeely was an assistant professor in Emory University's Nell Hodgson Woodruff School of Nursing and is currently a gerontological nurse practitioner in private practice. Her research collaborators are in the Emory School of Medicine and the Atlanta Veterans Administration Medical Center.

INTERVIEWER: How did you happen to become a nurse researcher?

RESEARCHER: Accidentally. It was the last thing I envisioned. I happened to have a specialization in a field [gerontology] where research was growing. I became recognized as an expert in the field. My supervisor told me one day to go to a meeting where my expertise was needed. The meeting turned out to be a planning meeting for the multidisciplinary [involving professionals from several fields] research I do now.

INTERVIEWER: How do you believe your research has contributed to better patient care?

RESEARCHER: There are so many things people do because they "know" they work. But this knowledge doesn't get communicated beyond the walls of the institution. With hard data that comes from research, the information can be published so others can know how to do it. This improves patient care.

INTERVIEWER: What are some examples?

RESEARCHER: This tai chi grant. They have been doing tai chi in China for hundreds of years. But thousands of testimonials to the benefits won't lead to its being recommended by medical professionals in this country. We have to study the effects systematically before it will be supported by the medical profession.

INTERVIEWER: How do you like your work as a nurse researcher?

RESEARCHER: It's intriguing. Everyone needs to realize the importance of getting hard data to support practice.

INTERVIEWER: What do you like best about your work?

RESEARCHER: The air of excitement and discovery that comes when we see that some of our ideas are working. Also, my association with other researchers and the opportunities for thinking.

INTERVIEWER: What do you like the least?

RESEARCHER: There is a lot of tedium. It's hard to realize how long it takes to get from idea to publication. You have to be "long-term" oriented.

INTERVIEWER: What would you like to say to nursing students?

RESEARCHER: I would tell them that nurses have a unique contribution to make to the multidisciplinary research team. The problems are complex and require complex approaches, including the nursing perspective.

These interviews demonstrate how two nurse researchers feel about the work they do. Nationwide there are hundreds of nurses who, like Killeen and McNeely, are excited about nursing research and the contributions it makes to improving nursing practice.

RELATIONSHIP OF NURSING RESEARCH TO NURSING THEORY AND PRACTICE

Relationships among nursing research, practice, and theory are circular. As mentioned earlier, research ideas are generated from three sources: (1) clinical practice, (2) literature, and (3) theory.

Questions about how best to deal with patient problems regularly arise in clinical situations. As shown in the example of Mrs. Abney, the elderly lady who could not find her room, problems often can be "solved" for the present. When the same questions recur, long-term answers may be needed. Research develops solutions that can be used with confidence in different situations.

Published articles about nursing research often generate interest in further studies. If there is published research literature on a particular nursing care problem, other researchers may be stimulated to investigate further and refine the solutions. This is how nursing knowledge builds.

Nursing theorists also generate research ideas. They piece together postulates or premises that "explain" what has been discovered. The explanation is "tested" to see if it is robust or strong enough to be useful. If so, there may be more implications for applications in clinical practice.

Nursing research journals are full of clinical studies that have made a difference in patient care. A few examples of changes in nursing practice stimulated by research include:

1. Improved care of patients with skin breakdown from pressure ulcers.
2. Decreasing light and noise in critical care units to prevent sleep deprivation.
3. Using caps on newborns to decrease heat loss and stabilize body temperature.
4. Positioning patients following chest surgery to facilitate respiration.
5. Scheduling pain medication more frequently following surgery.
6. Preoperative teaching to facilitate postsurgery recovery.

Nursing research findings not only improve patient care, but also affect the health care system itself. For example, research studies have demonstrated the cost-effectiveness of nurses as health care providers. This is discussed further in Chapter 16.

Another contribution of nursing research to practice is in the area of power. A person who possesses knowledge that is useful to others has power. Nurses gain much knowledge through clinical practice. Yet practical knowledge, as important as it is, lacks the power of research-validated knowledge. Research can be used to demonstrate, for example, that one nursing action is more effective than another. When knowledge from practice is validated through research, that knowledge is more powerful. Thus, it could be said that research *empowers* practice.

A final point about the influence of research on practice has to do with professionalism. In Chapter 6, the characteristics of professions were given. One of the criteria commonly mentioned is a scientific body of knowledge that is expanded through research. Nursing research enhances the status of nursing as a profession by expanding nursing's scientific knowledge base.

A brief example that may clarify the interplay between nursing research, practice, and theory is found in Box 12–2.

BOX 12–2
Relating Nursing Research to Practice and Theory

Behavior theory suggests that behavior can be modified with reinforcement (reward or punishment). Incontinence is behavior characterized by involuntary urination before the patient can get to the bathroom or get positioned on a bedpan or with a urinal. Some researchers wondered, "Can incontinence be modified with positive reinforcements such as a special treat or additional time in the tele- vision room?" Specifically, they believed that patients could be "taught" to control urination if effective reinforcers were applied. Several subsequent studies suggest that patients can learn to control incontinence in specific situations. In this case, a theory—behavior theory—was useful in planning research, the results of which enable nurses to improve the clinical nursing care of incontinent patients.

COLLABORATION IN NURSING RESEARCH

The history of nursing research spans almost 40 years. Beginning in the 1960s with awareness of the need for a nursing body of knowledge based on research, nursing research today has matured to the level of collaboration with other disciplines to generate knowledge that would be limited if done only by members of one discipline. The Open Letter to Nursing Students from nurse researcher Larry Scahill (Box 12–3) and a discussion of research partnerships featuring Judith Noble Halle (Goldsmith, 1995) illustrate the effectiveness and excitement of collaborative research relationships.

Halle, a doctoral student at the University of California at Los Angeles School of Nursing, works with women who are experiencing difficult pregnancies. Halle's concern is for the health of the infant, and she is doing physiological research to develop methods for preventing brain damage owing to a lack of oxygen at birth. Her research is based on a major finding of a physician with whom she collaborates. Other major collaborators include another nurse, Christine Kasper, who administers a nursing cell physiology laboratory, and the director of a pediatric neurosurgery research laboratory.

According to Kasper, "Many of the unique questions that nurses ask when they begin to address new areas of research are supported by existing fields of science, such as cell physiology, or the behavioral sciences. Rather than reinventing the wheel, collaborating with scientists outside of nursing contributes to nursing science, and nursing contributes to others" (Goldsmith, 1995, p. 7).

SUPPORT FOR NURSING RESEARCH

Nursing research is expensive, and support takes many forms. It can include encouragement, consultation, computer and library resources, money, and release time from researchers' regular work responsibilities. Each of these forms of support is important, but none alone is adequate. Early in the development of nursing research, encouragement was often the only support available, and not all nurse researchers had that. Gradually over the years, funding sources have developed, but financial support is still difficult to obtain, particularly for new researchers.

The National Institute of Nursing Research (NINR) was created in 1992 from what had been the National Center for Nursing Research (NCNR), part of the National Institutes of Health. The purpose of the NINR is to provide structure for selecting scientific opportunities and initiatives and to promote depth in developing the knowledge base for nursing practice. In the years of NCNR/NINR's existence, its budget has quadrupled, but it still is able to fund only a small portion of the proposals it receives. To establish priorities for funding, the National Nursing Research Agenda (NNRA) was launched in 1987. The research priorities in the first phase of the NNRA were selected in 1988 and included:

- Low birth weight: mothers and infants
- Human immunodeficiency virus (HIV) infection: prevention and care
- Long-term care for older adults
- Symptom management: pain

Child psychiatry is in the midst of tremendous change. Previous assumptions about the etiology of child psychiatric disorders are collapsing under the weight of new research findings. These findings emerge from several related fields, including neuroanatomy, developmental neuroscience, pharmacology, genetics, molecular biology, and epidemiology. Because no one discipline can embrace all of these fields, research in child psychiatry is multidisciplinary. Although nursing education does not prepare students for careers in basic biological research, nurses can and do collaborate in clinical research. What is clinical research in child psychiatry and what part do nurses play in clinical research?

Clinical research refers to research endeavors that are closely connected with care of patients. In child psychiatry, this might include a medication trial in children with depression, an evaluation of a cognitive-behavioral intervention program in attention-deficit hyperactivity disorder, a neuroimaging study of brain volumes in Tourette's syndrome, or a family genetic study in obsessive-compulsive disorder. Each of these research studies requires comprehensive assessment of subjects, careful management of the data collected, and analysis of results.

As with other fields of research, clinical research usually involves a question about the relationship between two things. The research question may emerge from theory or from clinical practice. For example, the question of whether the vulnerability for obsessive-compulsive disorder is inherited originated in part because clinicians noticed that it recurred in families at higher than expected rates. To investigate the relationship between childhood obsessive-compulsive disorder and family history, researchers interview family members to ascertain the frequency of obsessive-compulsive disorder in the family and the pattern of inheritance. By contrast, the neuroimaging study of Tourette's syndrome evolved from a theory that specific brain structures play a central role in this disorder.

Another area of increasing importance in child psychiatry is psychopharmacology. The proliferation of pharmacologic agents for the treatment of psychiatric disorders of childhood offers hope for children afflicted with mental illness. Despite the promise of this growing list of medications, however, the scientific support for their use is surprisingly scarce. Indeed, only a few of the drugs commonly used in child psychiatry have clearly demonstrated efficacy. To demonstrate that a medication is effective for a given set of psychiatric symptoms, there must be a clear relationship between the treatment and a positive clinical outcome. For example, it has been shown that children treated with fluoxetine (Prozac) for depression achieve better results compared with those who received placebo. For some, studies of this sort are unacceptable because a child may receive a placebo rather than the active treatment. In the absence of clear evidence that a given medication is effective in children, others raise ethical concerns about exposing children to psychotropic medications. Thus, an additional benefit of placebo-controlled trials is that the effectiveness of the medication is closely monitored.

Research involves the systematic investigation of the relationship between two or more phenomena. Research in child psychiatry is expanding and embraces a wide range of disciplines from basic scientists to clinicians. Especially relevant for nurses is clinical research, such as placebo-controlled medication trials. These studies require careful assessment, close monitoring during the trial, and accurate assessment of outcome. The future of child psychiatry will increasingly rely on neuroscience, psychopharmacology, and clinical measurement. Nurses interested in these fields can consider a career in clinical research in child psychiatry.

Larry Scahill, M.S.N., M.P.H.

- Nursing informatics: enhancing patient care
- Health promotion for older children and adolescents

The NNRA, Phase 2, began in 1995 with the following priorities for the five-year period:

- Community-based nursing models (1995)
- Effectiveness of nursing interventions in HIV/AIDS (1996)
- Cognitive impairment (1997)
- Living with chronic illness (1998)
- Biobehavioral factors related to immunocompetence (1999)

These new priority areas were to be refined by a multidisciplinary Priority Expert Panel.

Several other federal agencies, although not giving priority to the funding of nursing research, do accept proposals that meet their funding guidelines when submitted by qualified nurse researchers. These include the National Institute on Aging, the National Cancer Institute, the National Institute of Mental Health, the National Institute of Alcohol Abuse and Addiction, the National Institute on Drug Addiction, and the Centers for Disease Control and Prevention.

Nursing associations also fund nursing research. The American Nurses Foundation, Sigma Theta Tau, and many clinical specialty organizations provide research awards. State and local nursing associations sometimes have seed money for pilot projects. Universities, schools of nursing, and large hospitals also may provide small amounts of research funds. Generally, however, finding adequate funding for large-scale studies continues to be a problem faced by nurse researchers.

ROLES OF NURSES IN RESEARCH

The *Code for Nurses* states: "The nurse participates in activities that contribute to the ongoing development of the profession's body of knowledge" (American Nurses Association, 1985). In an ideal world, every nurse would be involved in research. In the real world, all nurses should, as a minimum, use research results to improve their practices. Professional nurses should not practice nursing without staying abreast of the current literature, especially studies done in their areas of clinical practice.

As seen in Table 12–2, in addition to using research to improve practice, all professional nurses can contribute to one or more aspects of the research process. Baccalaureate nurses can read, interpret, and evaluate research for applicability to nursing practice. Through clinical practice, they can identify nursing problems that need to be investigated. They can participate in the implementation of scientific studies by helping principal researchers collect data in clinical settings or elsewhere. This beginning level of researcher must know enough about the purpose of the research to follow the research protocols explicitly or know when it is necessary to deviate from the protocol for a patient's well-being. Baccalaureate nurses also can help disseminate research-based knowledge by sharing useful research findings with colleagues.

TABLE 12–2
Levels of Educational Preparation and Levels of Participation in Nursing Research

Level of Preparation	Level of Research Participation
Student nurse	Consumer
BSN nurse	Problem identifier
	Data collector
MSN nurse	Replicator
	Concept tester
Doctoral nurse	Theory generator
Postdoctoral nurse	Funded program director

BSN, Bachelor of science in nursing; MSN, master of science in nursing.

The master's prepared nurse may be ready to replicate studies that have been previously conducted. Researchers cannot be sure that their findings are what they seem to be until studies are repeated with similar results. Nurse researchers have learned that it is not necessary (or even desirable) always to generate a totally new and disconnected idea to do research. As mentioned earlier, to be most useful, research must be based on a conceptual framework and related to previous research.

Depending on education, clinical and research experiences, and interests, some nurses at the master's level are better prepared to conduct research than are others. In addition to education and experience, a crucial factor is the support system the nurse has available. To do research, nurses need time, money, consultation, and subjects. With rich resources in a research environment, master's prepared nurses can and do make vital research contributions.

Usually, to be a nationally recognized researcher and obtain federal funding for a research program, nurses need doctoral and even postdoctoral preparation. Researchers across the United States in all professions compete for a limited pool of research dollars available each year. Only those nurses with strong academic and experiential backgrounds and the best proposals succeed in obtaining federal funding.

Nurses who aspire to careers as competitive nurse researchers should plan a specific program of research. This means limiting one's research to a defined set of phenomena. For example, May Wykle (Wykle, 1986; Dunkle and Wykle, 1988; Fitzpatrick, Wykle, and Morris, 1990), who is at Case Western Reserve, has a research program producing stimulating studies about persons who care for their elderly dependent relatives. Sandra Dunbar of Emory University is focusing her research program on circadian rhythms, which are physiological patterns occurring approximately every 24 hours, in various populations. These researchers realize that only by becoming specialists in a particular area of research can they receive the kind of funding they need to support their research and the national recognition it takes to get the results of their studies published so that they can have the desired impact—improvement in nursing care.

SUMMARY

The scientific method is the name given to a systematic, orderly process of solving problems. It has been used for centuries and is applicable in many different situations. Knowledge can be categorized as either pure knowledge—that is, knowledge that is not immediately useful—or applied knowledge—that is, knowledge that can be used in a practical way.

Much of the scientific knowledge we take for granted today was discovered through use of the scientific method. This method has been particularly useful in the fields of medicine and health care, and human existence has been profoundly affected by discoveries made through its use.

The scientific method uses two types of logic: inductive and deductive reasoning. A combination of both types of reasoning is necessary to combine the theoretical and the practical aspects of the scientific method. For safety reasons, there are limitations on the use of the scientific method with human beings.

Nursing research was defined as the systematic investigation of phenomena related to improving nursing care. The major steps in the research process were reviewed: identification of a research problem, review of the literature, formulation of the research question, design of the study, implementation, drawing conclusions based on findings, discussion of implications, and dissemination of findings. Examples of significant contributions of selected nurse researchers were highlighted. The circular relationship of nursing research to nursing theory and practice was described. Sources of funding for nursing research were identified. The research roles of nurses with differing educational backgrounds were described.

REVIEW AND DISCUSSION QUESTIONS

1. Why is nursing called an applied science? Tell why you agree or disagree with this description.
2. Name and describe the two types of reasoning that are used in the scientific method. Explain why neither alone is adequate to advance knowledge.
3. List and discuss each step of the scientific process.
4. Explain why a purely experimental model is an inadequate one for nursing.
5. Go to the college library and see which nursing research journals are in the collection. Thumb through some recent issues and notice the types of studies reported.
6. Read a research article that interests you. See if you can identify each of the steps in the research process. If not, what is missing? Discuss with your teacher and class what the significance of the missing steps might be.
7. Find out what research is being done in your school or hospital. If possible, talk with those involved, including data collectors, data analysts, research directors, subjects, families of subjects, and nurses who work on units where research is being conducted. What do they know about the research? What are their concerns? What do they hope will be learned from the research?

8. Obtain job descriptions for nurses at varying experience levels at different agencies. Are research functions included in the job descriptions? If not, what research functions do you think might appropriately be included?
9. Of the following studies, identify which are nursing research and which are not, giving your rationale for each:
   a. The investigation of optimum staffing patterns in a long-term care facility.
   b. A study of effective methods of clinical supervision of nursing students.
   c. A comparison of two behavioral techniques for managing incontinence in spinal cord–injured patients.

REFERENCES

American Nurses Association (1985). *Code for nurses with interpretive statements*. St. Louis: Author.

Dunkle, R. E., and Wykle, M. L. (1988). *Decision making in long-term care: Factors in planning*. New York: Springer.

Fitzpatrick, J. J., Wykle, M. L., and Morris, D. L. (1990). Collaboration in care and research. *Archives of Psychiatric Nursing*, 4(1), 53–61.

Flexner, S. B., Stein, J., and Su, P. Y. (Eds.). (1980). *The Random House dictionary*. New York: Random House.

Friends of the NINR. (1995). *Nursing research: Advancing science for health*. Washington, D.C.: Author.

Goldsmith, J. (1995). Newborn research depends on partnerships. *Sigma Theta Tau International Reflections*, 21(3), 6–8.

Kuhn, T. S. (1970). The structure of scientific revolutions. In O. Nurath (Ed.), *International encyclopedia of unified science* (2nd ed., vol. 2). Chicago: University of Chicago Press.

Medoff-Cooper, B., and Ray, W. (1995). Neonatal sucking behaviors. *Image: Journal of Nursing Scholarship*. 27(3), 195–200.

Pinch, S. J. (1994). Women in research. *ANA Center for Ethics and Human Rights Communique*, 3(3), 4–5.

Polit, D. F., and Hungler, B. P. (1995). *Nursing research: Principles and methods* (5th ed.). Philadelphia: J.B. Lippincott.

Ware, C. F., Panikkar, K. M., and Romein, J. M. (1966). *The twentieth century: History of mankind, cultural and scientific development* (vol. 6). New York: Harper & Row.

Wykle, M. L. (1986). Mental health nursing: Research in nursing homes. In M. S. Harper and B. Lebowitz (Eds.), *Mental illness in nursing homes: A research agenda* (pp. 221–234) (Publication No. 86–1459). Rockville, MD: U.S. Department of Health and Human Services.

CHAPTER 13

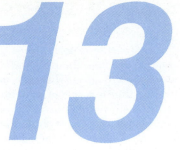

Jennifer E. Jenkins

The Health Care Delivery System

OBJECTIVES

- Describe the four types of services provided by the health care delivery system.
- Differentiate between the activities of health promotion and illness prevention.
- Explain the organizational structure of a typical health care facility.
- Describe how health care agencies are classified.
- Identify the roles of key members of the health care team.

VOCABULARY

authority
capitation
chief executive officer
chief nurse executive
chief of staff
continuous quality
  improvement (CQI)
cross-functional team
decentralization
dietitian
for-profit agency
gatekeeper
governmental (public)
  agency

health promotion
home health agency
illness prevention
institutional structure
interdisciplinary team
long-term care
managed care
multiskilled worker
not-for-profit agency
paramedical
patient-focused care
primary care
re-engineering
rehabilitation services

secondary care
self-directed work teams
shared governance
social services
subacute care
tertiary care
therapists
voluntary (private)
  agency
whole system shared
  governance

The health care delivery system in the United States has traditionally been a system of illness care delivery. It is complex, which makes it difficult for patients to negotiate. It is extremely expensive, with multiple types of financing. The technology and sophisticated procedures available are the best in the world, but many people do not have access to even the most basic care. It is a system in crisis.

It will be different in the future. Health care reform is evolving. Reform will take place before the year 2000 and affect the professional careers of today's students. This chapter describes the health care delivery system of the present and makes some predictions about the future.

The words *health care delivery system* speak to the nature of change in how the health and illness needs of patients will be met in the twenty-first century. Most planners believe that one of the essential parts of an improved health care system is an emphasis on prevention and the active participation of patients in their own health choices. Although scientists continue to search for and find cures to many illnesses, health care services increasingly emphasize the importance of holism or treating the whole person, not just the diseased part. A part of this paradigm is an increasing collaboration between health care professionals and governmental officials, who are working together to return the environment to a healthier balance, thus reducing pollution-related disease. This collaboration will not be easy and may experience many setbacks, but it is integral to increasing health and decreasing future health care costs.

The delivery system of the future will be more efficient than the current one. Life-threatening illnesses and injuries will continue to be treated in centers where technology and intensive care are available. People with noncritical injuries and illnesses will be cared for in homes or at work, in the schools, and in community-based facilities such as neighborhood clinics. Health care workers will be educated to provide holistic, efficient, and cost-effective care.

A system that answers the following questions will ensure that these objectives for the future are met:

1. What services does the patient need and want?
2. Who can best provide these services (patient, health care worker, family, others)?
3. Where is the most effective and efficient place to provide these services?
4. How will these services affect the quality of care, the cost, and both patient and health care worker satisfaction?

The U.S. government has not yet devised a definitive national health policy. An important first step, however, has been taken. As discussed in Chapter 10, in 1990, a consortium of nearly 300 national health organizations, the U.S. Public Health Service, and state health departments joined to draft goals and objectives for improving the health of U.S. citizens by the year 2000. The resulting report, *Healthy People 2000: National Health Promotion and Disease Prevention Objectives*, sets out three main goals (Box 13–1) (U.S. Department of Health and

---

BOX 13–1

Healthy People 2000 Goals

1. Increase the span of healthy life for Americans.
2. Reduce health disparities among Americans.
3. Achieve access to preventive services for all Americans.

(Reprinted with permission of U.S. Department of Health and Human Services. [1990]. *Healthy people 2000: National health promotion and disease prevention objectives.* Washington, D.C.: Author.)

Human Services, 1990). How well these goals are met will be determined by the commitment of health care providers and citizens and the degree to which government officials (elected and appointed) can continue to focus on desired health outcomes rather than becoming sidetracked with political maneuvering. With this brief look at the future, let us now take a look at the health care delivery system you will encounter and build a framework for understanding tomorrow's system.

TYPES OF HEALTH CARE SERVICES

There are four major types of health services: health promotion, illness prevention, diagnosis and treatment, and rehabilitation and long-term care. Each is briefly explained.

Health Promotion

Health promotion services assist patients to remain healthy, prevent diseases and injuries, and promote healthier lifestyles. These services require patients' active participation and cannot be performed solely by a health care provider. Health promotion services are based on the assumption that patients who participate in certain lifestyle changes are likely to avoid heart attacks, lung cancers, and other lifestyle-related diseases.

An example of health promotion services is prenatal classes. By learning good nutritional habits, an expectant mother can take care of both herself and her baby during pregnancy and after delivery. This increases the chances of a normal pregnancy and the birth of a healthy baby. Other examples include aerobic exercise classes and "stop-smoking" classes aimed at increasing the health of an individual's cardiovascular and respiratory systems.

Illness Prevention

When risk factors, such as a family history of heart disease, are identified, **illness prevention** services assist patients in reducing the impact of those risk factors on their health and well-being. These services also involve the patients' active participation.

Prevention services differ from health promotion services in that they address health problems *after* risk factors are identified, whereas health promotion services seek to *prevent* development of risk factors. For example, a health promotion program might teach the detrimental effects of alcohol and drugs on the person's health to prevent the person from using alcohol and drugs. Illness prevention services are used when the patient has been using alcohol or drugs and is at risk for developing health problems as a result. In reality, the boundary between health promotion and illness prevention is often blurred. Box 13–2 gives examples of activities in these two areas.

BOX 13-2
Illness Prevention and Health Promotion Activities

Illness Prevention
- Periodical histories and physical examinations
- Identification of familial and environmental risk factors
- Community health programs
- Promotion of healthy lifestyles to counteract risk factors
- Occupational safety programs (use of eye guards for work that endangers the eyes)
- Environmental safety programs (proper disposal of hazardous waste)
- Legislation that prevents injury or disease (seat-restraint laws)

Health Promotion/Maintenance
- Health education programs (prenatal classes)
- Exercise programs
- Health fairs
- Wellness programs (worksite/school)
- Proper nutrition
- Learning how to balance one's life

Diagnosis and Treatment

Traditionally in the U.S. health care system, there was heavy emphasis on diagnosis and treatment. Early diagnosis, that is, detecting disease as soon as the first signs occur, has been the focus of most physicians' efforts. Modern technology has enabled the medical profession to refine the acts of diagnosing illnesses and disorders and to treat them more effectively.

Health care technology has given physicians many treatment options to cure illnesses and disorders that have plagued humans for thousands of years. As a result, much human suffering has been avoided. Newer scientific advances permit many tests and treatments to be performed noninvasively, that is, without cutting into the body. Examples include the use of ultrasound to examine unborn fetuses to determine if they are developing normally and lithotripsy, which disintegrates kidney stones so they can be expelled in the urine. The future promises more "high-tech" noninvasive technologies.

On the negative side, high-tech services can lead patients to feel dehumanized. This occurs when the caregivers focus on machines rather than on patients. Nurses must remember that patients benefit most when they understand their diagnoses and treatments and when they can be active participants in the development and implementation of their own treatment plans.

Rehabilitation and Long-Term Care

Rehabilitation services are those that help restore the patient to the fullest possible level of function and independence following injury or illness. Rehabilitation programs deal with conditions that leave patients with less than full functioning, such as strokes, broken bones, or severe burns. Both patients and their families must be active participants in this care if it is to be successful. Rehabilitation services should begin immediately after the patient's condition has stabilized after an injury or stroke. These services may be provided in institutional settings such as hospitals, in special rehabilitation facilities, in long-term care facilities such as nursing homes, and in the home and the community. The objectives are to assist patients to achieve their potential and to return them to a level of functioning that permits them to be contributing members of society again.

Long-term care is care provided in residential facilities such as assisted living homes, skilled and intermediate nursing homes, and personal care homes. Each facility is tailored to provide services that the patient or family cannot provide while maintaining the highest possible patient control. With the aging of the population, and with more patients surviving severe trauma and disease with impairments in physical or mental functioning or both, these long-term care facilities are expected to experience rapid growth in the future.

ORGANIZATION AND STRUCTURE OF HEALTH CARE AGENCIES

The health care delivery system consists of agencies such as hospitals, clinics, associations, long-term care facilities, and home health services that provide any of the four major types of health services.

Institutional Structure

Institutional structure means how an agency is organized to do what it is intended to do. The institutional structure of most agencies includes a governing body, a board of trustees, also called a board of directors.

BOARD OF TRUSTEES

In the past, board members were often chosen from two groups: community philanthropists, who were expected to donate generously to the facility, and physicians who practiced in the institution. Boards were large, met infrequently, and had mainly ceremonial functions.

As the health care environment became more complex, board members were chosen to represent various business and political interests of the community. They were expected to bring knowledge and expertise from the larger business world as well as have an appreciation and understanding of health care agencies and how they operate.

Boards now tend to be smaller and carry significant responsibility for the mission of the organization, the quality of services provided, and the financial status of the organization. Boards are not involved in the day-to-day running of the agency, but they are responsible for establishing policies governing operations and for ensuring that the policies are executed. They delegate responsibility for running the agency to the chief executive officer (CEO).

CHIEF EXECUTIVE OFFICER

The **chief executive officer** is the individual responsible for the overall operation on a daily basis. He or she usually has a master's degree in business or hospital administration. The CEO's responsibilities include making sure that the institution runs efficiently, is cost-effective, and carries out the policies established
by the board. The CEO usually sits on the board of trustees and reports to the
board. The CEO in larger organizations is often assisted by a chief operating
officer (COO). Both of these positions are increasingly occupied by nurses with
advanced degrees and experience in administration, business, and health care
policy. Boards, who are responsible for hiring CEOs, have found that the broad,
holistic education and experience of nurses prepares them unusually well for
these positions.

MEDICAL STAFF

A medical staff consists of physicians who may be either employees or independent
practitioners. In either case, they must be granted privileges by the board of
trustees to see patients at that particular institution. They may not simply decide
to admit patients to an institution. This credentialing process is performed by a credentials committee, composed of members of the medical staff. They are charged
with the responsibility of assuring the board of trustees that every physician admitted to the medical staff of that facility is a qualified and competent practitioner
and that over time, each one keeps his or her skills and knowledge updated.

The medical staff, also through its credentials committee, is often charged
with the responsibility for credentialing nonphysician providers who admit or
consult with patients. These include advanced practice nurses, psychologists,
optometrists, podiatrists, and others.

In large organizations, medical staffs are usually organized by service (*e.g.*,
Department of Surgery, Department of Medicine, Department of Pulmonary
Medicine). A **chief of staff** is usually elected by the entire medical staff. Together with the chiefs of the various services, the chief of staff makes important decisions about medical policy for the institution. Bylaws govern these activities.
The actions of the medical staff must be approved by the board of trustees, to
whom the physicians are responsible.

Service on committees of the medical staff is a time-consuming activity that often goes unappreciated by others. It should be recognized that physicians who
dedicate their personal time to these activities are committed to the institution
and to the quality of medical care provided within it.

NURSING STAFF

The senior administrative nurse in an organization is known as the **chief nurse
executive,** vice president for nursing, or director of nursing. Once excluded
from broad institutional decision making, nurse executives of today are often
members of the board of trustees. Many organizations now consider the nurse
executive and the chief of the medical staff of equal importance.

The educational preparation for nurse executives includes a master's degree in nursing administration, business administration, or a new, joint MSN/MBA. Nurse executives are responsible for overseeing all of the nursing care provided in the institution and serve as clinical leaders as well as administrators. Increasingly the nurse executive is the chief of patient care or clinical services administrator. With the need to coordinate patient care and outcomes among all disciplines, the nurse as patient care executive can effectively lead and direct these efforts.

The nursing staff consists of all the registered nurses, licensed practical nurses/licensed vocational nurses, and nursing assistants employed by the department of nursing. They are usually organized according to the units on which they work.

Each patient care unit has its own budget and staff for which the manager is responsible. The manager, who is usually a nurse, is also a communication link between the staff and the next level of management.

In large or networked organizations, there may be an additional level of management between the nurse executive and the manager of a unit. These are middle-managers, known as clinical directors or supervisors. In most cases, they are nurses, but they may come from other clinical disciplines or from a business background. They have responsibility for multiple units or for specific projects or programs. These directors ensure that nursing and all other services they manage are integrated with other hospital services. They serve as the communication link between the unit managers and the executive staff.

Some nurses combine direct patient care responsibilities with research, education, and management responsibilities. They include nurse educators, nurse researchers, clinical nurse specialists, infection control nurses, and others. Nurses in these roles support direct care nurses and serve as expert resources to them in their area of specialization.

OTHER HEALTH CARE TEAM MEMBERS

Physicians, nurses, and all the other individuals who work with patients are called the health care team, or **interdisciplinary team.** They are supported in their work by a number of other departments, such as dietetics, housekeeping, laundry, and many others. Some key health providers are discussed later in this chapter.

Health care organizations are complex facilities. The way they are organized varies. Each has an organizational chart that shows its unique structure and explains lines of authority. It is informative when considering employment in a health care organization to examine the organizational chart to see how nursing is governed and relates to management and the board of directors.

Accreditation

As you learned in Chapter 2, schools of nursing may choose to participate in a process called accreditation. Health care organizations, too, are accredited. Their accrediting body is the Joint Commission on the Accreditation of Healthcare Organizations (JCAHO). JCAHO accreditation is important and requires that a number of standards are met in every department. The goal of accreditation is to improve patient outcomes. The way most organizations have chosen to work toward improvement in patient outcomes is through a process called **continuous quality improvement** (CQI).

CONTINUOUS QUALITY IMPROVEMENT/TOTAL QUALITY MANAGEMENT

In the 1940s, W. Edwards Deming (1982, 1986) proposed that groups of employees, rather than managers, be allowed to make decisions about how work was to be done. He called the employee groups *quality circles*. Deming's ideas were discussed in the United States but did not receive widespread acceptance here. There was interest in Deming's ideas elsewhere, however. The Japanese government asked him to help them rebuild their workplaces, which were devastated by World War II, and Deming went to Japan.

By the 1970s, consumers worldwide recognized that certain Japanese-made products were superior to their American-made counterparts. American businesses began to discuss and imitate Japanese management techniques. These were really Deming's ideas brought back through Japan.

Today's health care systems have borrowed management concepts from industry and are interested in CQI, also called total quality management (TQM). Rather than trying to identify mistakes after they have occurred, these systems focus on establishing procedures for assuring high-quality patient care.

Using quality improvement concepts, groups of employees from different departments decide how care will be provided. They decide what outcomes are desired and design systems and assign roles and activities to create those outcomes. Every effort is made to anticipate potential problems and prevent their occurrence. Management delegates authority to the providers of services to plan and carry out quality improvement programs. CQI/TQM programs reinforce the belief that quality is everyone's responsibility (Fig. 13–1).

Nurses are actively involved both in quality improvement and in accreditation processes, but these activities are not the responsibility of nursing alone. They are institutionwide initiatives, and everyone at all levels gets involved. Working together to improve patient care in the institution builds cooperation among departments and clinical disciplines and boosts morale.

New Organization and Structure

Nurses and all other health care workers are being transformed by the CQI/TQM movement. Putting quality improvement programs into place requires reorganization of whole systems.

RE-ENGINEERING

By the 1990s, businesses, including health care, were so complex, bureaucratic, and convoluted that many were failing to deliver high-quality products and ser-

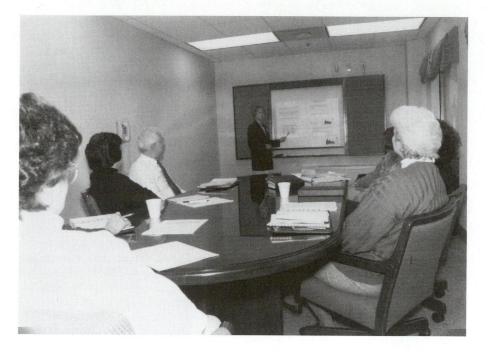

F I G U R E   1 3 – 1
This group of professionals works together to implement continuous quality improvement processes in an acute care hospital with the goal of improving efficiency and patient care while reducing costs. (Photo by Kelly Whelen.)

vices consistently. In health care, for example, it was not unusual for a patient staying five to seven days in a typical hospital to travel by wheelchair or stretcher eight or nine miles during their stay. A simple laboratory test might require 40 to 60 separate activities or tasks before results could be reported. Excessive and duplicative paperwork and trivial tasks burdened care providers and left patients dissatisfied and angry. The patient was no longer the center of the system. At times, it seemed patients and families were nuisances that got in the way of bureaucratic activities.

With the advent of CQI teams, it became evident that the system was not only sick, it was in danger of dying. A dramatic new paradigm was needed. It came in the form of re-engineering and patient-focused care.

Re-engineering is the "fundamental rethinking and radical redesign of business processes to bring about dramatic improvement in performance" (Hammer and Stanton, 1995). **Patient-focused care,** also known as patient-centered care, means placing the patient at the center of activity and designing processes around the patient that efficiently and effectively attain desired patient outcomes.

Re-engineering and patient-focused care are accomplished by **cross-functional teams,** who are involved with all aspects of achieving a specific patient-focused outcome. The cross-functional teams are composed of people from all parts of the organization who contribute to a particular process and outcome. They redesign, from scratch, how the work will be done, who will do it, in what time frame, and in what location. Staff are cross-trained to be able to complete several different tasks, each of which was formerly performed by a different worker. Workers who are cross-trained to perform different tasks are also known as **multiskilled workers.**

For example, consider a patient who is to be admitted for same-day surgery. In the past, an admissions clerk would take demographic and financial information and create a chart. A nurse would take a history and record clinical information. A laboratory technician would draw blood and a radiology technician would take a chest x-ray. An electrocardiogram technician would get an electrocardiogram and a nursing assistant would prepare the skin over the operative site. Often the patient would travel to different locations for all of these activities. It was an expensive, time-consuming, and exhausting process for the patient.

In a re-engineered patient-centered scenario, the patient would be met at the same-day surgery site by the nursing case manager. The nursing case manager would collect all pertinent demographic, financial, and clinical information and enter it into a computer. The computer would be programmed to respond to key data and to individualized information specific to this patient. It would then produce an individualized interdisciplinary plan of care. The plan would outline key

RESEARCH NOTE

Nursing administrators are faced daily with ethical dilemmas as costs are trimmed and quality of care is challenged. Borawski sought to explore these ethical dilemmas by replicating a previous study.

Nurse administrators in 159 acute care hospitals in North Carolina were asked to complete a descriptive survey. Of survey instruments, 104 (65 percent) were returned, and 102 of those were usable. This represents a 64 percent response rate.

Respondents identified ethical dilemmas in 15 different areas of their work. There were seven areas in which greater than 50 percent of the respondents voiced ethical dilemmas. They were staffing level or ratio of licensed to unlicensed personnel (84 percent), developing or maintaining standards of care (76 percent), allocation or rationing of scarce resources (75 percent), incompetent physicians (66 percent), demotion or termination of employees (63 percent), employee relations (60 percent), and incompetent nurses (56 percent).

Because of the design of the study, exploration of how demographics may have affected the results was not possible. There is also a concern that the wording of the questionnaire may have biased subjects toward socially acceptable responses.

As re-engineering and restructuring decrease the options for nurse administrators, it becomes an increasing challenge to match diminishing resources with increasing patient needs. This study points out the high level of concern felt by key nurse executives in acute care facilities. The outcomes of decisions related to cost reduction should be carefully monitored to ensure that they do not adversely affect quality of care.

(Adapted with permission of Borawski, D. B. (1995). Ethical dilemmas for nurse administrators. *Journal of Nursing Administration*, 25(7/8), 60-62.)

steps and activities for the patient, which would be negotiated with the patient so that optimal outcomes could be reached. The nurse would draw the blood, get an electrocardiogram and chest x-ray, and prepare the operative site. Alternatively a cross-trained technician, working in partnership with the nurse, would perform these tasks. The patient would have all these things performed in one location. Time, personnel costs, and equipment usage would be minimized. In this system, accountability and outcomes are easily tracked, and continual improvement of the system and processes can be made. Patient satisfaction is typically higher than with the older fragmented, bureaucratic methods.

When done well, re-engineering addresses the purpose of the business; the organizational culture needed for success, processes, and performance; and the people, knowledge, and skills needed to accomplish the redesigned work. When done poorly, re-engineering is often a euphemism for downsizing or staff reductions or layoffs. Although it is true that in redesigning the work, fewer people may be needed, staff reduction is not the only goal of re-engineering. The Research Note discusses re-engineering and ethical dilemmas.

Downsizing without work redesign simply leaves fewer people to accomplish already inefficient and ineffective work. Unfortunately, many companies, both in and outside health care, take this shortsighted approach to re-engineering. The result is poor morale, loss of competent staff, lower-quality outcomes, patient dissatisfaction, and loss of market share. Box 13–3 lists key components for successful re-engineering.

Tomorrow's health care workers are facing a different work environment. It is unlikely that they will have one, two, or even three jobs during their careers. They will probably have seven to ten different jobs during an average work career. Even when employed in the same position, they should expect that it will undergo major evolution and change. How can you thrive in this constantly changing environment? The following suggestions should help you keep your options open, even as the health care system changes.

- Take every opportunity to learn new skills.
- Read widely both inside and outside your field.
- Identify emerging trends and new opportunities.
- Find new ways to apply your knowledge and skills.

BOX 13–3
Keys to Successful Re-engineering

- Strong leadership
- Support from the top (financial, cultural, time, resources)
- Team members who love ambiguity, creativity, risk taking, and holism
- An irreverence for the past
- Optimism, persistence

- Ability to answer the questions:
  - —What is our business?
  - —What culture do we want?
  - —How do we need to do our work?
  - —What people do we want to work with?

- Volunteer for community activities that will stretch your skills, help you learn new skills, and help you meet people who can be helpful to you.
- Keep your resume current, but do not change jobs too often because that implies instability.

DECENTRALIZATION

The key to the new organization and structure is **decentralization.** Rather than decision-making authority being closely held by a few top executives or managers, decisions are made by those most affected by the decision. This does not only mean fewer layers in an organizational chart, but also refers to the philosophy that all professionals should be encouraged to use their talents fully.

Decentralization empowers staff, allowing them to exercise their own good judgment rather than waiting to be told what to do. For empowerment to be effective, the board of trustees and top executives must clearly articulate their vision, goals, and expectations so that each member of the organization knows where the organization is going and what his or her part in it is. In the most decentralized model, employees at all levels are involved in the process of developing the hospital's vision and goals.

Decentralization and empowerment involve the development and use of many skills. These include consensus decision making, positive discipline, developing worker independence and interdependence, negotiation, collaboration, and critical thinking.

One area that can be unclear in decentralized decision making is **authority.** The question of who has the final say for decisions is sometimes in doubt when so many people have responsibility. The knowledge, experience, and maturity of individuals as well as deadlines, legal considerations, institutional and regulatory body policies, and other factors must be considered to determine how much authority can be delegated to any person or group. Four levels of decision making and authority to be considered before delegating are outlined in Box 13–4.

FORMS OF DECENTRALIZATION

In addition to Deming's quality circles, a number of other decentralized models exist.

Shared Governance. **Shared governance** is founded on the philosophy that employees have both a right and a responsibility to govern their own work and time within a financially secure, patient-centered system. A common structure used for shared governance in nursing is the council model shown in Figure 13–2.

In the council model, there is a coordinating council made up of the chief nurse executive and the chairpersons of four subcouncils (clinical practice council, education council, administrative affairs council, and quality of care/research council). The coordinating council coordinates nursing activities, sets broad goals and objectives, and facilitates communication about nursing's vision. This group also ensures that successes are shared and that learning rather than punishment is the result of risk taking.

BOX 13–4
Levels of Authority

**Level I: Gather Data/
Complete Tasks**
In this level, people have limited knowledge or skill and do not make the decisions.

**Level II: Gather Data/Complete Tasks
Plus Make Recommendations to the
Decision Maker(s)**
As people gain experience and knowledge, they begin to learn how things fit together, and they are asked for recommendations. This does not mean that they make the decisions but contribute to the idea generation and options the decision maker has to choose from.

**Level III: Gather Data/Complete Tasks
Plus Make Recommendations*:
Decide and Act**
The delegator is interested in building the delegatee's confidence in decision mak-

ing. The delegatee is authorized to make the decision and take action. The asterisk (*) indicates, however, that the delegatee must consult or negotiate with someone or communicate information to someone or a group before the decision is made. It does not mean that the delegatee can take the decision-making authority back just because he or she would make a different decision. The asterisk (*) simply means that the delegatee must know the parameters and limitations placed on the decision.

**Level IV: Act on Your Own
or On Another's Behalf**
At this level of authority, the delegator is comfortable with the skill level of the delegatee. The delegatee is given full authority and responsibility for the decision-making process. This includes evaluating the effectiveness and appropriateness of the decision (accountability).

The other councils have the responsibility, authority, and accountability within their designated areas—clinical, administrative, education, and quality of practice—for setting the standards, policies, procedures, and behaviors necessary for nursing to carry on its work. Each council works closely with the others to ensure that decisions are well thought out. At the patient care unit level, a unit committee (or council) is elected by the staff to represent all jobs and shifts on that unit. This group is authorized to translate the organizational council decisions at the unit level.

To show how the council model of shared governance works, the clinical practice council might set a standard that all patients know their nurse's name and what they can expect from the nurse. The unit committees would then decide how that will be done and report back to the practice council on how they plan to implement the new standard on their particular units.

The council model is only one of several possible ways departments in hospitals are structured to perform professional governance functions.

Whole System Shared Governance.   At the organizational level, **whole system shared governance** is being implemented by some progressive organizations. This is driven by the need for organizational structures and operational systems that can link large, complex, or multisite systems made up of many smaller agencies or departments.

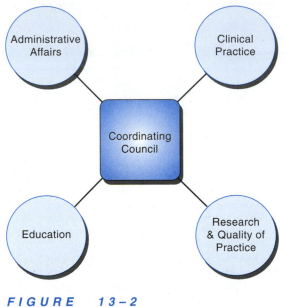

F I G U R E   1 3 – 2
Council model for shared governance. (Reprinted
with permission of Jenkins, J. E. [1991]. Shared
governance: The missing link. *Nursing Management,*
22[8], 30.)

These whole-system approaches involve people at all levels from the board of directors to front-line caregivers. Councils are commonly formed to represent patient care providers, operations, governance, and medical practice. In this system, nursing continues with its own or a modified model and is represented on the systems councils.

Self-Directed Work Teams.   Another method of decentralizing decision making is through **self-directed work teams.** These are cross-functional groups of people united around common goals and outcomes. They may exist for long periods of time or may be formed and disbanded as soon as they achieve their objectives.

Self-directed work teams work well because they put the people who do the work in the position to make decisions about how the work will be done. They are empowered by their managers, who provide them the information, support, coaching, and training necessary to be successful.

In all these decentralized models, the management role changes from supervisor to facilitator, mentor, coach, and supporter. Levels of authority are clearly defined so that everyone knows who has final say, who has influencing power, who has recommending power, and whose power is limited simply to gathering pertinent information.

This change in organizational behavior from bureaucratic to decentralized models will have lasting impact on the health care system and society. Employees and managers who experience the success of these strategies are unlikely to revert to centralized, hierarchical organizations. Fewer middle managers and more intergroup collaboration provide flexibility, lower costs, and improve quality. Unfortunately, however, this also means fewer jobs for middle managers. Under the old systems, middle managers were a large group of employees and many were nurses.

CLASSIFICATIONS OF HEALTH CARE AGENCIES

There are many agencies involved in the total health care delivery system. Organizations that deliver care can be classified in several ways: as governmental or voluntary agencies, as not-for-profit or for-profit agencies, and by the level of health care services they provide.

Governmental or Public Agencies

There are many **governmental (public) agencies** that contribute to the health and well-being of U.S. citizens. All are primarily supported by taxes, administered by elected or appointed officials, and tailored to the needs of the communities served.

LOCAL AGENCIES

Local agencies serve one community, one county, or a few nearby counties. They provide services to both paying and nonpaying citizens. Public health departments are examples of local governmental agencies found in almost every county in the United States. All citizens, whether or not they can pay, are eligible for health care through local public health departments. These services usually include immunizations, prenatal care and counseling, well-baby and well-child clinics, sexually transmitted disease clinics, tuberculosis clinics, and others. Public health nurses sometimes make home visits as well.

STATE AGENCIES

State health agencies oversee programs that affect the health of citizens across the state. Examples of state governmental health agencies include state departments of health and environment, departments that regulate and license health professionals such as state boards of nursing, and those that administer Medicaid insurance programs for the poor. These agencies are not typically involved in providing direct patient care but support local agencies that do provide direct care.

With increasing influence from managed care organizations (discussed later), the federal government seems inclined to transfer responsibility for managing governmental health care funds to the states. This move is justified by the rationale that states may be able to exercise more flexibility in designing and administering health care programs tailored to the needs of citizens. The danger does exist that traditional "safety nets" of federal mandates for services for the poor, elderly, or disadvantaged could be lost. If so, the long-term outcome would be patients who put off seeking care until they are so sick that they are even more expensive to treat, thus defeating the purpose of state control.

FEDERAL AGENCIES

Federal agencies focus on the health of all U.S. citizens. They promote and conduct health and illness research, provide funding to train health care workers, and assist communities in health care services planning. They also develop health programs and services and provide financial and personnel support to staff them. They establish standards of practice and safety for health care workers and conduct national health education programs on subjects such as the benefits of nonsmoking, prevention of acquired immunodeficiency syndrome (AIDS), need for prenatal care, and many others. Examples of federal agencies are the U.S. Public Health Service (PHS), the National Institutes of Health (NIH), the U.S. Department of Health and Human Services (DHHS), the Occupational Safety and Health Administration (OSHA), and the Centers for Disease Control (CDC).

A little known but important branch of the PHS is the Indian Health Service, which provides health care to Native Americans who live on federal reservations. In addition, the federal government operates hospitals providing direct care to active duty military personnel, their dependents, and veterans.

Voluntary or Private Agencies

Citizens often voluntarily support agencies working to promote or restore health. When an agency providing health care is supported by private volunteers, it is called a **voluntary (private) agency.** Support is generally through private donations, although many of these agencies apply for governmental grants to support some of their activities.

Voluntary agencies often begin when a group of individuals band together to address a health problem. All their services may initially be performed by volunteers. Later, they may obtain enough donations to hire personnel, staff an office, and expand services. They may be able to secure ongoing funding through grants or organizations such as the United Way. Examples of voluntary health agencies are the Visiting Nurses Association, the American Heart Association, Hospice, the American Cancer Society, and the Mental Health Association (Fig. 13–3).

Not-for-Profit and For-Profit Agencies

Another way to classify health service delivery agencies is by what is done with the income earned by the agency. A **not-for-profit** agency is one that uses profits to pay personnel, improve services, advertise services, provide educational programs, or otherwise contribute to the mission of the agency. A common misconception is that not-for-profit agencies do not ever make a profit. The reality is that they may make profits, but the profits must be used for the improvement

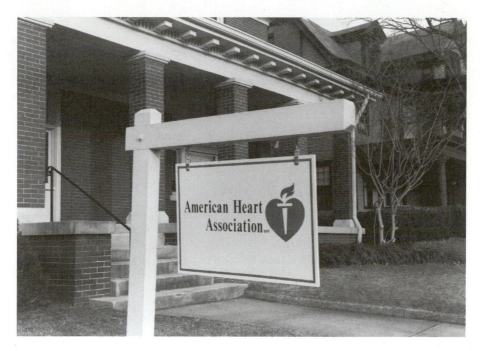

F I G U R E   1 3 – 3
Private, not-for-profit agencies provide a variety of health-related services to citizens of their communities. (Photo by Kelly Whalen.)

of the agency. Most voluntary agencies, such as the ones listed previously, are not-for-profit, as are many private hospitals.

Proprietary agencies, or **for-profit agencies,** may distribute profits to partners or shareholders. The growth in for-profit health care agencies has mushroomed over the past decade. Health care is big business and has the potential to be very profitable.

For-profit agencies include numerous home health care companies that send nurses and other health personnel to care for patients at home. There are also several large national chains of for-profit health care providers that have demonstrated that it is possible to provide quality patient care and make a profit while doing so. As the 1990s draw to a close, the home health and long-term care industries are undergoing consolidation, and many large for-profit chains are buying them and forming large regional and national networks. An issue hotly debated is that for-profit health care organizations do not typically treat nonpaying patients. These people must go to publicly funded facilities that are rapidly becoming overburdened with patients who are unable to pay their bills.

Level of Health Care Services Provided

A third way health care services are classified is by the level of health care services provided.

PRIMARY CARE SERVICES

Care rendered at the point at which a patient first enters the health care system is considered **primary care.** This may be in a student health clinic, health centers in the community, an emergency department, physicians' offices, nurse practitioners' clinics, health clinics at work sites, and many more. Aydelotte (1983, p. 812) defined the major goals of the primary health care system as providing:

1. Entry into the system.
2. Emergency care.
3. Health maintenance.
4. Long-term and chronic care.
5. Treatment of temporary malfunctioning that does not require hospitalization.

In addition to treating common health problems, primary care centers are, for many citizens, where much of the prevention and health promotion work takes place. These centers are plagued by many problems, such as lack of adequate financing, staffing, space, and community support. The unfortunate truth is that preventive services are not well reimbursed by insurance, which prevents people from seeking them and contributes to growing health costs. This pattern is changing in large part by the increasing influence of managed care, which is discussed later. Box 13–5 contains examples of primary care agencies.

SECONDARY CARE SERVICES

Secondary care involves assisting in the prevention of complications from disease, treating temporary dysfunction requiring medical intervention such as hospitalization, evaluating long-term care or chronic patients who may need treatment changes, and providing counseling and therapy that are not available in primary care settings (Aydelotte, 1983). Although hospitals have traditionally been associated with this level of care, agencies that increasingly provide secondary health services are **home health agencies,** ambulatory care agencies, skilled nursing agencies, and surgical centers. These agencies offer skilled personnel, easy access, convenient parking, compact equipment and monitoring systems, medications and anesthesia services, and a financial reimbursement program that rewards shorter lengths of stay and home or community care. It is expected that the trend toward providing community-based secondary care will continue well into the next century.

TERTIARY CARE SERVICES

Tertiary care services are those provided to acutely ill patients, to those requiring long-term care, and to those needing rehabilitation services. Tertiary care also includes provision of care to the terminally ill. It usually involves many health professionals working together on interdisciplinary teams to design treatment plans.

BOX 13-5
Examples of Primary Care Agencies

Ambulatory care centers. These centers provide a variety of services ranging from diagnostic to therapeutic; nurse practitioners and clinical nurse specialists may have pivotal roles in providing services in these centers.

Crisis centers and hotlines. Hospitals and communities typically offer services to assist citizens experiencing things such as suicide, acquired immunodeficiency syndrome (AIDS), herpes, abuse, psychiatric crisis, and so on; hotlines generally provide information and support; crisis centers may provide telephone hotlines, direct counseling, limited first aid, ongoing support, and guidance.

Day care centers. Formerly thought of for children only, these now also serve the elderly and medically or emotionally impaired; usually open during daytime hours, some may offer extended hours when there is a need; they also provide respite care for families who need a break from caring for family members in the home or who need help while they work.

Employment settings. As managers and employees recognize the benefits of healthy employees, nurses are in demand to run employee health clinics at the worksite; services may include histories and physical examinations, health teaching and promotion, health screens, and occupational safety programs.

Home health care agencies. A fast-growing service, nurses and other health care team members (social workers, physical therapists, respiratory therapists, pharmacists, and others) provide services traditionally provided in the home and hospital; even acute care services (home ventilators, intravenous therapy, chemotherapy) are provided.

Managed care organizations. To hold down health care costs, many businesses use managed care organizations to provide health care to employees at a prearranged fee; examples of these are:

- Health maintenance organizations (HMOs)—group health agencies providing basic and supplemental services to enrollees at a fixed rate; clients generally may not have much choice as to which physician will care for them; preventive care is stressed.
- Preferred provider organizations (PPOs)—groups of physicians/hospitals that provide services at a discounted rate; the client chooses which physician in the group he or she wishes to see.
- Individual practice associations (IPAs)—"middlemen" in the system; clients pay the IPA for services at a fixed rate, and the IPA pays the providers; profits are shared with the providers, and losses are absorbed by the IPA.

Neighborhood health centers. These centers are usually found in areas where citizens are underserved, financially stressed, and at risk; a variety of health care workers provide basic health care and social services support; a new addition to this category is a health care center run primarily by volunteers to provide health services to the "working poor" (those who have jobs but cannot afford health care insurance).

Physicians' offices. In general, people seek the services of the physician when they are ill; nurses working in these settings register clients, give medications, take vital signs, assist with examinations, and provide information and education.

Support groups. These groups assist individuals with ongoing coping and lifestyle changes; Reach for Recovery assists women who have had mastectomies; Alcoholics Anonymous helps alcoholics stop drinking through a 12-step program; the Dream Machine helps children who are terminally ill have one of their wishes come true. Some of these are well funded by agencies, and others are purely voluntary.

Examples of tertiary agencies are specialized hospitals such as trauma centers and specialized pediatric centers; long-term care facilities offering skilled nursing, intermediate care, and supportive care; rehabilitation centers; and hospices, where care is provided to the terminally ill and their families in the hospital, in the home, or in special centers.

SUBACUTE CARE SERVICES

A growing segment of health care, **subacute care** services, emerged in the 1990s. According to the JCAHO, this is defined as:

> goal-oriented, comprehensive, inpatient care designed for an individual who has had an acute illness, injury, or exacerbation of a disease process. It is rendered immediately after, or instead of, acute hospitalization to treat one or more specific, active, complex medical conditions or to administer one or more technically complex treatments in the context of a person's underlying long-term conditions and overall situation. Generally, the condition of an individual receiving subacute care is such that the care does not depend heavily on high-technology monitoring or complex diagnostic procedures.
>
> Subacute care requires the coordinated services of an interdisciplinary team, including physicians, nurses, and other relevant professional disciplines who are knowledgeable and trained to assess and manage these specific conditions and perform the necessary procedures. It is given as part of a specifically defined program, regardless of the site.
>
> Subacute care is generally more intensive than traditional nursing facility care and less intensive than acute inpatient care. It requires frequent (daily to weekly) patient assessment and review of the clinical course and treatment plan for a limited time period (several days to several months), until a condition is stabilized or a predetermined treatment course is completed (JCAHO, 1995, p. 3).

Subacute care falls between hospital care and long-term care. In the mid-1990s, this was one of the fastest-growing segments of the health care delivery system and provided employment opportunities for nurses and other health care team members who lost jobs when hospitals downsized. The goal is to provide lower-cost health care and create a seamless transition for patients moving through the health care system.

IMPACT OF MANAGED CARE

A new paradigm is emerging in the health care industry—**managed care.** Interestingly, it is one that has *health*, not illness, as one of its primary goals. As the 1990s progressed, the rising cost to employers of providing health care benefits to their employees, growing taxpayer unrest about the rising cost of tax-funded health care programs, and concern about ineffective and inefficient health care systems lent strong impetus to the managed care model. Already strong in traditionally progressive markets such as California, Oregon, and Minnesota, the movement took off elsewhere in the 1990s.

Managed care, in contrast to the fee-for-service system, is an organized system in which a defined group of people receive health care services for a predetermined fixed fee. The fee is usually negotiated for a period of one to three years. A managed care system includes a full range of integrated health care services, facilities, and products and has the patient's access to services coordinated and managed by a primary care provider. The primary care provider, sometimes called a **gatekeeper,** is responsible for all referrals for tests as well as to services of specialists.

Most managed care systems manage costs by use of a payment system called **capitation.** Under this system, fees are paid per person or *per capita*, and a primary care provider assumes financial responsibility for coordinating patient care within the capitated rate for all his or her patients. The provider is given a maximum amount of money per person no matter how many or how few services are used. Keeping patients healthy means the primary care provider gets to keep more of the fee. Some people worry that this will discourage gatekeepers from ordering diagnostic tests and referring patients to specialists, even when indicated.

Hallmarks of good managed care systems include well-defined clinical standards, pathways, and procedures; incentives to reduce health care expenditures; discounted fees and services from providers; quality functional outcomes measured regularly; and lower levels of hospital usage by patients.

Managed care organizations can drive costs down. They enroll people and provide care for a set price. They save money by limiting options in types of care, limiting numbers and type of providers, and using standards of care to guide providers in rendering the most cost-effective care. Concerns about the quality of care notwithstanding, managed care is expected to grow (Fig. 13–4).

Future growth for managed care will depend on several factors. First, there must be increased interagency cooperation to streamline and redesign care delivery and improve patient satisfaction. Second, growth will depend on improving the actual health of enrollees. By switching to a prevention paradigm, the high costs of illness care can be managed and reduced. How well managed care ultimately performs will depend on its ability to change the health care delivery system so that it embraces health promotion and illness prevention as well as providing high-quality, cost-effective illness care.

HEALTH CARE TEAM

At one time, physicians and nurses were the only members of the health care team. As health care became more complex and technology expanded, a number of other health disciplines developed. Today, there are many different health care team members who come from a variety of backgrounds. Deciding which of these various personnel need to be involved in the care of a patient depends on the patient outcomes that must be achieved.

Once physicians were the only coordinators of patient care. In contemporary practice, the coordination of services is likely to be governed by an individual known as a case manager. Case managers, who most often are nurses, recognize the contribution of each discipline in achieving the desired outcomes and bring a team together to plan, deliver, and evaluate the desired outcomes in the most

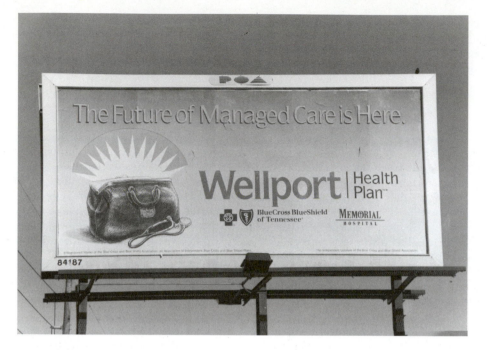

FIGURE   13–4
Managed care has created a highly competitive health care market, as this billboard demonstrates. (Photo by Kelly Whalen.)

cost-effective manner. The role of the nurse as case manager is discussed more fully in Chapter 14.

Key Members of the Health Care Team

In addition to nurses, there are dozens of health care workers who serve from time to time on interdisciplinary health care teams. Several of the key members who are most likely to be involved in the care of patients are mentioned.

PHYSICIANS

Physicians have completed college and three to four years of medical school and are licensed by a state board of medical examiners. Although it is not required to practice medicine in all states, most physicians have also completed a residency in a hospital setting, and many do postgraduate work in a specialty area.

Physicians are responsible for the medical diagnosis and medical therapies designed to restore health. Although physicians have traditionally been involved mainly in restorative care, many are coming to recognize the value of illness and injury prevention and health promotion. These activities have not been reimbursed by most insurance companies, and there has been little financial incentive to do so. Changes in some physician reimbursement plans, however, have dramatically increased reimbursement for preventive care.

DIETITIANS

Many patients require management of their nutritional intake as part of the healing process. Others need to know how to prepare and eat a healthy diet. **Dietitians** have baccalaureate degrees and may have completed internships. They understand how the diet (oral or intravenous) may affect a patient's recovery and promote and maintain health. They focus on the therapeutic value of foods and on teaching people about therapeutic diets and healthful nutrition.

PHARMACISTS

Pharmacists prepare and dispense medications, instruct patients and other health workers about the medications, monitor the use of controlled substances such as narcotics, and work to reduce medication errors. The number and complexity of drugs available today require special education and training in their preparation, dispensing, monitoring, and evaluation of actions and effects on patients.

Pharmacists may pursue either a bachelor's degree in pharmacy, which takes five years, or a doctor of pharmacy, which takes six years. Depending on state licensing requirements, they may also be required to do an internship. They are assisted by pharmacy technicians.

PARAMEDICAL PERSONNEL

A number of personnel are educated to assist physicians in the diagnosis of patient problems. This connection with medicine identifies them as **paramedical** staff.

Laboratory technologists handle patient specimens such as blood, sputum, feces, urine, and body tissues to be examined for cancer or other abnormalities (Fig. 13–5). Laboratory technologists carefully subject these body substances to various tests to determine whether or not the patient needs treatment. Technologists have at least a bachelor's degree and are often assisted by laboratory technicians, who have two-year degrees. They must pass a licensing examination to practice.

Radiologic technologists perform x-ray procedures. Although patients still need routine x-rays, technology in this field has become sophisticated. Subspecialties such as computed tomography (CT), magnetic resonance imaging (MRI), and positron-emission tomography (PET) have evolved. These are all ways of "seeing" what is going on inside the body without surgery. All require specially educated technicians who operate multimillion-dollar equipment. Although some radiology technicians are still trained "on the job," most are educated in formal

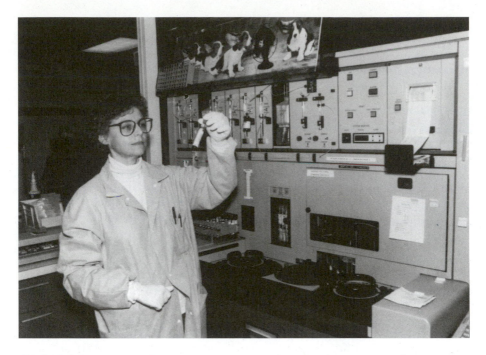

F I G U R E   1 3 – 5
A laboratory technologist examines a patient specimen for abnormalities and prepares a
report for the treatment team. (Photo by Kelly Whalen.)

programs lasting from one to four years. Radiologic technologists have a bachelor's degree. They must be registered with the state in which they practice.

RESPIRATORY TECHNOLOGISTS

Acutely ill or injured patients often require assistance in breathing. Respiratory technologists operate equipment such as ventilators, oxygen therapy devices,
and intermittent positive-pressure breathing machines. They also perform some
diagnostic procedures such as pulmonary function tests and, in some facilities,
blood gases. With the increase in respiratory care in the home and community,
these health care team members are working closely with home health agencies
and community health centers. They must complete either a two-year (technician) or four-year (technologist) educational program and in some states must
complete an internship.

SOCIAL WORKERS

The impact of illness and injury on patients and their families can often be profound. Financial problems may arise if the breadwinner cannot work or if in-

surance benefits are inadequate. Interruption of the normal family relationships may produce family crises. Lack of knowledge about community support systems may hinder the discharge of a patient from the hospital, home health care, or long-term care facility.

The **social services** worker is specifically educated and trained to assist patients and their families with these and many other life and social challenges. They hold either a bachelor's or master's degree. Social workers serve as liaisons between hospitalized patients and the resources and services available in the community. In addition, social workers frequently are called on to assist other health care personnel to cope more effectively with the stresses associated with caring for patients in crisis.

THERAPISTS

Several types of **therapists** help patients with special challenges. Physical therapists, or physiotherapists, assist patients to regain maximum possible physical activity and strength. They focus on assessing preillness or preinjury function, current damage, and potential for recovery. They then develop a long-term plan for gradual return to function through exercise, rest, heat, and hydrotherapy. Physical therapists, who have a minimum of a bachelor's degree, also supervise physical therapy assistants, who hold associate degrees.

Occupational therapists work with physical therapists to develop plans to assist patients in resuming the activities of daily living after illness or injury. They may help patients learn how to cook, take care of their own hygiene, or drive a specially equipped car with the physical capacity left to them. In addition, they assist patients to learn skills to return to previous employment or retrain patients for new employment options. Occupational therapists have bachelor's degrees. Other types of therapists include recreational therapists, art and music therapists, and massage therapists.

ADMINISTRATIVE SUPPORT PERSONNEL

In all organizations, there are administrative functions that must be performed: answering phones, directing visitors, scheduling patient tests, payroll, billing, filing insurance claims, filing forms, paying bills, system support, and others. These activities require considerable time. By hiring administrative staff, the clinical staff is freed to concentrate on direct patient care services.

Keeping complete and accurate medical records is an extremely important administrative function that ensures proper insurance billing and legal protection of the hospital and its staff. Registered records administrators are vital members of the administrative staff (Fig. 13–6). At one time, these professionals worked in what was known as the medical records department. Medical records departments are now referred to as "health information services."

The administrative staff ensures that the operations of the facility run smoothly and that clinicians have the resources necessary to meet patient needs. They also educate the clinical staff on the financial realities of the environment and work with the staff to find ways to provide quality care at the lowest possible cost.

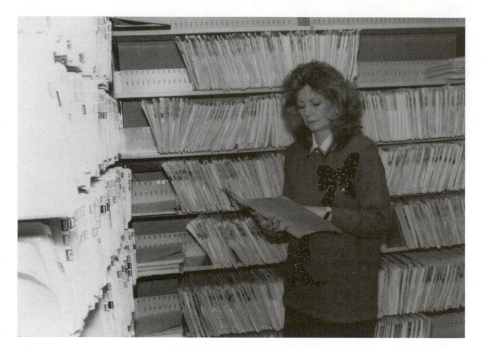

FIGURE   13-6
This registered records administrator is a highly trained professional whose work is vital to the health care agency by which she is employed. (Photo by Kelly Whalen.)

SUMMARY

The health care delivery system in the United States is a fragmented and complex system that provides illness prevention, health promotion and maintenance, diagnosis and treatment, and rehabilitative and long-term care. Health care agencies are classified as governmental or voluntary, for-profit or not-for-profit, or according to level of care provided. The interdisciplinary health care team consists of an array of professionals. Each member has an important part to play in ensuring the best patient outcomes. The trend to managed care will play a major role in the re-engineering of health care systems in the future and will affect professional nursing in many ways, most of which are yet unknown.

REVIEW AND DISCUSSION QUESTIONS

1. Using the yellow pages of your telephone directory or a directory of social services, identify local health services falling in the categories of health promotion, illness prevention, diagnosis and treatment, rehabilitation, and long-term care. Judging from the numbers of each, where does the health care emphasis in your community seem to be?

2. Obtain the organizational chart of a health care facility. Examine it to see how nursing fits into the overall structure. Who reports to the nurse executive, and to whom does the nurse executive report? What other administrative staff members are on the same level with the nurse executive? Are nursing decisions centralized or decentralized?

3. Hold a panel discussion on reimbursement. Invite representatives from government, a managed care organization, an insurance company, a major employer, and a nonprofit charity to discuss how managed care has affected their organizations.

4. Interview a nurse and one or more nonnurse health professionals. Ask them to share some of their experiences as members of interdisciplinary health care teams during downsizing or restructuring of their institutions. What impact have these initiatives had on the way they care for patients?

5. Go to the library and scan the local newspaper for the past month for articles about local health care institutions. Look also for their advertisements. What are the major activities they are initiating? Do the local hospitals seem to be joining one another in collaborative projects, or are they still engaging in fierce competition?

REFERENCES

Aydelotte, M. K. (1983). The future health care delivery system in the United States. In N. L. Chaska (Ed.), *The nursing profession: A time to speak.* New York: McGraw-Hill.

Borawski, D. B. (1995). Ethical dilemmas for nurse administrators. *Journal of Nursing Administration,* 25(7/8), 60–62.

Deming, W. E. (1986). *Out of the crisis.* Cambridge, MA: Massachusetts Institute of Technology, Center for Advanced Engineering Study.

Deming, W. E. (1982). *Quality, productivity, and competitive position.* Cambridge, MA: Massachusetts Institute of Technology, Center for Advanced Engineering Study.

Hammer, M., and Stanton, S. (1995). *The reengineering revolution.* New York: Harper Business.

Joint Commission on Accreditation of Health Care Organizations (JCAHO) (1995). *Survey protocol for subacute programs.* Oakbrook Terrace, IL: Author.

Jenkins, J. E. (1991). Shared governance: The missing link. *Nursing Management,* 22(8), 26–28, 30.

U.S. Department of Health and Human Services (1990). *Healthy people 2000: National health promotion and disease prevention objectives.* Washington, D.C.: Author.

14

Jennifer E. Jenkins

Nursing Roles in the Health Care Delivery System

OBJECTIVES

- Differentiate among four historical nursing care delivery systems.
- Discuss the purpose of differentiated levels of practice.
- Describe the five professional accountabilities.
- Discuss a variety of roles for the nurse in the health care delivery system.
- Identify skills the nurse needs when working with interdisciplinary teams.
- Recognize the legal responsibilities of registered nurses in supervising unlicensed personnel.

VOCABULARY

accountability	collaboration	patient advocate
ancillary workers	delegate	primary nursing
autonomy	differentiated practice	professional
case management	entrepreneur	accountabilities
nursing	functional nursing	supervision
change agent	interdisciplinary team	team nursing

Chapter 13 covered aspects of the health care delivery system, discussed the organizational structure of health agencies, and reviewed the various roles of members of the health care delivery team. This chapter takes a closer look both at nursing from an historical perspective and at how nursing is integral to the health care delivery team today and into the future.

TYPES OF NURSING CARE DELIVERY SYSTEMS

As seen in Chapter 1, pre–World War I nurses cared for the sick in the patients' homes. As hospital care improved and nursing education evolved, more sick people were treated in hospitals. Providing care to groups of patients rather than individuals required nurses to be efficient and use their time effectively. Various types of care delivery systems were designed to meet the goals of efficient and effective nursing care. Several types of patient care delivery systems are in use today. Four historical systems—functional nursing, team nursing, primary nursing, and case management nursing—are reviewed.

Functional Nursing

By the 1930s, advances in medical technology had evolved to a point at which hospital treatment surpassed that which could be provided at home. As more patients were admitted to hospitals, more nurses were employed to care for them.

The functional approach to nursing care grew out of a need to provide care to large numbers of patients. It focused on organizing and distributing tasks, or functions, among the personnel. Trained nurses provided care that required higher skill levels, and untrained workers with little skill or education performed many less complex tasks.

In **functional nursing,** personnel worked in isolation, each performing his or her tasks. The goal of functional nursing was efficient management of time, tasks, and energy. Although this practice saved hospitals money, patient care was fragmented, and patients had to relate to numerous personnel. There was no one person they could call, "My nurse."

Today, functional nursing is still used in some settings. It is particularly useful when there are few personnel available, such as at night, on weekends, and on holidays. It often is combined with another method, however, and is rarely used as the sole care delivery method (Bernhard and Walsh, 1990). Table 14–1 lists advantages and disadvantages of functional nursing.

Case Study: Functional Nursing

A registered nurse (RN) on the evening shift at a local nursing home has been assigned to administer special skin care treatments to bed-bound patients, change dressings, and give all medications. A licensed practical nurse (LPN) monitors all patient temperatures and blood pressures, weighs patients, records the amount they eat and drink, and monitors the blood sugar of diabetic patients. The nursing assistants have each been assigned a different group of patients for whom they are responsible dur-

TABLE 14–1
Advantages and Disadvantages of Functional Nursing

Advantages	Disadvantages
Efficient—can complete many tasks in a reasonable time frame	Care is fragmented—emphasis on task, not person
Workers do only tasks they are educated to do	Patients do not know who their nurse is
Promotes organizational skills—each worker must organize his or her own work	RNs have little time to talk with patients or render personal care
Promotes worker autonomy	

ing the shift. They help these patients with personal hygiene; see that they receive their meals and snacks; and assist them with eating, toileting, and other tasks. Because it is evening, the head nurse is not there. In her place is a charge nurse, who signs all charts, indicating that care was administered; talks with physicians and family members; and orders supplies and medications.

As they go about their work, there is little interaction among the personnel. Often they can be heard telling a patient who asks for something, "I'm not assigned to do that tonight. I'll tell the other nursing assistant that you need something."

Team Nursing

In response to the frustration some nurses felt when using the functional approach to patient care, Lambertson (1953) designed **team nursing.** She envisioned nursing teams as democratic work groups with different skill levels represented by different team members. They were assigned as a team to a group of patients.

Team nursing has been widely used in hospitals and long-term care facilities. The members of the team are often an RN, who serves as team leader, an LPN, and one or more certified nursing assistants.

The team leader is ultimately responsible for all the care provided but **delegates** (assigns responsibility for) certain patients to each team member. Each member of the team provides the level of care for which they are best prepared. The least skilled and experienced members care for the patients who require the least complex care, and the most skilled and experienced members care for the sickest patients who require the most complex care.

Team nursing allows the team leader to shift, match, and redistribute patient assignments to team members according to their level of education and expertise. For example, because of the acuity level (extent of illness) of a group of patients, a team leader may "trade" another team leader a nursing assistant for an additional RN. The nursing assistant works on the team with less acutely ill patients, and the team with the sickest patients has an extra RN.

Team nursing enables the RN team leader to supervise, coordinate, and manage the care given to all the team's patients for the assigned shift (Fig. 14–1). Often the team approach is closer to functional nursing because the team leader delegates without overseeing the care given by team members or patient outcomes. The team leader reports to the head nurse.

Case Study: Team Nursing

The team leader for 12 patients on a medical-surgical unit during the night shift has one LPN and one certified nursing assistant (CNA) on his team. First, the RN team leader makes visits to all patients' rooms to assess their conditions.

Based on those assessments, he assigns the LPN to five patients. Three patients had surgery within the past three or four days and are recovering without complication. The other two have routine conditions.

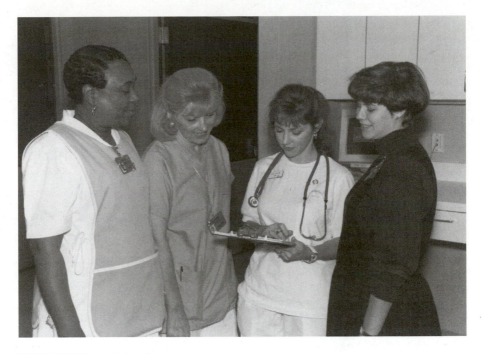

F I G U R E   1 4 – 1
A registered nurse team leader coordinates patient care with other team members.
(Photo by Kelly Whalen.)

The nursing assistant is assigned to two patients who are ready for discharge tomorrow, two more who are within two days of discharge, and one newly admitted patient who will have surgery tomorrow.

One patient has had surgery that day and has intravenous fluids as well as a lot of pain. There is a family member spending the night with him. The team leader takes this patient himself but does not overload himself with patients because he needs the flexibility to assist where needed and to supervise the other team members. During the night, the team leader also develops and updates nursing care plans on all the team's patients.

In team nursing, the RN team leader oversees all care for a particular shift, makes assessments, and documents responses to care. The LPN team member provides direct care by performing treatments and procedures and reports patient responses to the team leader. The CNA provides routine direct, personal care.

Similar to functional nursing, team nursing has both advantages and disadvantages (Table 14–2).

Advantages and Disadvantages of Team Nursing

Advantages	Disadvantages
Potential for building team spirit	Constant need to communicate among team members is time-consuming
Provides comprehensive care	
Each worker's abilities are used to the fullest	All must promote teamwork or team nursing is unsuccessful
Promotes job satisfaction	Team composition varies from day to day, which can be confusing and disruptive
Decreases nonprofessional duties of RNs	

Primary Nursing

Developed by Manthey (1980), **primary nursing** was designed to promote the concept of having an identified nurse for every patient during the patient's stay on a particular unit. The goal of primary nursing is to deliver consistent, comprehensive care by identifying *one* nurse who is responsible, has the authority, and is accountable for the patient's nursing care outcomes for the time the patient is on that unit.

In primary nursing, each newly admitted patient is assigned by the head nurse, or the staff, to a primary nurse. Primary nurses assess their patients, plan their care, and write the plan of care. They care for their patients when they are at work and delegate responsibility to associate nurses when they are off duty. Associate nurses may be other RNs or LPNs.

Patients are divided among primary nurses in such a manner that each nurse is responsible for the care of a group of patients 24 hours a day. Unless there is a compelling reason to transfer a patient, the primary nurse cares for the patient from admission to discharge from the unit. These nurses know their patients well and can enjoy a feeling of accomplishment and completion when the patients leave the hospital.

Primary nursing is similar to practice in other professions because there is a continuing relationship between the professional nurse and the patient. It promotes both **autonomy** and **accountability** because one nurse is responsible for all the nursing care for the patient. The primary nurse may be assisted by other care providers (RNs, LPNs, aides, technicians) but retains accountability for care outcomes 24 hours a day for the time the patient is on the unit. The primary nurse communicates effectively with associate nurses caring for the patient on other shifts and with primary nurses on other units when the patient transfers (e.g., operating room, intensive care unit).

Case Study: Primary Nursing

A primary nurse in a rehabilitation hospital is assigned a new patient. He is a 25-year-old man who sustained a spinal cord injury in a diving accident. He has been in a trauma intensive care unit, and now that his condition has stabilized, he has been transferred. He is paralyzed from the shoulders down.

TABLE 14–3
Advantages and Disadvantages of Primary Nursing

Advantages	Disadvantages
High patient and family satisfaction	Difficulty hiring all RN staff
Promotes RN responsibility and authority	Nurses do not know other patients—cannot "cover" for each other
Patient knows nurse well, and nurse knows patient well	Stress of round-the-clock responsibility
Cost-effective	Heavy responsibility, especially for new nurses
Promotes professionalism	
Promotes job satisfaction and sense of accomplishment for nurses	

In addition to providing direct care and writing the care plan, the primary nurse assesses that the patient's wife of two months has few sources of emotional support and is growing anxious about the future. In addition, she feels guilty about her anger and frustration over this dramatic change in their life plans.

The primary nurse acknowledges and discusses these feelings. She explains that patients and family members often have angry feelings under similar circumstances. She refers the couple to a rehabilitation psychologist who works with them in replanning and reprioritizing their life goals.

Primary nursing has several advantages. A major advantage is that owing to the amount of time they spend with patients, primary nurses are in a position to deal with the entire person—physical, emotional, social, and spiritual. Other advantages and disadvantages of primary nursing are listed in Table 14–3.

Case Management Nursing

The most recent evolution in nursing care delivery systems is **case management nursing.** In many ways, it is a return to the type of nursing practiced before patients were cared for primarily in hospitals. Begun in the late 1980s as another attempt to improve the cost-effectiveness of patient care, case management ensures that patients receive the services they need from the entire health care team in an efficient manner while holding costs down (Fagin, 1990). In most case management systems, nurses serve in the role of case manager.

Nursing case management evolved from several different models, two of which are often referred to as *within the walls* case management and *beyond the walls* case management. Although different in scope, the principles for both are the same. Nurses are coordinators, integrators, and collaborators ensuring that the desired health care needs of and outcomes for the patient are met while using the fewest resources. Key skills for nurses in these roles include critical thinking, communication, advocacy, negotiation, holistic planning and evaluation, and the ability to set both long-term and short-term goals. Additionally, facility in using modern technologies such as computers, modems, facsimile machines, and cellular phones is a necessity.

The New England Medical Center and the Center for Case Management in Boston, Massachusetts, developed a within-the-walls nursing case manager role for select patients—about 20 percent of the hospital population—whose care was either complex or required the use of many health care resources (Bower, 1992). These nursing case managers are primary nurses on various units, usually medical-surgical units. They not only care for these patients while on their assigned units, but also manage the plans of care from admission to discharge, crossing interdepartmental lines. Although the nursing case managers do not physically provide care in all units, they actively collaborate with primary nurses assigned to the patients in those units. This model is similar to that of a family practice physician who coordinates medical care for a hospitalized patient but defers to the expertise of a specialist physician if the patient is in the intensive care unit.

In this nursing model, Critical Paths are used for all patients. A Critical Path, such as the Sickle Cell CareMap shown in Chapter 5 (see Fig. 5–1) is an interdisciplinary agreement showing who will provide care in a given time frame to achieve agreed-upon outcomes. The use of Critical Paths is intended to standardize patient care and allow hospitals to plan staffing levels, lengths of stay, and other factors that heretofore could not be anticipated. Variances in the path are identified. Using continuous quality improvement methodology, health care team members review data periodically to determine if variations are patient induced, staff induced, or system induced. Once identified, they attempt to plan solutions to reduce variances.

Another form of case management nursing began at Carondelet St. Mary's Hospital and Health Center in Tucson, Arizona (Bower, 1992). Often known as beyond the walls case management, the nurse case managers work about 30 percent of their time in the hospital and 70 percent outside the hospital. Similar to their counterparts in New England, they are partners with their patients. Also similar to the New England model, this model reflects a professional practice model of nursing using principles of shared governance; acuity-based billing for nursing care; and salaried, rather than hourly, pay status for the case managers. The nurse case manager in this "multi-setting case management model" is part of a large network (i.e., hospital, clinic, home health agency, long-term care) and may provide services anywhere in the system (Fig. 14–2).

Other case management models may be found in health maintenance organizations (HMOs), managed care organizations (MCOs), third-party payers (e.g., insurance companies), public health departments, physicians' offices, home health agencies, and long-term care facilities. As can be seen from the type of activities they engage in, case managers do complex and challenging work. In most cases, these are nurses with at least five years of clinical experience. Occasionally, social workers, psychologists, rehabilitation counselors, or other professionals may also serve as case managers. All case managers, regardless of their discipline, work to reduce the cost of providing services through coordination of care providers across the continuum of care. They work closely with equipment suppliers to get the best price on medical equipment and supplies. As seen in the Research Note in Chapter 13, concern continues about whether the emphasis on cost reduction has an effect on quality of care. In the end, reasonable cost and high quality must both be provided if adequate resources are to be available for health care in the future.

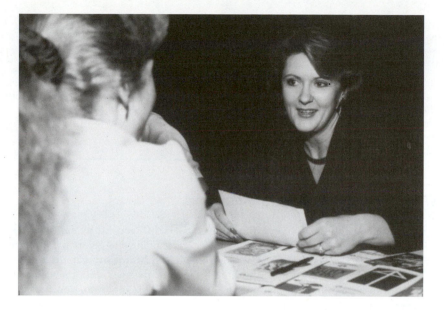

FIGURE   14–2
The nurse case manager continues to work with the patient after discharge.
(Photo courtesy of Memorial Hospital, Chattanooga, TN.)

Case Study: Case Management Nursing

An RN case manager is working with a patient scheduled for a modified mastectomy the following day. He explains the sequence of events to the patient and family and tells them what to expect. He gives the patient and family a tour of the hospital, including the surgical suite and postanesthesia care unit.

As her case manager, he follows the patient after surgery and may or may not provide direct nursing care. He makes sure a "Reach to Recovery" volunteer from the American Cancer Society is called in to see his patient before she leaves the hospital and that she has a follow-up home visit planned with the volunteer. He talks with the patient's family members, especially her spouse, to help them understand their own feelings and anticipate those of the patient.

Before discharge, he provides any discharge planning or teaching she may need. He makes sure she has a follow-up appointment scheduled with the surgeon and that she has transportation to the appointment. After discharge, he makes a home visit with the patient to check on her progress and report back to the physician. If indicated, he refers her to an ongoing support group, such as Y-ME.

Advantages and disadvantages of case management nursing are shown in Table 14–4.

TABLE 14–4
Advantages and Disadvantages of Case Management Nursing

Advantages	Disadvantages
Nurse has increased responsibility	Requires additional training
Promotes collaboration with other health professionals	Requires nurses to be off unit for periods of time
Cost-effective	Time-consuming
Eases patient's transition from hospital to community services	

Differentiating Levels of Practice

A continuing issue in the delivery of nursing care is differentiating among the levels of nursing practice. Historically, nurses with different levels of education were used interchangeably in hospitals. Nursing graduates qualify for the same license, and in many settings, diploma, associate degree, and baccalaureate nurses all function under the same job description. This sometimes creates a discrepancy between the competencies nurse managers expect of new graduates and their actual competencies.

The goal of **differentiated practice** is to define two levels of practice. This implies that there are also two levels of education and could lead to two levels of licensure. This is a difficult issue with which nurses have been struggling for years.

Clearly differentiating two levels of practice would promote understanding of nursing practice in terms of technical skills needed to provide care, interpersonal skills needed for care, and leadership skills to manage care. In the mid-1980s, the W. K. Kellogg Foundation funded the South Dakota Statewide Project for Nursing and Nursing Education. This project lasted for two years. The project participants described the differentiated associate degree in nursing (ADN) and bachelor of science in nursing (BSN) competencies as follows:

> The BSN cares for focal clients who are identified as individuals, families, aggregate, and community groups. The level of responsibility of the BSN is from admission to postdischarge. The unstructured setting is a geographical and/or situational environment that may not have established policies, procedures, and protocols and has the potential for variation requiring independent nursing decisions. The ADN cares for focal clients who are identified as individuals and members of a family. The level of responsibility of the ADN is for a specified work period and is consistent with the identified goals of care. The ADN is prepared to function in a structured health care setting. The structured setting is a geographical and/or situational environment where the policies, procedures, and protocols for the provision of health care are established and there is recourse to assistance and support from the full scope of nursing expertise (Primm, 1988, p. 2).

Table 14–5 compares selected competencies of ADN and BSN nurses.

Only one state, North Dakota, has adopted a model of differentiated nursing education and practice. There, associate degree nursing graduates are LPNs and

TABLE 14–5
Comparison of Differentiated ADN and BSN Competencies

ADN	BSN
Clients	
Individuals and family members	Individuals; families; aggregate and community groups
Level of responsibility	
For a specified work period	From admission to postdischarge
Type of setting	
Structured; other personnel available	Unstructured; other personnel may not be available

ADN, Associate degree in nursing; BSN, bachelor of science in nursing.
Data from Primm, P. (1987). Differentiated practice for ADN and BSN prepared nurses. *Journal of Professional Nursing*, 3(4), 218–225.

baccalaureate nursing graduates are RNs. Although this model has been in place since the early 1990s, other states have been slow to follow. This is an issue that creates great division within the ranks of nursing itself. To deliver high-quality care in the future, however, it will be necessary to differentiate among nurses with regard to the level of care they are best prepared to provide. This issue should become an increasing focus of attention by professional nursing associations in the future.

Five Professional Accountabilities

In all settings, professional nurses must have five **professional accountabilities** for which they are responsible. These accountabilities are described in Box 14–1 and include the areas of practice, quality improvement, research, education, and management. Each accountability takes on more or less importance depending on the role a nurse assumes. For example, staff nurses' accountabilities are primarily in the areas of clinical practice and quality improvement. They also may have secondary accountabilities in other areas; for example, they may advise managers about management of resources, precept new orientees, and join a research discussion group to learn about research being done by other nurses.

Nurse managers have primary accountability to manage resources so that the clinical staff has what they need to provide care. They also advise the clinical staff in areas of practice and quality improvement. They collaborate with nurse educators on staff orientation and continuing education programs. They may work with nurse researchers to identify needs for research to define new and better nursing practices.

Novice nurses usually concentrate on the accountabilities central to their jobs. Later, as they gain confidence and competence, they gradually expand their scope to include all five professional accountabilities.

B O X 1 4 – 1
Five Professional Accountabilities Inherent in the Role of the Professional Nurse

Practice
- Define standards of care (patient outcomes).
- Define standards of practice (interventions).
- Define standards of performance (job/position descriptions and expectations).
- Management of interdisciplinary collaborative relationships.
- Define career advancement criteria.
- Select and manage the conceptual framework and/or care delivery system.

Quality Improvement
- Develop measurement tools and methods for applying to:
  Standards of care
  Standards of performance
  Standards of practice
  Career advancement
- Develop and administer the nursing plan for continuous quality improvement referring to the appropriate group(s) or individual(s) for resolution of variances.
- Integrate unit-based quality improvement activities.

Research
- Review the literature for nursing research pertinent to current work environment.
- Identify opportunities for nursing research.
- Develop mechanisms and forums for validating current practice.
- Develop mechanisms for studying ways to improve care through new nursing interventions and/or new ways of applying existing interventions.

- Disseminate information on nursing research to the nursing staff.
- Review requests for nursing research and approve as appropriate, ensuring safety of clients and staff, full disclosure, and minimized risk.

Education (Competency)
- Foster a positive environment for learning and teaching.
- Evaluate need for and develop competency-based educational programs (orientation, inservice, continuing education).
- Measure the outcomes of nursing education programs.
- Manage the relationship between schools of nursing and the care facility.
- Monitor effectiveness of nursing's communication and develop interventions for improvement as needed.
- (Recognize that both the individual and the corporation have responsibility for insuring competency).

Management
- Coordination, allocation, and management of human, fiscal, material, support, information, and system resources needed to deliver care to patients and to foster healthy, productive working relationships.

(Adapted with permission of Porter-O'Grady, T. (1992). *Shared governance implementation manual.* St. Louis: Mosby Year Book; Jenkins, J. (1991). Professional governance: The missing link. *Nursing Management,* 22(8), 26–28, 30.)

NURSE'S ROLE ON THE HEALTH CARE TEAM

Nurses fulfill a number of roles on the health care team. They are perhaps the most flexible of health professionals and do a number of things well. This section provides an overview of several aspects of the nursing role.

Provider of Care

Nurses provide direct, hands-on care to patients in all health care agencies and settings. As providers, they take an active role in illness prevention and health promotion and maintenance. They offer health screenings, home health services, and an array of health care services in schools, workplaces, clinics, physicians' offices, and other settings. They are instrumental in the high survival rates in trauma centers and newborn intensive care units. Nurses with advanced nursing degrees are increasingly providing care at all levels of the health care system. Their breadth and depth of knowledge, their ability to care holistically for patients, and their natural partnership with physicians are making them some of the most sought after care providers.

Educator

Nurse educators teach patients and families, the community, other health care team members, students, businesses, and government. In hospital settings as patient and family educators, nurses provide information about illnesses and teach about medications, treatments, and rehabilitation needs. They help patients understand how to deal with the life changes necessitated by chronic illnesses (Fig. 14–3). Nurses also teach how to adapt care to the home setting when that is required.

In community settings, nurses offer classes in injury and illness prevention and health promotion. Often, these classes are jointly taught with other health care team members. For example, a nutritionist and a nurse may teach a group of expectant parents how to prepare formula and feed their infants. Nurses also have a responsibility to understand and teach how a healthful or unhealthful environment may affect both the short-term and long-term health of the community.

Nurses are often the key educators on the health care team. They teach other team members about the patient and family and why different interventions may have varying degrees of success. Nurses help other team members find cost-effective, quality interventions that are desired and needed by the patient rather than wasting resources on ineffective, inefficient, undesired, or unneeded services.

Nurses also serve as teachers of the next generation of nurses. Nursing students need educators who set high standards and ideals and who help students understand the ethical choices that all health care providers must make.

Counselor

People who experience illness or injury often have strong emotional responses. It is clear that the relationship between emotions, the mind, and the body is crit-

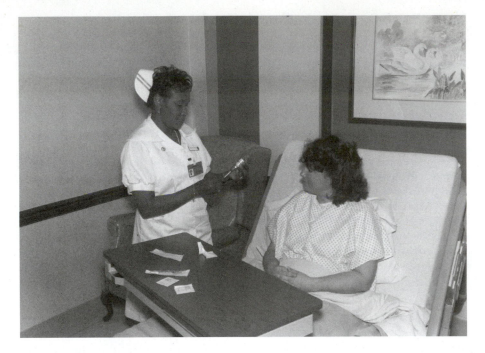

F I G U R E   1 4 – 3
A nurse educates a newly diagnosed diabetic patient about her insulin injections.
(Photo by Kelly Whalen.)

ical to promotion of and restoration to health. As counselors, nurses provide basic counseling and support to patients and their families.

Using therapeutic communication techniques, nurses encourage people to discuss their feelings, to explore possible options and solutions to their unique problems, and to choose for themselves the best alternatives for action. They also serve as bereavement counselors to terminally ill patients and their families. Nurses may, with advanced education and certification, provide psychotherapy services, which extend beyond the basic counseling role.

The nurse's role as counselor often overlaps with the roles of social workers, psychiatrists, spiritual advisers, and mental health specialists. Because nurses are with patients more, they have opportunities to respond to the emotional needs of patients as they occur.

Manager

The effective management of nursing resources is essential. With budgets ranging from hundreds of thousands to many million dollars, nurse managers of patient care units in hospitals manage "businesses" larger than many small companies. Nurse managers must have strong leadership, financial, marketing, systems, and organizational behavior skills.

Chief nurse executives may manage more than 1000 employees and multimillion-dollar budgets. They interact with other top executives and community leaders, often sitting on the health care organization's board of directors. Nurse executives must ensure the quality of nursing care within financial, regulatory, and legislative constraints. As noted in Chapter 13, nurses frequently serve as patient care executives, chief operating officers, and chief executive officers.

All nurses are managers, however. The bedside staff nurse must manage the care of a group of patients and decide what priorities are, which staff members to assign to patients, and how to accomplish all the activities during an 8- or 12-hour period. Nurses are also involved in case management or managed care. In this role, nurses review patient cases and coordinate services so that quality care can be achieved at the lowest cost. With health care costs escalating, managed care is one way to distribute scarce resources to the greatest number of patients.

Researcher

As discussed in Chapter 12, whether research is a nurse's primary responsibility or not, all nurses should be involved in nursing research. Nurse researchers investigate whether current or potential nursing actions achieve their expected outcomes, what options for care may be available, and how best to provide care. Nursing research looks at patient outcomes, the nursing process, and the systems that support nursing services. Participation by all nurses in research is essential to the growth and development of the nursing profession. See Research Note.

Collaborator

With so many health care workers involved in providing patient care, **collaboration** among the professions is important. The collaborator role is an important one for nurses to ensure that everyone has the same patient outcomes in mind. Collaboration requires that nurses understand and appreciate what other health professionals have to offer. They must also be able to interpret to others the nursing needs of patients. More about collaboration with professional colleagues is in Chapter 18.

An often overlooked collaborative function of nurses is collaboration with patients and families. In planning nursing care, patients should always be involved to the full extent of their interests and abilities. Involving patients and their families in the plan of care from the beginning is the best way to ensure their cooperation, enthusiasm, and willingness to work toward the best patient outcomes.

Change Agent (Intrapreneur)

When changes are needed in the nursing system, nurses themselves can serve as agents of change. Most professional nursing education programs include change theory as part of their management courses, and graduates are prepared to become change agents in their work settings. The role of **change agent** is one that

RESEARCH NOTE

McLaughlin and colleagues looked at how restructuring has affected nursing care services in acute care hospitals. Several components were assessed: nursing care delivery models, registered nurse skill-mix trends, assignment of nonnursing personnel to the nursing department, use of unlicensed assistive personnel, and registered nurse role changes.

Methods used in this study included literature review and a descriptive cross-sectional, investigator-designed survey instrument. The sample was 295 hospitals whose chief nurse executives were members of the California Organization of Nurse Executives. Unique specialty hospitals were excluded. Forty-nine hospitals responded.

Respondents reported that restructuring had the following effects in their settings:

- Changes in nurse manager responsibilities.
- Use of a variety of nursing care delivery systems.
- Decrease in the use of registered nurses.
- Increase in the use of nonnursing personnel by the nursing department.

- Widespread use of patient acuity systems to determine personnel needs.
- Increased use of unlicensed assistive personnel.
- Moderate to profound changes in the registered nurse role.
- Key registered nurse roles reported included team leading, delegation, allocation of personnel, evaluation of patient outcomes and team performance, patient care management, and the assignment of unit tasks and duties.

Restructuring of the health care delivery system has many implications for nurses. Nurses need to anticipate changes, prepare for changes in knowledge and skills, and work with other disciplines to ensure that patient care outcomes are maintained at a high level.

The authors caution that their sample was restricted to one state and the number of hospitals participating was limited. They therefore recommended that other studies be done to validate their results.

(Adapted with permission of McLaughlin, F. E., Thomas, S. A., and Barter, M. (1995). Changes related to care delivery patterns. *Journal of Nursing Administration*, 25(5), 35–46.)

requires a combination of tact, energy, creativity, and interpersonal skills. Change is often resisted, particularly if people are comfortable with the "old way" and believe it works. The role of change agent within a health care organization has been dubbed *intrapreneurship* (Manion, 1990) in the belief that it requires the same kind of initiative and risk taking that entrepreneurship requires (Box 14–2).

Entrepreneur

Nurse **entrepreneurs** are becoming more common. As you learned in Chapter 5, nurses now have businesses of their own that provide direct patient services in hospitals, community settings, businesses, schools, homes, and many other settings. Nurse entrepreneurs provide consultation and education services to nurses and other health team members. They provide services to businesses by con-

---

BOX 14-2
Self-Assessment: How Intrapreneurial Are You?

If you answer "yes" to more of these questions than you answer "no," you have the personality characteristics to become an intrapreneur.

- Do you like to spend time thinking of ways to make things work better?
- Are you willing to take risks that you view as reasonable?
- Do you enjoy ambiguity because it stimulates your creativity?
- Do you think of new ideas while driving to work, taking a shower, or exercising?
- When you have a new idea, can you visualize the steps to take to get it done?
- Do you have more energy than most people you know?
- Do you like the challenge of new tasks and projects?
- Are you willing to work extremely hard at problems or tasks when you

believe you can make a difference in how they turn out?
- Are you good at influencing others to accept new ways of doing things?
- Do you have a good sense of humor? Can you laugh at yourself?
- Do you like to consider the possibilities rather than the limitations in a situation?
- Can you mobilize the necessary resources (time, energy, people, materials) when a job needs to be done?
- Can you work collaboratively with others on your ideas?
- Do you learn from your failures?
- Have you found ways to give yourself positive feedback so you are less reliant on the feedback of others?

(Adapted with permission of Manion, J. (1991). Nurse intrapreneurs: The heroes of health care's future. *Nursing Outlook*, 39(1), 18-21.)

---

ducting worksite wellness programs and by advising human resource staff on how to provide high-quality health benefits to employees while reducing their costs.

PATIENT ADVOCATE

Because hospitals and the entire health care system are so complex, patients sometimes "fall through the cracks." Others need someone to help them negotiate their way through the system. They need to know how to cut through the levels of bureaucracy and red tape to get what they need when they need it.

Health care institutions often have special positions for **patient advocates.** Nurses who occupy these positions must value patient self-determination, that is, patient independence and decision making. In this role, nurses sometimes help patients bend the rules when it is in the patient's best interests and no one else will be harmed by doing so. Patient advocates are nurses who realize that policies are important and govern most situations well but that policies occasionally can, and should, be broken. For example, special care units often have strict visiting hours. Family members may be allowed in to see the patient for only 10 minutes each hour. If a patient's recovery will be faster if the family is present, the nurse, serving as a patient advocate, will allow the family members

---

B O X 1 4 – 3
Nursing Roles

- Provider of care
- Teacher
- Counselor
- Manager
- Researcher

- Collaborator
- Change agent
- Entrepreneur
- Patient advocate

---

more generous visitation than the policy provides. Box 14–3 lists the roles nurses fulfill.

TEAM-BUILDING SKILLS

For years nurses have tried to implement care teams that included all disciplines providing care to a particular patient to discuss, agree on, and deliver complex care to patients. Too often, nurses were frustrated in achieving success because of a variety of problems: a lack of skill in developing and managing teams; a lack of incentive for other health care team members to participate; and a failure of the system to sanction, support, create, and encourage opportunities for this.

Because of the emphasis on continuous quality improvement, re-engineering, restructuring, and changing reimbursement patterns, nurses now find themselves at the center of **interdisciplinary teams.** These teams often have their performance reviews or compensation (or both) linked directly to achieving quality patient outcomes at the lowest cost.

Nurses managing interdisciplinary teams must know how to manage people as equals and not as subordinates because other team members are frequently experts in their fields (radiology technicians, physicians, social workers, physical therapists, laboratory technicians, and so on). In many settings, there is no permanent team leader. The member who has the most relevant expertise becomes the team leader until other needs emerge. Then leadership changes. Nurses must be prepared to participate both as leaders and as members of these teams and to assume and relinquish the leadership role to meet best the needs of patients and the team.

Most members of such teams, including nurses, are cross-trained to perform duties not traditionally associated with their scope of practice. The goal with cross-training is to have personnel who are flexible in meeting patient needs. Managing this diverse group requires tact, diplomacy, a genuine respect for the contribution of each team member, flexibility, and the ability to "think outside the box." The last-mentioned quality is demonstrated when a person's mind is open to solutions that are nontraditional and challenge current thinking and practice. For many nurses who have fought hard for their "turf," sharing it with others is intimidating. For others, it is a freeing experience that permits them to experience truly collaborative relationships on equal footing with other professionals (Fig. 14–4).

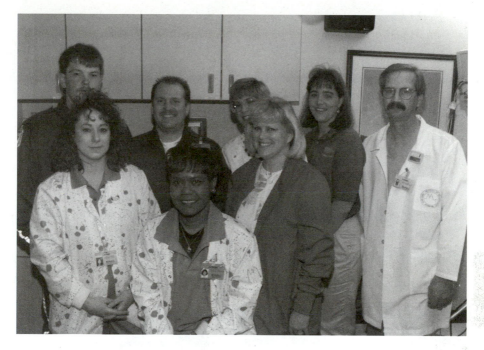

F I G U R E   1 4 – 4

Working with this emergency department interdisciplinary team—composed of a nurse, physician, emergency medical technicians, radiology technician, respiratory therapist, physical therapist, medical technician, and nursing assistant—requires the nurse to use all of her team-building skills. (Photo by Kelly Whalen.)

LEGAL ISSUES IN THE DELIVERY OF NURSING CARE

As the need for **ancillary workers** such as nursing assistants increased, nurses were asked to supervise more unlicensed assistive personnel. In making assignments and delegating tasks to these workers, nurses must determine what the workers can safely and effectively do. Nurses should consider the following questions: What can I legally delegate to unlicensed personnel? What is my responsibility to them, to the patient, and to the facility?

Licensed nurses are responsible and accountable for actions that require nursing assessment and judgment. These actions are clearly identified in each state's nurse practice act. It is not currently the responsibility of unlicensed workers to recognize that they should or should not perform a patient care activity. In the future, boards of nursing may choose to prosecute nonlicensed health care workers for their actions, but at present, they clearly hold RNs responsible for the actions of unlicensed personnel.

Most state nurse practice acts, through the rules and regulations developed to clarify them, make statements about the responsibilities of RNs where unlicensed personnel are concerned. For example, the *Administrative Rules of the Ten-*

nessee Board of Nursing (1995) state that "failing to supervise persons to whom nursing functions are delegated or assigned" constitutes negligence on the part of RNs. **Supervision,** the initial direction and periodic inspection of the actual accomplishment of a task, is an important activity for professional nurses and is closely related to **delegation.** If nurses delegate responsibility to other health care personnel, they are legally responsible for providing adequate supervision as well. Delegation to another person does not absolve RNs from accountability for the nursing care of all patients under their care. You may want to review the summary of the *American Nurses Association Guide to Safe Delegation* in Chapter 4 (see Box 4–4). More about the complex legal responsibilities of RNs is found in Chapter 20.

SUMMARY

There are a number of systems of nursing care delivery, each of which has advantages and disadvantages. Functional nursing, team nursing, primary nursing, and case management nursing were reviewed in this chapter. Each was presented in its theoretical or pure form, but in reality, there are many variations in use today.

Either satisfaction or frustration can result from the match between nurses' expectations and the system of care. When interviewing for a position, nurses must assess the delivery system carefully to make sure it is congruent with their values about nursing practice. In addition, nurses must understand the laws regulating delegation of nursing tasks and supervision of unlicensed personnel.

Nurses often serve as liaisons between the health care system and patients and their families. In doing so, they use a variety of roles, such as provider of care, teacher, counselor, manager, researcher, collaborator, change agent, and patient advocate in meeting patients' needs.

As members of interdisciplinary care teams, nurses are often leaders. Equally important is the flexibility to allow others to assume leadership when their expertise is needed. Respect for the contributions of each member is paramount in working effectively with interdisciplinary teams.

REVIEW AND DISCUSSION QUESTIONS

1. Compare and contrast the four types of nursing care delivery systems from the viewpoint of the patient. If you were a consumer of nursing care, which system would you prefer? Why?
2. Look at the same question from the standpoint of the nurse. Which system would you find most satisfying in terms of your practice? Which would you like least?
3. Talk to a practicing nurse and find out which system(s) he or she has used to deliver care. What were the strong and weak points?
4. Obtain your state's nurse practice act and read the passage relating to registered nurses' responsibilities for unlicensed personnel. Initiate a class discussion of the implications for professional nurses.

5. Interview nurses in practice in your community to determine how they apply the five professional accountabilities on a daily basis. Which roles emphasize different accountabilities?
6. From your own experiences as a consumer of nursing care, identify all the nursing roles you have encountered. Share these with at least one classmate.
7. If possible, interview nurses from different countries. How does their approach to providing nursing care differ from nursing in the United States? In what ways is it similar?

REFERENCES

Bernhard, L. A., and Walsh, M. (1990). *Leadership: The key to the professionalism of nursing.* (2nd ed.) St. Louis: Mosby Year Book.

Bower, K. A. (1992). *Case management by nurses.* Washington, D.C.: American Nurses Publishing.

Fagin, C. M. (1990). Nursing's value proves itself. *American Journal of Nursing,* 90(10), 17–30.

Jenkins, J. (1991). Professional governance: The missing link. *Nursing Management,* 22(8), 26–28, 30.

Lambertson, E. (1953). *Nursing team organization and functioning.* New York: Columbia University.

Manion, J. (1990). *Change from within: Nurse intrapreneurs as health care innovators.* Kansas City, MO: American Nurses Association.

Manthey, M. (1980). *The practice of primary nursing.* Boston: Blackwell Scientific Publications.

McLaughlin, F. E., Thomas, S. A., and Barter, M. (1995). Changes related to care delivery patterns. *Journal of Nursing Administration,* 25(5), 35–46.

Porter-O'Grady, T. (1992). *Shared governance implementation manual.* St. Louis: Mosby Year Book.

Primm, P. L. (1988). Differentiated nursing care management/patient care delivery system. *Kansas Nurse,* April 1988, 2.

Primm, P. L. (1987). Differentiated practice for ADN and BSN prepared nurses. *Journal of Professional Nursing,* 3(4), 218–225.

Tennessee Board of Nursing. (1995). *Administrative rules.* Nashville, TN: Author.

15

Barbara R. Norwood

Essentials of the Nursing Process

OBJECTIVES

- Explain the purpose of the nursing process.
- Identify the steps in the nursing process.
- Explain the difference between subjective and objective patient data.
- State nursing diagnoses using the PES format.
- Discuss two frameworks for prioritizing nursing diagnoses.
- Differentiate between short-term and long-term patient goals.
- Determine the difference between psychomotor, cognitive, and affective goals.
- Explain how outcome criteria are used to evaluate goals.
- Differentiate between nursing orders and medical orders.
- Explain the differences between independent, interdependent, and dependent nursing actions.
- Describe evaluation and its importance in the nursing process.
- Identify three types of nursing care planning formats.

VOCABULARY

affective goal
analysis
assessment
cognitive goal
consultation
defining characteristics
dependent intervention
evaluation
implementation
independent intervention
interdependent
  intervention

long-term goal
North American Nursing
  Diagnosis Association
  (NANDA)
nursing diagnosis
  (diagnoses)
nursing order
nursing process
objective data
outcome criteria
patient interview
planning

primary source
protocol
psychomotor goal
secondary source
short-term goal
signs
subjective data
symptoms
tertiary source

The **nursing process** is a method used by nurses in solving patient problems in professional practice. It is an outgrowth of the scientific method and can be used as a framework for approaching almost any problem. Yura and Walsh (1983) defined the nursing process as "a designated series of actions intended to fulfill the purposes of nursing—to maintain the patient's wellness—and, if this state changes, to provide the amount and quality of nursing care the situation demands to direct the patient back to wellness." They went on, "if wellness cannot be achieved, then [the purpose of the nursing process is] to contribute to the patient's quality of life, maximizing his resources as long as life is a reality" (p. 71).

The nursing process as a method of clinical problem solving is taught in nursing curricula across the United States, and many states refer to it in their nursing practice acts. It is now so widely accepted that the Joint Commission on the Accreditation of Healthcare Organizations (JCAHO) expects there to be evidence in each patient's record that nurses used the elements of the nursing process as the basis for clinical decision making (Joint Commission of Accreditation of Healthcare Organizations, 1992).

Somehow over the course of its development and widespread usage, the nursing process became, for some people, imbued with mystery. Exactly why is not clear, but the reality of this phenomenon is best illustrated by the popularity of lapel pins a few years ago that read, "And on the eighth day God created the nursing process, . . . and nobody has rested since." These buttons were once in vogue at nursing conferences and workshops during the time that members of the profession were adjusting to using the nursing process.

If you are a beginning student who is not sure about the value of the nursing process, read the letter in Box 15–1. It is from a student nearing graduation and describes her thoughts about the nursing process and how they have changed since she first began using it. If you are already a registered nurse who is back in school pursuing a bachelor's degree, read this chapter's Research Note to find out how other nurses feel about the nursing process.

To demystify the nursing process, let's look at a daily decision that you and most other people face each and every day: how to dress for the day. Before putting on your clothes, there are several factors you need to consider. What is the temperature expected to be? Will it be clear, raining, or snowing? How much time will be spent outdoors? Are there any activities planned that require special dress? Next, you probably look at the possible clothing choices. Some clothes may be out of season, others need repairs, and some don't fit quite right. After considering the environmental factors, the day's activities, and mood, you select the day's clothing. After dressing, you may look in a mirror to evaluate how you look. You may then modify your outfit based on your image in the mirror. At this point, you have solved the problem of clothing yourself. You have identified a problem, considered various factors related to the problem, identified possible actions, selected the best alternative, evaluated the success of the alternative selected, and made adjustments to the solution based on the evaluation. This is the same general framework nurses use in solving patient problems.

NURSING PROCESS IN HISTORICAL PERSPECTIVE

For individuals outside the profession, nursing is commonly defined in terms of tasks (*i.e.*, giving injections or starting intravenous infusions). Even within the profession, the intellectual basis of nursing practice was not fully recognized until the 1960s, when nursing educators and leaders began to identify and name the

BOX 15–1
Letter to Beginning Nursing Students

Dear Nursing Students:

I recall sitting in my first nursing class wondering how long my professor would lecture about the "nursing process." I didn't want to learn about problem-solving techniques. I didn't want to get bogged down in all the time-consuming paperwork. I wanted to save lives. You know what I mean—I was only interested in learning about the diseases, traumas, and surgeries I was sure I would be dealing with on a daily basis. What *was* all this assess, diagnose, plan, etc., stuff? I was impatient to be finished with this material and thought that once I got through the exam covering the nursing process, I would be home free. I was so naive!

I can also remember the day I realized that the nursing process had become as natural to me as walking and talking. It was during my acute care rotation when I walked into a patient's room to find him experiencing respiratory difficulty. I im-

mediately assessed the patient and began to take steps to alleviate his distress. I admit I felt a little anxious, yet I was able to take the necessary steps to bring the situation under control. If not for my knowledge of the nursing process, I am positive that I would have been unable to organize my thoughts and actions in an efficient manner while under pressure.

So my message to you is this: Relax and don't resist learning the nursing process. I guarantee this tool will help you feel more self-confident and better able to organize your time and thoughts.

Good Luck!

Elizabeth Baird
Senior Nursing Student
The University of Tennessee
at Chattanooga

(Courtesy of Elizabeth Baird.)

RESEARCH NOTE

What do nurses who provide direct patient care have to say about the nursing process? This question was posed by Patricia A. Martin and five of her colleagues as they conducted a multifaceted study of the use of the nursing process. A survey instrument entitled the "Dayton Attitude Scale Toward Care Planning" was developed and sent to more than 3000 nurses practicing in nine acute care hospitals in midwestern metropolitan areas. A total of 1096 surveys were returned. Statistical analysis of the surveys revealed that a relatively positive attitude existed toward the nursing process and nursing diagnosis. Nurses with BSNs and nurses who

had been practicing longer had higher positive attitudes than other nurses. The most common barrier to using the nursing process was lack of time, with 30 percent stating that they did not like the way care planning was done in their facility. The study suggests that improving the systems for implementing care planning would increase both the use of and positive attitudes toward the nursing process.

(Adapted with permission of Martin, P., Dugan, J., Freundl, M., Miller, S., Phillips, R., and Sharritts, L. [1994]. Nurses' attitudes toward nursing process as measured by the Dayton Attitude Scale. *The Journal of Continuing Education in Nursing*, 25[1], 35-39.)

components of nursing's intellectual processes. This marked the beginning of the nursing process.

During the 1970s and 1980s, debate about the use of the term *diagnosis* began. Up until that time, diagnosing was considered to be within the sphere of practice of physicians only. Nurses were not considered competent to diagnose patients. All this began to change in 1973 when the National Group for the Classification of Nursing Diagnosis, now called the **North American Nursing Diagnosis Association (NANDA)** published its first list of nursing diagnoses. The purpose of this group was (and is) to identify terminology and definitions that may be used and tested as nursing diagnoses.

Nursing's professional organizations have supported the use of the nursing process over the years. For example, in 1980, the American Nurses Association (ANA) in its publication entitled *Nursing: A Social Policy Statement* defined nursing in terms of diagnosis and treatment. In 1990, the American Association of Critical Care Nurses identified nursing diagnosis as the framework for conceptualizing the practice of nursing (American Association of Critical Care Nurses, 1990). In 1991, the ANA published the revised *Standards of Clinical Nursing Practice,* in which they defined competent nursing care as involving assessing, diagnosing, identifying outcomes, planning, implementing, and evaluating. The nursing process proved so useful in improving the consistency and quality of nursing care that, as mentioned earlier, the JCAHO included nursing diagnosis as one of six elements of nursing care that had to be documented for institutions to achieve accreditation (Joint Commission of Accreditation of Healthcare Organizations, 1992).

The 1995 revision of *Nursing's Social Policy Statement* includes the following statements (p. 9):

> Nurses identify the human responses to actual or potential health problems they observe and name their conceptualization of the diagnosis using a variety of classification systems. Diagnoses facilitate communication among health care providers and the recipients of care and provide for initial direction in choice of treatments and subsequent evaluation of the outcomes of care.

The *Statement* goes on to describe nursing assessments, interventions, and evaluation of outcomes—all of which are steps in the nursing process. Clearly the nursing process is a cornerstone of nursing practice and should be well understood by every nurse.

STEPS IN THE NURSING PROCESS

As in the scientific method, a series of steps is involved in the nursing process. This chapter discusses each of the steps and gives an example of the use of the nursing process in a clinical situation.

Step 1: Assessment

Assessment is the beginning step in the nursing process. During this step, information or data about the individual patient, family, or community are gathered.

Data may include physiological, psychological, sociocultural, developmental, spiritual, and environmental information. Patient resources such as financial or material resources that are available also need to be assessed and recorded in whatever format is in use. Each institution usually has a slightly different instrument for recording assessment data.

TYPES OF DATA

There are two different types of data that nurses obtain about patients: subjective and objective. **Subjective data** are obtained from patients as they describe their needs, feelings, strengths, and perceptions of the problem. Subjective data are frequently referred to as **symptoms.** Examples of subjective data are statements such as "I am in pain" and "I don't have much energy." The source for these data can only be the patient. Subjective data should include physical, psychosocial, and spiritual information. For nurses to be successful in obtaining subjective data, some of which are quite private, patients must view nurses as trustworthy.

The second type of patient data is **objective data.** These are data that the nurse obtains through observation, examination, or consultation with other health care providers. These data are factual, not colored by patients' perceptions, and include patient behaviors observed by the nurse. Objective data are frequently called **signs.** An example of objective data that a nurse might gather includes observing that the patient, who is lying in bed, is diaphoretic, pale, tachypneic, and holding his hand to his chest.

Objective data and subjective data usually are congruent; that is, they usually are in agreement. In the situation just mentioned, if the patient told the nurse, "I feel like a rock is sitting on my chest," the subjective data would substantiate the nurse's observations (objective data) that the patient is having chest pain. There are times, however, when subjective and objective data are in conflict. An example of incongruent subjective and objective data would be an emaciated teenager stating, "I'm too fat."

SOURCES OF PATIENT DATA

Patient data can be obtained from many sources (Fig. 15–1). The patient is considered the only **primary source.** Sources of data such as the nurse's own observations or reports of family and friends of the patient are considered **secondary sources. Tertiary sources** of data include medical records and information gathered from other health care providers such as physical therapists, physicians, or dietitians.

METHODS OF COLLECTING PATIENT DATA

A number of methods are used when collecting patient data. An important one is the **patient interview.** This usually involves a face-to-face interaction with the patient and requires the nurse to use the skills of interviewing, observation, and listening. The environment in which the interaction occurs or other internal and

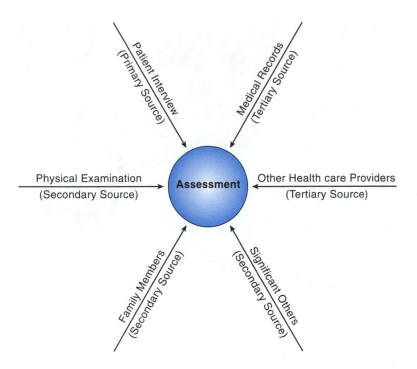

Patient Interview (Primary Source)

Medical Records (Tertiary Source)

Physical Examination (Secondary Source)

Assessment

Other Health care Providers (Tertiary Source)

Family Members (Secondary Source)

Significant Others (Secondary Source)

F I G U R E   1 5 – 1
Sources of patient data.

external factors can influence the amount and the type of data obtained. For example, when interviewing a patient who is having difficulty breathing, the data obtained may be limited. Likewise, if the interview takes place in a cold, noisy, or public place, the type of data obtained may be affected.

A second method of obtaining data is through consultation. **Consultation** is discussing patient needs with health care workers and others who are directly involved in the care of that patient. Nurses also consult with patients' families to obtain background information and their perceptions about the patients' needs.

Physical examination is the third method for obtaining data. Nurses utilize physical assessment techniques of inspection, auscultation, percussion, and palpation to obtain these data (Fig. 15–2).

ORGANIZING PATIENT DATA

Once patient data have been collected, they must be sorted or organized. A number of methods have been developed to assist nurses in organizing patient data. They include Abdellah's 21 nursing problems, Henderson's 14 nursing problems, Yura and Walsh's human needs approach, and Gordon's 11 functional health patterns. Contemporary nursing theorists continue to develop other organizing frameworks, including those of Madeleine Leininger, Sister Callista Roy, Dorothy Orem, and others (Marriner-Tomey, 1994). Nurses choose differ-

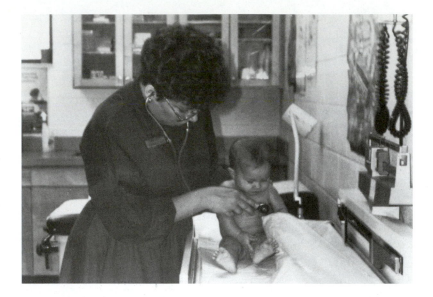

FIGURE 15–2
Physical examination is one source of objective assessment data. (Photo courtesy of the University of Akron, Akron, OH.)

ent methods of organizing patient data depending on personal preference and the method used in the agencies where they are employed.

CONFIDENTIALITY OF PATIENT DATA

A word of caution is needed in regard to patient data. Earlier, it was mentioned that patients confide personal information to nurses only if they believe the nurse is trustworthy. Patients need to know and trust that nurses share such information only with the other treatment team members. Nurses must respect patients' privacy rights and should never discuss patient information with anyone who does not have a work-related need to know.

A complicating factor in ensuring patients' privacy in this age of computer technology is that vast amounts of patient data may be stored and retrieved relatively easily. Although the issues of computer confidentiality and access to data have yet to be resolved, each nurse should commit himself or herself never to violate a patient's privacy by revealing patient information except to other members of that patient's treatment team.

Step 2: Analysis

As mentioned, during the data-gathering phase of the nursing process, nurses obtain a great deal of information about their patients. These data must be validated, then compared with norms to sort out data that might indicate a problem or identify a pattern. Next, the data must be clustered or grouped so that problems can be identified and their cause discerned. This process is known as data **analysis** and results in the identification of one or more nursing diagnoses. Knowledge from the biological sciences, social sciences, and nursing enables nurses to analyze relationships among various pieces of patient data.

NURSING DIAGNOSIS

Nursing diagnosis was defined by Gordon (1976) as "actual or potential health problems which nurses, by virtue of their education and experience, are capable and licensed to treat" (p. 1299). In 1990, NANDA defined nursing diagnosis as "a clinical judgment about individual, family, or community responses to actual or potential health problems/life processes . . . (which) provide the basis for selection of nursing interventions to achieve outcomes for which the nurse is accountable" (North American Nursing Diagnosis Association, 1990).

NANDA DIAGNOSES

NANDA has worked for two decades to develop a comprehensive list of nursing diagnoses. NANDA is a group of nursing educators, theorists, and practitioners from the United States and Canada who first met in 1973 to develop standard terminology, content, and format for nursing diagnoses. The group has continued to meet every two years to revise the original list of approved diagnoses. After each revision, new diagnoses are tested by nurses in practice settings to evaluate their appropriateness and usefulness. This is a continuing process. NANDA membership is open to all nurses interested in advancing nursing diagnosis. Box 15–2 contains the 1994 list of NANDA nursing diagnoses.

All nursing diagnoses must be supported by data, which NANDA refers to as **defining characteristics.** These defining characteristics are also known as signs and symptoms. Remember that a sign is observable, whereas a symptom is reported by the patient.

WRITING NURSING DIAGNOSES

A format that can be used to write the diagnostic statement is called the *PES format* and was developed by Gordon (1987) (Box 15–3). In this format, the *P* stands for the concise description of the problem using the NANDA diagnostic label, for example, ineffective breathing pattern. The *E* part of the statement stands for etiology and begins with the words *related to.* These related factors are conditions or circumstances that can cause or contribute to the development of the problem. To follow the example, "ineffective breathing pattern related to anxiety" explains that the cause of the ineffective breathing pattern is the patient's high anxiety level. If the cause were decreased energy or fatigue rather than anxiety, the nurse would need to select different nursing actions to solve the problem.

The last part of the diagnostic statement is *S*, which stands for signs and symp-

BOX 15–2
1994 NANDA Diagnoses

Activity/Rest
- Activity intolerance
- Activity intolerance, risk for
- Disuse syndrome, risk for
- Diversional activity deficit
- Fatigue
- Sleep pattern disturbance

Circulation
- Adaptive capacity intracranial, decreased
- Cardiac output, decreased
- Dysreflexia
- Tissue perfusion, altered (specify): cerebral, cardiopulmonary, renal, gastrointestinal, peripheral

Ego Integrity
- Adjustment, impaired
- Anxiety (specify level)
- Body image disturbance
- Coping, defensive
- Coping, ineffective individual
- Decisional conflict (specify)
- Denial, ineffective
- Energy field, disturbance
- Fear
- Grieving, anticipatory
- Grieving, dysfunctional
- Hopelessness
- Personal identity disturbance
- Posttrauma response
- Powerlessness
- Rape-trauma syndrome
- Rape-trauma syndrome: compound reaction
- Rape-trauma syndrome: silent reaction
- Relocation stress syndrome
- Self-esteem, chronic low
- Self-esteem disturbance
- Self-esteem, situational low
- Spiritual distress
- Spiritual well-being, potential for enhancement

Elimination
- Bowel incontinence
- Constipation
- Constipation, colonic
- Constipation, perceived
- Diarrhea
- Incontinence, functional
- Incontinence, reflex
- Incontinence, stress
- Incontinence, total
- Incontinence, urge
- Urinary elimination, altered patterns
- Urinary retention (acute/chronic)

Food/Fluid
- Breast-feeding, effective
- Breast-feeding, ineffective
- Breast-feeding, interrupted
- Fluid volume deficit [active loss]
- Fluid volume deficit [regulatory failure]
- Fluid volume deficit, risk for
- Fluid volume excess
- Infant feeding pattern, ineffective
- Nutrition, altered: less than body requirements
- Nutrition, altered: more than body requirements
- Nutrition, altered: risk for more than body requirements
- Oral mucous membranes, altered
- Swallowing, impaired

Hygiene
- Self-care deficit (specify): feeding, bathing/hygiene, dressing/grooming, toileting

Neurosensory
- Confusion, acute
- Confusion, chronic
- Infant behavior, disorganized
- Infant behavior, disorganized, risk for
- Infant behavior, organized, potential for enhancement
- Memory, impaired

(continued)

BOX 15–2   *(Continued)*

- Peripheral neurovascular dysfunction, risk for
- Sensory-perceptual alterations (specify): visual, auditory, kinesthetic, gustatory, tactile, olfactory
- Thought processes, altered
- Unilateral neglect

Pain/Comfort
- Pain [acute]
- Pain, chronic

Respiration
- Airway clearance, ineffective
- Aspiration, risk for
- Breathing pattern, ineffective
- Gas exchange, impaired
- Spontaneous ventilation: inability to sustain
- Ventilatory weaning response, dysfunctional

Safety
- Body temperature, altered, risk for
- Environmental interpretation syndrome, impaired
- Health maintenance, altered
- Home maintenance management, impaired
- Hyperthermia
- Hypothermia/infection, risk for
- Injury, risk for
- Perioperative positioning injury, risk for
- Physical mobility, impaired
- Poisoning, risk for
- Protection, altered
- Self-mutilation, risk for
- Skin integrity, impaired
- Skin integrity, impaired, risk for
- Suffocation, risk for
- Thermoregulation, ineffective
- Tissue integrity, impaired
- Trauma, risk for
- Violence, risk for: directed at self/others

Sexuality (Component of Ego Integrity and Social Interaction)
- Sexual dysfunction
- Sexuality patterns, altered

Social Interaction
- Caregiver role strain
- Caregiver role strain, risk for
- Communication impaired, verbal
- Community coping, enhanced, potential for
- Community coping, ineffective
- Family coping ineffective: compromised
- Family coping ineffective: disabling
- Family coping, potential for growth
- Family process, altered: alcoholism
- Family processes, altered
- Loneliness, risk for
- Parent/infant/child attachment, altered, risk for
- Parental role conflict
- Parenting, altered
- Parenting, altered, risk for
- Role performance, altered
- Social interaction, impaired
- Social isolation

Teaching/Learning
- Growth and development, altered
- Health-seeking behaviors (specify)
- Knowledge deficit [learning need]
- Noncompliance [compliance altered] (specify)
- Therapeutic regimen: community, ineffective management
- Therapeutic regimen: families, ineffective management
- Therapeutic regimen: individual, effective management
- Therapeutic regimen: individual, ineffective management

(From Doenges, M. and Moorhouse, M. [1995]. *Nurse's Pocket Guide: Nursing Diagnoses with Interactions*, 5th ed. Philadelphia: F. A. Davis. Used by permission.)

B O X   1 5 – 3
Writing Nursing Diagnoses

P = Problem
E = Etiology
S = Signs and Symptoms (defining characteristics)

---

toms or as NANDA calls them, defining characteristics. Thus, the complete diagnostic statement for the diagnosis could be, "ineffective breathing patterns related to anxiety as manifested by dyspnea, nasal flaring, shallow and rapid respirations, and use of accessory muscles of respiration."

PRIORITIZING NURSING DIAGNOSES

After diagnoses are identified, the nurse must put them in order of priority. There are two common frameworks used to establish priorities. One of these considers the relative danger to the patient. Using this framework, diagnoses that are life-threatening are the nurse's first priority. Next come those that have the potential to cause harm or injury. Last in priority are those that are related to the overall general health of the patient. Thus, a diagnosis of "ineffective airway clearance" would be dealt with before "sleep pattern disturbance," and "sleep pattern disturbance" would have priority over "knowledge deficit."

Another framework that may be used to prioritize diagnoses is Maslow's (1970) hierarchy of needs (see Fig. 10–3). When this framework is used, there is an inverse relationship between high-priority nursing diagnoses and high-level needs. In other words, highest priority is given to diagnoses related to basic physiological needs. Diagnoses related to higher-level needs such as love and belonging or self-esteem, although important, have lower priority.

Except in life-threatening situations, nurses should take care to involve patients in identifying priority diagnoses. Because varied sociocultural factors have a great impact on the manner in which patients prioritize problems, nurses must not only be aware of these factors, but also take them into consideration when planning patient care.

MEDICAL AND NURSING DIAGNOSES

Nursing diagnosis is different from medical diagnosis and was never intended to substitute for it. Rather than focusing on what is wrong with the patient in terms of a disease process, a nursing diagnosis identifies the problems the patient is experiencing *as a result of* the disease process.

An important difference between nursing diagnosis and medical diagnosis is that nursing diagnoses cover patient problems that nurses can legally treat. It would do little good for nursing diagnoses to include "appendicitis" because appendicitis is a medical diagnosis requiring surgery, and it is not legal for nurses to perform surgery. An appropriate nursing diagnosis for a patient after an appendectomy might be: "ineffective airway clearance related to incisional pain." Because it is legal in all states for nurses to provide comfort measures and to assist patients to cough and deep breathe, this would be both appropriate and a legal nursing diagnosis.

Step 3: Planning

Planning is the third step in the nursing process. **Planning** begins with the identification of patient goals. These are goals that are used by the patient and the nurse to guide the selection of interventions and to evaluate patient progress.

Just as nursing diagnoses are written in collaboration with the patient, goals should also be agreed on by both nurse and patient unless collaboration is impossible, such as when the patient is unconscious. In that event, family members or significant others can collaborate with the nurse. Goals give the patient, family, significant others, and nurse direction and make them active partners.

WRITING PATIENT GOALS AND OUTCOMES

The terms *goal* and *objective* are frequently used interchangeably. These terms are statements of what is to be accomplished and are derived from the diagnoses. Because the problem or diagnosis is written as a patient problem, the goal should also be in terms of what the patient will do rather than what the nurse will do. The goal begins with the words "the patient will" or "the patient will be able to." The goal sets a general direction, includes an action verb, and should be both attainable and realistic for the patient.

Outcome criteria are specific and make the goal measurable. Outcome criteria define the terms under which the goal is said to be met, partially met, or unmet.

Each diagnosis has at least one patient goal, and each patient goal may have several outcome criteria. Effective outcome criteria tell under what conditions, to what extent, and in what time frame the patient is to act. A sample patient goal with outcome criteria might be: "The patient will demonstrate effective bowel elimination as evidenced by having one soft, formed stool every other day without the use of laxatives or enemas within two weeks." It is easy to see that this goal is written in terms of what the patient will do (have a bowel movement at least every other day), is measurable (one soft, formed stool), gives conditions (without the use of laxatives or enemas), and has a specified time frame for accomplishment (two weeks).

Types of Patient Goals.
There are three types of patient goals: psychomotor, cognitive, and affective goals. A goal that requires motor skills or actions by the patient is a **psychomotor goal,** for example, "The patient will walk 10 feet in the hallway with a walker three times per day within one day after surgery." **Cognitive goals** deal with a desired change in a patient's knowledge level. An example of a cognitive goal might be: "The patient will list three effects of a high choles-

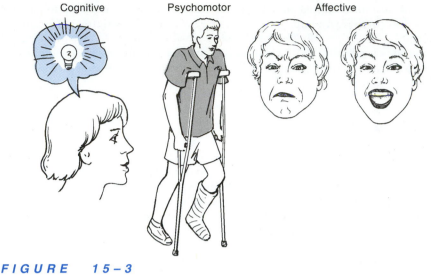

Cognitive   Psychomotor   Affective

F I G U R E   1 5 – 3
Types of goals.

terol level on the heart prior to discharge from the hospital." **Affective goals** involve a change in mood, values, attitudes, or belief systems. An example of an affective goal is: "The patient will express an increased sense of well-being after participating in an exercise program for one month." A single patient may have a combination of psychomotor, cognitive, and affective goals (Fig. 15–3).

Establishing Realistic Time Frames for Patient Goals. One aspect of goal setting not yet discussed is the estimated length of time needed to accomplish the goal. **Short-term goals** may be attainable within hours or days. They are usually specific and are small steps leading to the achievement of broader, long-term goals. For example, "The patient will lose two pounds" is a short-term goal, and the time limit for accomplishment can be brief, perhaps a week or 10 days.

Long-term goals usually represent major changes. A goal such as "The patient will lose 75 pounds" may take months or perhaps even years to accomplish, and the time frame should be set accordingly.

It is extremely important to assist patients to set realistic goals for themselves. Setting their sights too high causes frustration and discouragement in patients, families, and nurses.

SELECTING INTERVENTIONS AND WRITING NURSING ORDERS

After short-term and long-term goals are identified through collaboration between nurse and patient, the nurse writes nursing orders. **Nursing orders** are actions designed to assist the patient in achieving a stated patient goal. Every goal has specific nursing orders. Nursing orders may be carried out by a registered nurse (RN) or delegated to other members of the nursing staff.

Nursing orders and medical orders differ. Nursing orders refer to interventions that are designed to treat the patient's response to an illness or medical treatment, whereas medical orders are designed to treat the actual illness or disease. An example of a nursing order is "Teach turning, coughing, and deep-breathing exercises prior to surgery." These activities are designed to prevent postoperative respiratory problems owing to immobility. They are appropriate nursing orders because prevention of complications owing to immobility is a nursing responsibility. Nursing orders may include instructions about consultation with other health care providers, such as the dietitian, physical therapist, or pharmacist.

Step 4: Implementation of Planned Interventions

When nursing orders are actually carried out, the fourth step of the nursing process, **implementation,** begins. Most people think of nursing as "doing something" for or to a patient. Notice, however, that in using the nursing process, nurses must do a great deal of thinking, analyzing, and planning before the first actual nursing action takes place.

Nurses who skip the essential first three steps of the nursing process and jump immediately into action are not behaving in a responsible, professional manner. Patients feel a greater sense of trust in a nursing staff if both physicians' orders and nurses' orders are carried out in an orderly, planned, and competent manner.

It is difficult to make general statements about this step in the nursing process because interventions vary widely, depending on the nursing diagnosis and patient goals. Typical nursing interventions include such actions as monitoring patients' responses to medications, patient teaching, and performing certain procedures, such as changing dressings on a wound.

Very sick patients require intense nursing care. As patients improve, however, they are gradually able to assume responsibility for self-care. It is important for nurses to allow patients to do as much for themselves as their illnesses allow. Patient independence is an important step in recovery.

To implement the plan of care, nurses must possess a triad of skills: thinking or cognitive skills, doing or psychomotor skills, and interpersonal skills. If any one set of skills is lacking, the nurse's ability to implement the nursing process is significantly decreased. Implementation involves performing actions, delegating, teaching, counseling, consulting, reporting, and recording, all while continuously assessing.

TYPES OF NURSING INTERVENTIONS

Nursing interventions are of three basic types: independent, dependent, or interdependent. **Independent interventions** are those for which the nurse's intervention requires no supervision or direction by others. Nurses are expected to possess the knowledge and skills to carry out independent actions safely. An example of an independent nursing intervention is teaching a patient how to examine her breasts for lumps. The nursing practice act of each state usually specifies types of independent nursing actions.

Dependent interventions do require instructions, written orders, or supervision of another health professional, usually a physician. These actions require knowledge and skills on the part of the nurse but may not be done without explicit directions. An example of a dependent nursing intervention is the administration of medications. Although a physician or advanced practice RN must order most medications, it is the responsibility of the nurse to know how to administer them safely and to monitor their effectiveness.

The third type, **interdependent interventions,** are actions in which the nurse must collaborate or consult with another health professional before carrying out the action. One example of this type of action is when the nurse implements orders that have been written by a physician in a protocol. **Protocols** define under what conditions and circumstances a nurse is allowed to treat the patient as well as what treatments are permissible. They are used in situations in which nurses need to take immediate action without consulting with a physician, such as in an emergency department, critical care unit, or home setting.

WRITING THE PLAN OF CARE

Some health care agencies use individually developed plans of care for their patients. The nurse creates and develops a plan for each patient. Others use standardized plans of care that are based on common and recurring problems. The nurse then individualizes these standard plans of care. One of the advantages of using standardized plans is that they can decrease the time spent in generating a completely new plan each time a patient is seen. These plans are easily computer-generated, with the nurse making selections from menus to individualize the plan to the particular patient (Fig. 15–4). The amount of time needed to update and document these plans is thereby vastly decreased. Computer use also facilitates data collection for research.

Because of the decreasing average length of stay for patients in health care facilities and the increasing focus on achieving timely patient outcomes in the specific time frame permitted by reimbursement systems, many agencies have adopted the use of multidisciplinary plans of care known as critical pathways, care tracks, or care maps. See Figure 5–1, which contains a CareMap for sickle cell anemia. Multidisciplinary care plans such as the CareMap are written in collaboration with physicians and other health care providers and establish a sequence of short-term daily outcomes that are easily measured. This type of care planning facilitates communication and collaboration among all members of the health care team. It also permits comparisons of outcomes between treatment plans as well as among health care facilities.

The development of appropriate plans of care depends on nurses' ability to think critically. Nurses must be able to analyze information and arguments, make reasoned decisions, recognize many viewpoints, and question and seek answers continuously. At the same time, nurses must be logical, flexible, creative, and take initiative.

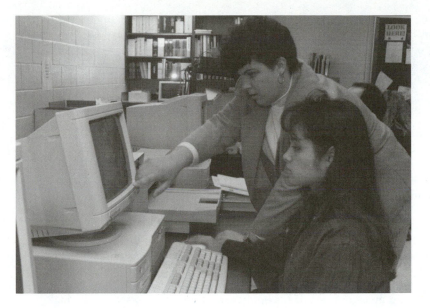

F I G U R E   1 5 – 4
In the learning laboratory, a student learns how to select nursing
interventions from a standardized plan of care. (Photo courtesy of the
University of Akron, Akron, OH.)

Step 5: Evaluation

The final step in the nursing process is **evaluation.** In this step, the nurse examines the patient's progress in relation to the goals and stated outcome criteria associated with the goals to determine if a problem is resolved, is in the process of being resolved, or is unresolved. In other words, the outcome criteria are the basis for evaluation of the goal. Evaluation may reveal that data, diagnosis, goals, and nursing interventions were all on target and that the problem is resolved.

Evaluation may also indicate a need for a change in the care plan. Perhaps inadequate patient data were the basis for the plan, and further assessment has uncovered additional needs. The nursing diagnoses may have been incorrect or placed in the wrong order of priority. Patient goals may have been inappropriate or unattainable within the designated time frame. It is possible that nursing actions were incorrectly implemented.

Evaluation is a critical step in the nursing process and one that is often slighted. It is not enough to continue to do the "right things" if the patient is not improving in the expected manner. If, on evaluation, the problem has not been resolved, the nursing care plan must be revised to reflect the necessary changes, and the process must begin again.

In addition to evaluating the individual plan of care, nurses are responsible for evaluating the quality of care that all patients receive. As discussed in chapter 13, many terms are currently used for this process including *total quality management (TQM)*, *continuous quality improvement (CQI)*, and *quality improvement (QI)*. Regardless of the terminology, the goal is the same: to improve health care and its delivery to patients.

CYCLIC NATURE OF THE NURSING PROCESS

Although the steps in the nursing process are discussed separately here, in practice they are not so clearly delineated. Nor do they always proceed from one to another in a linear fashion. As seen in Figure 15–5, the nursing process is cyclic in nature, meaning that nurses are continuously going from one step to another and then beginning the process again. Often a nurse performs two steps at the same time, for instance, observing a wound for signs of infection (assessment) while changing the dressing on the wound (intervention).

Now that you have reviewed the steps in the nursing process, let us look back at the opening scenario. The problem that was identified was the necessity to don appropriate clothing. Data, both objective (the temperature outdoors) and subjective (the mood one is in), were gathered. Selection was made and implemented, and an evaluation of the implementation was carried out by looking into the mirror. This comparison reveals that problem solving is something each person does every day. The use of the nursing process simply provides professional nurses with a patient-oriented framework with which to solve clinical problems.

An example of using the nursing process in a clinical situation is found in Box 15–4. This case study demonstrates how the nursing process becomes so ingrained that experienced nurses go through the steps almost automatically.

S U M M A R Y

The nursing process is a systematic problem-solving process that is based on the scientific method. It is used by nurses when delivering patient care. The steps in this process are assessment, analysis, planning, implementation, and evaluation.

The activities of each step were outlined and discussed. The nursing process is cyclic and dynamic, or ever-changing. Similar to any new behavior, nurses initially find that using the nursing process feels awkward or slow. After practice, however, most find it becomes a natural yet organized way to approach patient care.

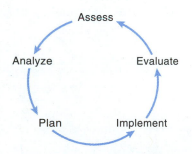

F I G U R E   1 5 – 5
The cyclic nature of the nursing process.

BOX 15–4
Nursing Process Case Study

You have just received a report from the day shift about Mr. Burkes. You were told that he had been admitted with a diagnosis of cancer of the tongue and that he had had a radical neck dissection. He has a tracheostomy and requires frequent suctioning. He is alert and responds by nodding his head or writing short notes.

When you enter his room, you note that he is apprehensive, tachypneic, and gesturing for you to come into the room. You auscultate his lungs and note coarse crackles and expiratory wheezes. You can see thick secretions bubbling out of his tracheostomy. He has poor cough effort.

Based on these data, you realize that a priority nursing diagnosis is *ineffective airway clearance*. You immediately prepare to perform tracheal suctioning. As you are suctioning, you watch the patient's nonverbal responses and note that he is less apprehensive when the suctioning is completed. You also auscultate the lungs and note decreased crackles and the expiratory wheezes are no longer present. Mr. Burkes writes "I can get my breath now" on his note pad.

I. Assessment
  A. Subjective data
  1. None owing to inability to speak
  B. Objective Data

   1. Tracheostomy with copious, thick secretions
   2. Tachypnea
   3. Gesturing for help
   4. Coarse crackles and expiratory wheezes
   5. Poor cough effort
II. Analysis
  A. Ineffective airway clearance related to copious, thick secretions
III. Plan
  A. Short-term goal: Patient will have patent airway as evidenced by absence of expiratory wheezes and crackles
  B. Long-term goal: Patient will have patent airway as evidenced by his ability to clear the airway without the use of suctioning
IV. Implementation
  A. Assess lung sounds every hour for crackles and wheezes
  B. Suction airway as needed
  C. Elevate head of bed to 45 degrees
  D. Teach patient abdominal breathing techniques
  E. Encourage patient to cough out secretions
V. Evaluation
  A. Short-term goal: Achieved as evidenced by decreased crackles and absent wheezes when auscultating the lungs

When all nurses use the nursing process, patient care is consistent, comprehensive, and coordinated. Through the use of the nursing process, nurses are able to work toward resolving patient problems in a systematic manner, thus advancing both the scientific base of nursing and professionalism.

REVIEW AND DISCUSSION QUESTIONS

1. Describe the steps in the nursing process and the activities of each step.
2. Describe a recent problem you needed to solve. Identify the steps that you used to solve the problem. Which of your steps resemble those in the nursing process?

3. Think of a recent conversation you have had and give examples of subjective and objective data from that conversation.
4. List a short-term personal goal and a long-term personal goal using all the essential elements of effective goals. Evaluate your progress toward these goals.
5. Compare the nursing process with the scientific method (chapter 12) and state how they are similar and how they differ.
6. Explain the difference between independent, dependent, and interdependent nursing interventions and give an example of each.
7. Describe the PES format for writing a nursing diagnosis.
8. Explain the difference between medical and nursing diagnosis.
9. Describe what is meant by the statement "the nursing process is a cyclic process."

R E F E R E N C E S

American Association of Critical Care Nurses (1990). *Outcome standards for nursing care of the critically ill.* Laguna Niguel, CA: Author.

American Nurses Association (1995). *Nursing's social policy statement.* Philadelphia: J.B. Lippincott Company.

American Nurses Association (1991). *Standards of clinical nursing practice.* Kansas City, MO: Author.

American Nurses Association (1980). *Nursing: A social policy statement.* Kansas City, MO: Author.

Doenges, M. and Moorhouse, M. (1995). Nurse's pocket guide: Nursing diagnoses with interactions. (5th ed). Philadelphia: F. A. Davis.

Gordon, M. (1987). *Nursing diagnosis: Process and application* (2nd ed.). New York: McGraw-Hill.

Gordon, M. (1976). Nursing diagnosis and the diagnostic process. *American Journal of Nursing,* 76(5), 1298–1300.

Joint Commission on Accreditation of Healthcare Organizations (1992). *Accreditation manual for hospitals.* Oakbrook Terrace, IL: Author.

Marriner-Tomey, A. (1994). *Nursing theorists and their work.* St. Louis, MO: Mosby.

Martin, P., Dugan, J., Freundl, M., Miller, S., Phillips, R., and Sharritts, L. (1994). Nurses' attitudes toward nursing process as measured by the Dayton Attitude Scale. *The Journal of Continuing Education in Nursing,* 25(1), 35–39.

Maslow, A. (1970). *Motivation and personality.* New York: Harper & Row.

North American Nursing Diagnosis Association (1990). *Taxonomy I revised: 1990—with official nursing diagnoses.* St. Louis: Author.

Yura, H., and Walsh, M. B. (1983). *The nursing process: Assessing, planning, implementing, evaluation.* (4th ed.) Norwalk, CT: Appleton-Century-Crofts.

C H A P T E R

16

Frances A. Maurer

Financing Health Care

O B J E C T I V E S

- Explain the economic principle of supply and demand and its relevance to health care costs.
- Cite examples of causes of health care cost escalation.
- Describe the major methods of payment for health care.
- Explain cost-containment efforts since 1975 and their impact on nursing practice.
- Describe the relationship between cost containment and quality management initiatives.
- Identify current and proposed strategies aimed at changing segments of the health care delivery system.
- Identify general guidelines for evaluating national health insurance proposals.

V O C A B U L A R Y

acuity
capitation
certificate of need (CON)
co-payment
cost containment
deductible
diagnosis-related groups (DRGs)
gatekeeper
Health Care Financing Administration (HCFA)
health care network

health maintenance organization (HMO)
Hill-Burton Act
Medicaid
Medicare
out-of-pocket payment
patient classification system (PCS)
personal payment
point of service (POS)
preferred provider organization (PPO)
premium

private insurance
professional review organization (PRO)
prospective payment system (PPS)
quality management
retrospective reimbursement
self-insurance
skill mix
third-party payment
universal care
worker's compensation

The public debate over financing health care in the United States has waxed and waned since the mid-1970s. The dilemma faced by the nation is how to provide high-quality health care services to all citizens while keeping costs down.

In 1994, the nation's health care expenditures reached $938 billion and consumed 13.9 percent of the gross domestic product (GDP), more than any other single entity. More than $2.5 billion per day was spent on medical care in the United States, a staggering amount. Estimates for the year 2005 indicate that health care costs are expected to reach $2.2 trillion (Burner and Waldo, 1995). If this trend is allowed to continue until the year 2010, one-third of all national resources will be spent on health care. Yet the health of American citizens is not as good as it should be. As a result, almost everyone agrees that there is a crisis in health care and that reform is needed.

Evidence of public concern about rising health care costs can be seen in the media. For example, the cover story entitled "MediScare" in the September 18, 1995, issue of *Newsweek* magazine featured the statement: "Young Versus Old: Who Will Carry the Burden?" (Fineman, 1995) Accompanying that statement was a cover photograph of a young man struggling to hold an older woman in a wheelchair over his head. Almost four years earlier, the November 25, 1991, issue of *Time* magazine also carried a cover story about health care costs, leading off with the statement: "There are two kinds of prices in America today: regular prices and health care prices" (Castro, 1991, p. 34). It seems that at a time when health care miracles are at an all-time high, public support for the system that created those miracles is eroding.

Most Americans believe that health care is a right, not a privilege. President George Bush, in his 1992 "State of the Union" address, affirmed that belief with his statement, "Good health is every American's right." President Bill Clinton reaffirmed that belief and attempted to make national health care reform his major domestic policy effort.

In September 1993, Clinton announced plans for national health care reform. According to a Gallup poll conducted at that time, 6 of every 10 Americans supported the President's plan. His plan, however, designed by a task force headed by Hilary Rodham Clinton, was heavily attacked by various special interest groups and failed to pass Congress. Since then, debate and confusion about the exact nature of reform and its impact on the population has reduced enthusiasm and public support for governmental action to change the health care structure.

Despite governmental inaction, major changes have been forced by business interests. Corporations and other large employers were in the vanguard of efforts to reduce health care costs, primarily because health care benefits have become a significant cost to employers. For example, during 1990, employee health care benefits consumed 26 cents of every dollar of business profits (Cuniff, 1991). General Motors alone spent $3.2 billion, more than it spent on steel, to provide health coverage for employees, their dependents, and retirees (Castro, 1991).

The cost-reduction strategies implemented by businesses placed limits on employees' treatment options and altered the payment structure of health care for many employed Americans. It seems that with or without planned, organized comprehensive change in the structure of the health care system, significant change will nevertheless continue. Finding a solution to the health care finance dilemma while maintaining quality and improving access to services is a challenge that will not easily be achieved.

Nurses and nursing practice are profoundly affected by financial issues. Therefore, students of professional nursing need to understand the overall economic context in which nursing care is provided. This chapter explores several major concepts necessary to understanding health care finance: basic economic theory, a brief historical review of the causes of health care cost escalation, current methods of payment, cost-containment efforts, the economics of nursing care, and the impact of cost containment on nursing care. Criteria to evaluate proposals for national health reform are summarized.

BASIC ECONOMIC THEORY

Nursing school curricula do not typically require undergraduates to take courses in economics, yet there is an urgent need for nurses to understand the economic context in which they practice. Economics influences the type and quality of health services provided as well as employment opportunities for nurses.

Supply and Demand

A basic economic theory is the *law of supply and demand*. According to this theory, a normal economic system consists of two parts: suppliers, who provide goods and services, and consumers, who demand and use goods and services. In a monetary environment, that is, one in which money is used as a unit of exchange, consumers exchange money for desired goods and services.

In an efficient marketplace, the market price of goods and services serves to create an equilibrium in which supply roughly equals demand, and demand roughly equals supply. When demand exceeds supply, prices rise. When supply exceeds demand, prices fall. The relationship between price and equilibrium can be seen at the clothing store. During an unusually mild winter, for example, the demand for heavy coats is likely to be low. Because demand is low, manufacturers cut back on production, and retailers stop ordering coats and place their current stock of coats on sale. If the sale price is low enough, however, people will continue to buy coats. Through fluctuations in supply and demand, created by price, equilibrium is approached. This example illustrates the principle of price sensitivity, that is, a change in demand for goods or services is a function of the change in the price of those goods or services (Feldstein, 1993). Figure 16–1 illustrates the relationships among price, supply, and demand.

Difficulty with Basic Economic Theory in Health Care

There are problems associated with applying basic economic theory in the health care market. This chapter highlights a few of those problems.

HEALTH CARE AS A RIGHT OR PRIVILEGE?

In a free market economy, consumption of any good or service is determined by an individual's ability to pay. In a pure free market, a portion of the population

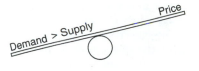 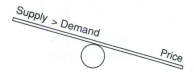

FIGURE 16–1
Price sensitivity in a normal economic environment.

would be denied health care if they were unable to pay. People who support this position consider health care a privilege. Others believe that everyone should have access to basic health care and consider health care a right.

Despite the United States's leanings toward a free market economy in general, health care is largely considered a right, not a privilege. Rather than allowing economically disadvantaged citizens to do without health services, the federal government has taken steps to ensure certain groups' access to health care services through publically funded programs such as **Medicare** and **Medicaid.** Although this is generally considered an ethical policy, it is nevertheless a policy decision that interferes with the functioning of free market principles.

PRICE SENSITIVITY IN HEALTH CARE

In pre–health insurance days when people paid their own medical bills, physicians and hospitals set their fees with some sensitivity to what patients could pay. When costs were high, patients complained. Health insurance created an indirect payment structure, **third-party payment,** that removed price sensitivity from the concern of most health care consumers because they pay only a small portion of the real costs; a third party (the employer, insurance company, or government) pays the rest. If someone other than the consumer pays, demand can increase because the consumer is insensitive to cost. This is an important point to keep in mind when reviewing the history of health care finance. History has demonstrated that when there is little or no out-of-pocket expense to the consumer, economic equilibrium is upset.

ADDITIONAL INFLUENCES ON THE HEALTH MARKET

Economists have identified a number of other factors that affect the health care market in ways that violate the assumptions surrounding an effective free market system. For example, consumers cannot always control demand for health care services. With other products, a consumer can delay a purchase until there is a sale or forego the purchase altogether. Health care is different because often health care needs are immediate. The consumer might suffer serious injury or even death by a delay in seeking services. Box 16–1 summarizes some of the other factors that reduce the efficient functioning of free market economics in the health care market.

BOX 16–1

Barriers to a Free Market Economy in Health Care

Poor Consumer Information

Individual consumers are not accustomed to "shopping" for the best available prices for medical services, supplies, and equipment. Even when the consumer is motivated to compare costs, getting that information from the suppliers of health care is difficult and time-consuming. Most consumers require services quickly and cannot afford long delays to seek information, even if they have the expertise to search out the needed information.

Ineffective Pricing System

When the price of services is based on "reasonable and customary costs of similar services" in an area, health care providers have an incentive to continue to increase their prices rather than compete by lowering prices. Eventually the new, higher price becomes the "reasonable and customary" price. Reform efforts have had some success at reducing the impact of this phenomenon by establishing prospective funding and capping reimbursement for the cost of selected services.

Health Care Providers' Interests Conflict with Consumers'

Health care providers have economic interests that can be in opposition to consumer interests. Physicians, for example, act both as suppliers of health care and demanders of patient services. When physicians are partners or stockholders in services, such as laboratories or radiographic facilities, they are more likely to order such tests, according to studies by the Department of Health and Human Services. Conversely, HMO or PPO physicians who receive incentives for not referring patients to specialists are less likely to do so.

Cost Efficiency Is Not Always a Motivator for Suppliers

Although businesses are expected to operate with cost efficiency, others, particularly some nonprofit organizations, may be influenced by other factors. By law, nonprofits cannot have a profit or surplus of funds at the end of the fiscal year, but there is no law that dictates how they spend their money. Most nonprofits operate efficiently and at the lowest cost to consumers; others have been found to use their funds to provide amenities and perks for staff and board members, such as plush exercise facilities, all-expense-paid trips, or purchase of private boxes at sports stadiums.

(Reprinted with permission of Maurer, F. A. (1995a). Financing of health care: Context for community health nursing. In Smith, C., and Maurer, F. A. (Eds.), *Community health nursing: Theory and practice*. Philadelphia: W.B. Saunders.)

HISTORY OF HEALTH CARE FINANCE

Before 1940, more than 90 percent of Americans either paid directly from their own pockets for health care or depended on charity care. Few had private health insurance. Public insurance programs, such as Medicare and Medicaid, had not yet come into existence (Eason, Lee, and Spickerman, 1988). Following World War II, most industrialized countries began publicly financed health care systems that provided care for all citizens to the extent each country could afford to do so. The United States, however, did not adopt a public, universal access system, choosing instead to continue the private, fee-for-service system.

Growth of Private Insurance

In 1943, the Internal Revenue Service (IRS) ruled that people did not have to pay income tax on health benefits paid by their employers. Providing employer-paid health benefits was a new way employers could reward employees without violating wage controls imposed during World War II to stabilize the economy. When states chose to grant tax-exempt status for hospital-owned and physician-owned private insurance companies, such as Blue Cross and Blue Shield, these private insurers grew dramatically. By 1960, two-thirds of nonelderly Americans had private health insurance, mostly paid for by employers.

Hill-Burton Act

In 1946, the U.S. Congress passed the Hospital Survey and Construction Act. Called the **Hill-Burton Act** after the congressmen who sponsored it, this law called for and funded surveys of states' needs for hospitals, paid for planning hospitals and public health centers, and provided partial funding for constructing and equipping them. Small towns, which could not have afforded community hospitals on their own, were encouraged by this legislation to build them, and many did. The scope of the Hill-Burton Act expanded until the late 1960s. With accessible, new, well-equipped hospitals in many towns and employer-paid health insurance a standard job benefit, the stage was set for dramatic increases in the utilization of hospitals and health care services.

Rise of Public Insurance Programs

The problem of paying for health care for the unemployed and the elderly was not solved by private insurance, and many continued to receive inadequate care. In 1965, Congress approved two public insurance programs to cover these groups: Medicare, which is for the elderly and certain disabled people, and Medicaid, which is for the poor. They were designed to ensure that citizens who were uninsured by employers and unable to afford their own private health insurance would be protected. At that point in time, a unique public-private partnership system of insurance that would care for all seemed to be in place. Unfortunately, that partnership has not lived up to anyone's expectations, and universal health care coverage for all Americans is still an elusive goal.

Retrospective Reimbursement

Originally, both public and private insurance plans were based on **retrospective** (after-the-fact) **reimbursement**. This meant that when Mrs. Johnson went to the hospital with pneumonia, a request for reimbursement for whatever services were rendered (chest x-rays, blood work, physical examinations, antibiotic therapy) was sent to the insurer. Depending on the terms of her insurance policy and the level of Mrs. Johnson's **deductible** (the portion she has to pay yearly before insurance coverage begins), the hospital was reimbursed for much, or even most, of the charges. **Co-payments** (the percent of charges the patient pays) were low, often as low as 10 percent. Using retrospective reimbursement, the cost of services to insured consumers of health care was extremely low or zero. Because neither the orderers of health care (physicians) nor the consumers (patients) were concerned about cost, the demand for health care services became virtually insatiable, driving costs up dramatically (Feldstein, 1993).

Cost-Containment Initiatives

From 1960 to 1993, state and federal government spending for health care more than doubled, rising from 5.3 percent of the GNP to 13.9 percent (Burner and Waldo, 1995). In the late 1960s, the Hill-Burton legislation was replaced with legislation calling for comprehensive health planning agencies. At least one agency per state was established and empowered to review the health care needs of communities. To build or expand existing facilities, a **certificate of need (CON)** had to be approved by the health planning agency. Use of existing facilities and needs of the public were examined closely before CONs were issued. The result of this attempt to cut costs was a dramatic slowing in the construction and expansion of hospitals and public health facilities nationwide (Lampe, 1987).

By 1975, additional serious cost-containment efforts were underway, stimulated by concerns about costs on the part of politicians, consumer groups, and employers. One important strategy was a move toward replacing retrospective payment for services to **prospective payment systems (PPS)**. In prospective payment systems, providers, such as physicians and hospitals, receive payment on a per-case basis, regardless of the cost to the provider to deliver the services. There is more about this and other cost-containment initiatives later in this chapter.

Continued Escalation of Health Care Costs

Despite comprehensive health planning efforts, health care costs continued to rise. In addition to the imperfect operation of a market economy in health care, other factors have affected costs. Some of the most important ones are inflation, improved technologies, increasing demand for health care services, and impact of fraud and abuse.

During the past 20 years, there were several periods of substantial inflation that affected the cost of all services, including health services. Inflation generally affects all business sectors but has tended to escalate faster in health care than in other segments of the economy.

Another reason for the rise in costs is related to the development of and demand for technology. Modern medical care depends on advanced technologies that were not even dreamed of a few decades ago. When the general public reads about these new advances, they want them to be available in their own commu-

---

BOX 16–2
Some Examples of Hospital Charges, 1995*

- Coronary bypass surgery for a 50-year-old man—$46,234.
- Bufferin tablet for a hospitalized patient—$1.50.
- Modified radical mastectomy—$9592.
- One day's intensive care for a crack baby—$2000.

- A 50-minute session with an elite psychotherapist—$175.
- Delivery of a baby by cesarean section—$7500.
- Cataract surgery for an 83-year-old grandmother—$2700.

*Does not include physician's charges.

---

nities. This leads to the proliferation of expensive machinery, often far more than a given community really needs. New technologies are extremely costly: A single x-ray machine can cost up to $250,000, and more advanced types of diagnostic imaging machines can cost up to $2 million each (Roddy, 1996, personal communication). Box 16–2 itemizes a sampling of hospital charges in 1995.

Demographics also play a role in escalating health care costs. The United States has experienced increases in both the aging and the nonelderly-but-uninsured populations. Medicare and Medicaid have improved access for the poor and elderly, two groups that previously had limited access because of inability to pay. Because older persons are more likely to have chronic illnesses, their demand for health care services exceeds that of younger segments of the population. The number of elderly is expected to continue to expand, thus increasing the demand for health care services. Although in 1996 only one in eight Americans was over 65 years of age, by 2030, this figure will increase to one in five, or 20 percent of the population (*CPR* [*Current Population Reports*], 1991).

Fraud and abuse of payment systems account for part of the problem as well. An estimated $75 billion of the United States's annual health expenditures may be due to fraud, including as much as 20 percent of all worker's compensation claims and 10 percent ($17 billion) in Medicare losses (Duston, 1996).

Health care providers such as physicians, clinics, and hospitals are on the honor system, but some intentionally cheat the system with "little fear of getting caught" (Duston, 1996, p. 2B). In June 1991, for example, a $1 billion scheme was uncovered in California. After offering free tests to learn patients' insurance information, sham "clinics" sent insurers phony bills without the awareness of the insured patients (Kerr, 1991). In February 1996, an expert in cardiac care devices testified before a Senate panel that hospitals and physicians "all around the country" defrauded Medicare and Medicaid billing systems by performing unapproved experimental procedures. This witness was willing to testify only if he was screened from view and his voice was electronically altered because he feared reprisals if his identity became known (Duston, 1996, p. 2B).

The result of upwardly spiraling costs, fueled by technology, demand for services, and fraud, is that health care costs accounted for an increasing portion of U.S. resources.

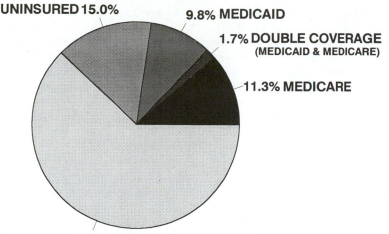

UNINSURED 15.0%   9.8% MEDICAID

1.7% DOUBLE COVERAGE
(MEDICAID & MEDICARE)

11.3% MEDICARE

62.2% PRIVATE INSURANCE

FIGURE   16–2
Source of financing for medical coverage: U.S. population 1993.
(Reprinted with permission of *Statistical Abstract of the United States.*
(1993). Washington, D.C.: U.S. Government Printing Office.)

CURRENT METHODS OF PAYMENT FOR HEALTH CARE

There are four major methods of payment for health services in use today: personal payment, Medicare, Medicaid, and private insurance. Worker's compensation is an additional mechanism for financing some health care services. Figure 16–2 represents the proportion each of the four major methods contributes to the purchase of health care.

Personal Payment

Personal payment for services is the least common method. Few people can afford **out-of-pocket payment** for more than the most basic health services. At today's prices, an illness or injury severe enough to require hospitalization can quickly exhaust a family's financial reserves, forcing them into bankruptcy. Generally, only those people without access to some form of private group insurance or public insurance rely on personal payment.

Medicare

Medicare, or Title XVIII of the Social Security Act, is a nationwide federal health insurance program established in 1965. Medicare is available to people aged 65 and over, regardless of the recipient's income. It also covers certain disabled individuals and people requiring dialysis or kidney transplants. Medicare has two separate but coordinated programs. The first, known as Part A, is a hospitalization insurance program. Part B is a supplementary medical insurance program that covers visits to physicians' offices and other outpatient services. Originally intended to be a no-cost or low-cost program for the elderly, the cost of participating in Medicare has risen steadily. By 1996, Part A required participants to pay a $736 deductible for hospitalization, and Part B required an annual $100 deductible and a monthly premium of $42.50 (*The Medicare Handbook*, 1996). Although originally designed to be all-inclusive, many elderly people now find they cannot afford to participate in Medicare. Ironically, some elderly are so poor that they qualify for Medicaid assistance in paying their Medicare premiums.

Medicaid

Medicaid, or Title XIX of the Social Security Act, is a group of jointly funded federal-state programs for low-income, elderly, blind, and disabled individuals. It, too, was established in 1965. There are broad federal guidelines, but states have some flexibility in how they administer the program. People must meet eligibility requirements determined by each state. Eligibility depends on income and varies from state to state. Rates of payment also vary, with some states providing far higher payments than others. The amount the federal government contributes to Medicaid varies from a minimum of 50 percent of total costs to a maximum of 75 percent. The differences in eligibility and payment rates lead to wide variations in the level of care provided to the poor in different states. In contrast to those on Medicare, people who receive Medicaid are not required to pay any fees to participate. Table 16–1 highlights the similarities and differences in the Medicare and Medicaid programs.

Private Insurance

Private insurance, also called voluntary insurance, is a system wherein insurance premiums are either paid by insured individuals or their employers or shared between individuals and employers. Periodic payments (**premiums**) are paid into the insurance plan, and certain health care benefits are covered as long as the premiums are paid. Early in the development of private insurance, many treatments were covered only if they were performed in an inpatient (hospital) setting. This was one of the features that tended to drive up the cost of services. Today most insurers stipulate that costs of hospitalization are reimbursable only if treatment *cannot* be performed on an outpatient basis.

Worker's Compensation

Worker's compensation constitutes a small proportion of insurance coverage. The program varies from state to state but generally covers only workers who are injured on the job. It usually covers both treatment for injuries and weekly

TABLE 16-1
Facts About Medicare and Medicaid

Medicare	Medicaid
Funded by	
Federal government	Federal and state governments
Administered by	
Federal government	State governments
Who is eligible?	
People over 65 and certain others	Poor and disabled (includes some elderly)
Level of benefits	
Same nationwide	Varies from state to state
Payment by recipients?	
Required	Not required
Coverage	
Hospitalization; outpatient care; no prescriptions or optical care	Comprehensive, including prescriptions and optical care

Data from *Health care expenditures and other data: An international compendium from the Organization for Economic Cooperation and Development.* (1989); and *Medicare and Medicaid statistical supplement.* (1995). Washington, D.C.: Health Care Finance Administration.

payments during the time the worker is absent from work for injury-related causes. In the case of accidental death, the worker's family receives compensation. Companies are required by law to contribute to a compensation fund from which money is withdrawn when accidental injuries or deaths occur (Black, 1988).

Significant Pool of Uninsured and Underinsured

The number of uninsured Americans is growing rapidly and is a grave national concern. In 1994, an estimated 39.7 million Americans, more than 17 percent of the population, had no health insurance (*AHA News,* 1996). In 1993, 51.3 million Americans, or one of every five citizens, was uninsured for some period during the year (Rowland et al, 1994). Because most nonelderly Americans are insured by job-related policies, they are at risk if they change or lose their jobs or if their employer chooses not to offer health insurance benefits. Although some uninsured people do not work, most do have part-time or full-time jobs. Davis and Schoen (1994) report that 84 percent of the uninsured are employed or are family members of employed individuals.

The uninsured are not alone in being at risk from escalating health costs. There are many more Americans who are underinsured and at substantial financial risk because their insurance plan either requires large out-of-pocket expenses or limits coverage for catastrophic illnesses. Estimates of the size of this at-risk group range from 30 to 60 million people (Jacobs, 1991; Knox, 1989).

COST-CONTAINMENT MEASURES REVISITED

Spiraling health care costs have caused both public and private insurers to examine their practices and to institute a variety of measures designed to reduce costs. This initiative is referred to as **cost containment.**

As discussed earlier, the 1970s saw attempts to control health care costs through legislation designed to regulate costs and monitor the quality of care. Comprehensive health planning agencies and CONs were two mechanisms used. Some states also practiced rate setting, in which the state set limits on reimbursements. Yet costs continued to rise. The retrospective payment method for Medicare and Medicaid had become uncontrollable. It was apparent that basic changes in payment mechanisms were required. Box 16–3 contains information about the dramatic increases in costs to taxpayers of Medicare and Medicaid since they were implemented in 1967.

The passage of the Tax Equity and Fiscal Responsibility Act (TEFRA) in 1982 stimulated a dramatic restructuring of health care delivery in the United States. Through this act, the federal government changed the payment method for Medicare from the retrospective system, which was uncontrollable, to a PPS based on **diagnosis-related groups (DRGs).** DRGs are described later in this chapter. Prospective payment was designed to create a more competitive environment and resulted in an emphasis on efficiency, cost-effectiveness, and financial accountability. It also stimulated competition among health care providers. For the first time, providers had incentives to operate in a cost-effective manner. Because PPS have the potential to encourage providers to undertreat patients to reduce costs, quality management initiatives were implemented to protect consumers.

BOX 16–3
Medicare and Medicaid Costs, 1967 and 1993

Medicare

1967*	**1993**
$5 billion	$151.1 billion

- Those helped = All elderly, regardless of family resources

Medicaid

1967*	**1993**
$2.3 billion	$12.8 billion

- Those helped in 1980 = 65 percent of the poor
- Those helped in 1993 = 36 percent of the poor
- Medicaid is the fastest-growing spending program in the United States

* First full year of operation for Medicare and Medicaid
(Data from *Health care expenditures and other data: An international compendium from the Organization for Economic Cooperation and Development.* (1989); and *Medicare and Medicaid statistical supplement.* (1995). Washington, D.C.: Health Care Finance Administration.)

Entire governmental agencies have been created to monitor and administer cost-containment programs. Private insurers have also gotten on the cost-containment bandwagon. There are several cost-containment entities of which students should be aware.

Federal Cost-Containment Programs

There are several main federal cost-containment programs that are noteworthy: the **Health Care Financing Administration (HCFA), professional review organizations (PRO)**, DRGs, and block grants. Each is reviewed briefly.

HEALTH CARE FINANCING ADMINISTRATION

HCFA is a federal cost-containment agency created to administer the Medicare and Medicaid programs. Briefly stated, HCFA's goals are:

1. To develop and establish standards to ensure that quality care is rendered to recipients of Medicare and Medicaid.
2. To improve the efficiency and responsiveness of Medicare and Medicaid and to promote beneficiary awareness.
3. To enforce standards for hospitals, nursing homes and other long-term care facilities, laboratories, clinics, and other health care facilities.

PROFESSIONAL REVIEW ORGANIZATIONS

PROs review every Medicare hospital admission to make sure that patients meet criteria for hospitalization and that their health care needs cannot be met on an outpatient basis or in a community-based setting. PROs also monitor all Medicare patients' lengths of stay. If a patient is hospitalized longer than the PRO determines is appropriate or if procedures are performed that the PRO determines are unnecessary, the hospital is denied reimbursement for the extra days and the unnecessary procedures (Dougherty, 1989). This causes hospitals to be careful about who they admit, how long they allow patients to stay, and what procedures are performed while patients are hospitalized.

DIAGNOSIS-RELATED GROUPS

A DRG is "a classification of diagnoses in which patients demonstrate similar resource consumption and length-of-stay patterns" (*St. Anthony's* . . . , 1994, p. iv). Diseases are grouped into 495 DRGs for Medicare reimbursement purposes (*St. Anthony's* . . . , 1994). For each DRG, the Medicare system has predetermined a fair price for hospital services based on averages. This represents the amount the hospital is paid by Medicare to treat patients in that particular DRG. If the hospital's costs exceed the pre-established reimbursement rate, it loses money. If the hospital is able to treat the patient successfully for less than the established reimbursement rate, it can keep the excess. This type of reimbursement system is an example of a prospective payment system (PPS).

BLOCK GRANTS

Combined with the enactment of DRGs and prospective payment, federal reform efforts in the 1980s included block grants to states. Block grants changed the funding mechanism the federal government employed to supply monies for combined federal-state programs. Instead of sharing the expense of a program, such as matching a state's expenditures on Medicaid, the block grant program gave the state a set amount of money. The state government then decided how to spend the federal and state dollars on behalf of Medicaid patients.

Since inception, block grants have reduced the proportion of health program costs paid by the federal government, while the states' shares have increased. At the same time, states have been mandated by federal requirements to provide specific health services to Medicaid patients, such as poor children and the elderly. Block grants have dramatically increased the number of dollars state budgets have been required to expend on health care, thereby forcing either tax increases or reductions in other state-funded programs. Reform proposals in the mid-1990s suggested even further reductions in federal block grants and simultaneous lowering of federal standards for mandated care. One proposal was to eliminate or reduce standards for nursing homes. If passed, this would free states to reduce health care services they provided. Concerned health professionals believed that under such a plan, the poor, especially children and the elderly, would be placed at particular risk (Berman, 1995).

Private Cost-Containment Programs

Private insurers have benefited from federal cost-containment initiatives because they tend to establish private reimbursement rates at the same level the federal government uses for reimbursing hospitals for Medicare DRGs. In addition, several other strategies focused around the managed care concept and designed to lower costs became popular with private insurers and employers.

In 1996, 100 million Americans were enrolled in some form of managed care program (Glieck, 1996). Managed care programs limit consumers' choices of treatment options or provider of care (or both) but are not intended to reduce quality of care. They include preferred provider organizations (PPOs), point of service (POS) providers, health maintenance organizations (HMOs), reduction or elimination of employer-provided health insurance, and health care networks.

PREFERRED PROVIDER ORGANIZATIONS

Preferred provider organizations are groups of physicians or institutions to which insurance companies direct their policyholders for care. These providers have agreed to provide services at discounted prices. Policyholders are provided a list of *preferred providers* from whom to choose. If they choose to use providers not on the list, they usually must pay a larger share of the costs of care. Insurers save money through PPOs because services are provided at discounted rates.

POINT OF SERVICE

Point of service is a hybrid of the PPO concept. It entails a provider network of physicians, but the consumer selects a primary care physician who acts as a **gatekeeper** in determining clients' needs for specific health services and referrals. Generally, consumers may seek care from other sources within or outside the provider network, but unless they have the express permission of the primary care physician, they incur additional costs in doing so. Some POS programs do not pay any part of services not approved by the primary physician. Some even pay physicians bonuses for reducing the number of services used by that physician's patients. Insurers save money through POS providers by discounted services, reducing services, and eliminating unnecessary specialist referrals.

HEALTH MAINTENANCE ORGANIZATIONS

Health maintenance organizations are networks or groups of providers who agree to provide certain basic health care services for a single predetermined yearly fee, called a **capitation** fee. The voluntarily enrolled participants in HMOs pay the same amount regardless of the amount and kind of services they actually receive. HMOs have an incentive to promote health maintenance and prevention of illness in the enrolled participants. HMOs benefit financially when their patients stay well because they receive the same fee whether patients use services or not.

REDUCTION OR ELIMINATION OF EMPLOYER-PROVIDED HEALTH INSURANCE

Unable to pay for employees' health care, some employers have left the system and insured their own employees (called **self-insurance**), scaled back or eliminated health benefits, limited the employees' choice of insurance plans, or passed more of the costs of insurance on to employees. In 1989, for example, 78 percent of all labor union strike activity was stimulated by employers eliminating previously provided health care benefits (Horine, 1990). Health insurance programs sponsored by employers continued to decline through the early 1990s.

HEALTH CARE NETWORKS

A **health care network** is a corporation with a consolidated set of facilities and services intended to provide comprehensive health care to its consumers. It is a private health care system. Referrals for almost all services are made within the network. Managed care and other cost-containment efforts are a significant part of any health network operation. A well-developed network includes the following components:

- A major hospital
- Several small hospitals
- A long-term care facility
- A rehabilitation center
- A home health care agency
- A subacute center (Nornhold, 1995).

Federal attempts at health care reform, although unsuccessful, spurred the formation of large health networks. Business interests, determined to survive in the changing health care market, merged and consolidated assets into larger systems. For example, early in 1996 Helix Health System and MedAtlantic Healthcare Group announced plans to merge and form BWHealth, which was expected to be one of the largest health care systems in the United States (Guidera, 1996).

Impact of Managed Care on Health Services

During the mid-1990s, the rapid growth of HMOs and related managed care organizations raised concerns that quality of care might suffer. Care decisions, formerly based on the needs of the patient, were increasingly influenced by business interests. Physicians, hospitals, and other providers were being forced to provide services for less. These conditions created shock waves in the health care industry, resulting in limits on choice and services, a drive to expand managed care to vulnerable populations, and physician gags and financial incentives to limit services.

LIMITS ON CHOICE AND SERVICES

By 1996, in an effort to lower health costs, many employers had limited employees' choice of health plans to the cheapest ones. A growing number of employers offered only managed care options. Some managed care plans moved to increase the cost (co-payments or deductibles) to consumers who used out-of-plan providers and services. Some plans refused to pay any part of out-of-plan services.

Managed care plans set stricter limits on the types of services covered than did other health insurance plans. Expensive, new therapies, such as bone marrow transplants for breast cancer, and costly treatments for rare conditions were often denied, as were referrals, especially outside the plan (Luciano, 1994; Larson, 1996). Routines services, such as hospitalization after childbirth, were also cut. News Note 16–1 describes Congressional reaction to such cuts. As managed care became widespread, concern also developed about managed care practices toward patients with psychiatric illnesses as denials and limits on coverage for chronic problems became routine (Sharpfstein, 1996).

NEWS NOTE 16–1
Getting Tough on Drive-Through Delivery

Government intervention is necessary to stop insurers from forcing mothers and newborns from the hospital too soon after delivery, Kathryn Moore, director of government relations for the American College of Obstetricians and Gynecologists, said Dec. 13 [1995].

Moore spoke at a panel discussion on the issue at a National Conference of State Legislatures meeting in Washington.

About half of the states have introduced or passed maternity-stay legislation since Maryland adopted the first such law earlier this year, Moore said.

The trend is a reaction to so-called "drive-through" deliveries—a growing insurer practice of limiting maternity-stay coverage to 24 hours or less after delivery. The obstetrician/gynecologist group and the American Academy of Pediatrics recommend 48-hour stays following a normal vaginal delivery and 96 hours for a cesarean section.

"We have a situation of insurers limiting consumers' coverage, of insurers pressuring doctors, ignoring medical guidelines and not producing any conclusive data that their practice is safe," Moore said.

Getting Tough

In some cases, insurers are overruling physicians' decisions to keep women in the hospital longer than their coverage allows, she said. Some insurers also threaten to cut physicians from the insurance panel unless they release women and infants early, she added.

State maternity-stay laws are a reaction to market forces' inability to change insurer practices, Moore said.

"Given all of these factors, government intervention is necessary," she said.

E. Neil Trautman, manager for health care policy for the U.S. Chamber of Commerce, disagreed.

"If we encourage the marketplace to respond to consumer demands, we can do better," he said.

The chamber opposes insurance-benefit mandates, Trautman said. Each mandate makes insurance less affordable and could price health coverage out of some Americans' reach, he added.

Supporters of maternity-stay legislation maintain that its price would be low.

According to Colleen Meiman, legislative assistant to Sen. Bill Bradley (D-NJ), maternity-stay legislation would only add $1.13 a year to insurance premiums. Bradley, along with Sen. Nancy Kassebaum (R-KS), sponsors federal maternity-stay legislation currently before Congress.

Bradley is looking for a measure to attach the legislation to a vote. Kassebaum said she prefers to hold hearings on the measure first and then bring it before the Senate next year.

Like the Bradley/Kassebaum bill, most maternity-stay legislation requires that insurers follow national guidelines. Many measures, including the federal proposal, permit early discharges if the physician and woman approve, and if follow-up care is provided.

Maryland has had trouble enforcing its new law, which took effect Oct. 1, 1995.

Insurers are forcing doctors to discharge women early with follow-up care, rather than giving physicians and women a choice, said Maryland Delegate Marilyn Goldwater (D-Bethesda). State lawmakers are trying to close that loophole, she said.—G.A.

(Reprinted with permission of Ashton, G. (1995). Getting tough on drive-through delivery. *AHA News*, 31(50), 3.)

DRIVE TO EXPAND MANAGED CARE
TO VULNERABLE POPULATIONS

Federal and state initiatives to reduce costs were aimed at enrolling large segments of the Medicare and Medicaid populations in managed care health plans.
The intent was to save costs related to the two programs. Critics were concerned
that these two vulnerable populations, who traditionally had poorer health status than employed adults, would not be well served by managed care. Pilot programs with Medicare HMOs reported that seniors were less satisfied and disen-
rolled more frequently than consumers covered by employer-provided managed
plans. States experimenting with using managed care to control Medicaid expenses reported that some plans practiced fraud and misrepresentation in efforts
to enroll Medicaid patients by overstating available benefits and services. In a
southeastern state, for example, one managed care organization offered a free
$10,000 life insurance policy to new enrollees during its first year of operation.
This practice was thereafter discontinued, but enrollees were not informed of the
change. In addition to these abuses, there was some evidence that Medicaid patients had difficulty negotiating the gatekeeping process to access services. They
often needed to call several times to succeed in getting an appointment or were
given appointments at geographically inaccessible sites (Khanna, 1995).

PHYSICIAN GAGS AND FINANCIAL INCENTIVES
TO LIMIT SERVICES

In 1996, a serious development involving managed care efforts to regulate dialogue between physicians and patients about treatment options came to light.
Physicians were sometimes discouraged or forbidden by their managed care contracts to mention treatment options that were expensive or not covered by a patient's managed care plan (Larson, 1996). Some plans offered physicians incentives for limiting services and referrals for their patients. U.S. HealthCare, for
example, offered physicians bonuses if they were able to reduce hospital stays,
limit emergency department use, and reduce referrals to specialists (Gray, 1996).
As seen in News Note 16–2, such bonuses placed physicians in conflict between
the best interests of patients and their own economic best interests. Physicians
who did not comply with gag requirements, called attention to bonus plans, or
exceeded average costs for services could be terminated by the plans (Gray, 1996;
Larson, 1996). These practices evoked concern by organized medicine, organized nursing, consumer groups, and in the U.S. Congress.

ECONOMICS OF NURSING CARE

Traditionally, nurses were unconcerned with the cost of care, believing all patients were entitled to high-quality nursing care regardless of ability to pay. Until fairly recently, few efforts were made to determine the actual cost of nursing
care. The average hospital bill included the cost of nursing services in the general category of "room rate," just as housekeeping services are included in the
room rate. In the past, the hospital census (number of patients) was used to de-

NEWS NOTE 16–2
HMOs "Dirty Secret" Threatens Practice, Consumer Safety

A dirty little secret in the managed care industry came under public scrutiny in December when U.S. Healthcare terminated one of its physician's contracts for violating its "gag rule." The gag rule, an increasingly used gambit among HMOs, is a clause that forbids health care practitioners from revealing certain sorts of information, including treatment options, to anyone, including patients.

David Himmelstein, MD, an associate professor at Harvard Medical School, signed on with U.S. Healthcare a year ago; he was fired when he voiced his concerns about the company's gag rule on *The Phil Donahue Show*. Specifically, the gag rule said that "physicians shall agree not to take any action or make any communication which undermines or could undermine the confidence of enrollees, potential enrollees, their employers, unions, or the public in U.S. Healthcare or the quality of U.S. Healthcare coverage." Further, the clause stated, "physicians shall keep the Proprietary Information and this Agreement strictly confidential."

The information that Himmelstein and other doctors can't share? How their pay will increase if they limit the treatments they provide or recommend. Himmelstein's HMO agreement promised him bonuses based on a formula for keeping his patients out of hospitals; if he exceeded his allotted hospitalization days, he would receive no money.

Nurses also are beginning to encounter these sort of clauses. At the year's end, *The New York Times* reported that one HMO had proposed a contract with its nurses that would pay bonuses to those RNs who helped move patients out of hospitals faster. Practices such as gag orders or monetary incentives can be violations of the professional and ethical integrity of nurses and, therefore, warrant vigilant attention. Nurses are encouraged to report such practices to their state nurses associations.

The American Nurses Association is closely monitoring these and other incidents. Upcoming issues of *The American Nurse* will include additional coverage on managed care rules and their impact on nurses.

(Reprinted with permission of *The American Nurse* (1996). 28(1), 8.)

---

termine the number of nurses needed. This worked fairly well when payment was retrospective. With the advent of prospective payment, however, it was imperative for hospitals to determine their staffing needs more efficiently.

It has long been recognized that different patients require different amounts of nursing time, depending in large part on how sick they are. Conner, working at Johns Hopkins Hospital in 1960, developed a **patient classification system (PCS)** that identified patients' needs for nursing care in quantitative terms. It was a new idea that patient needs were quantifiable, were predictable, and could help hospitals determine the need for nursing resources. For the first time, patient needs, as opposed to hospital census, could be used as criteria for determining the number of nurses needed (DiVestea, 1985). Since that time, different PCSs have been developed, most of which depend on patient **acuity,** or degree of illness, and the resulting amount and complexity of nursing care required.

Initiatives called *costing nursing services* are underway to determine the cost of nursing care precisely. It is believed that this will solve one dilemma of contemporary nurses who find themselves torn between two conflicting goals: first, their own desire to provide comprehensive patient care in the tradition of the past, when cost was no object, and second, pressure from financial managers to provide only services that are reimbursible under insurance regulations.

Not knowing the exact costs of nursing services limits nurses' ability to determine what high-quality nursing care costs and to calculate the number of hours of nursing care it takes to maintain it for each DRG. Determining the best skill mix, that is, the ratio of registered nurses to licensed practical nurses and nursing assistants on each hospital unit, is also impaired when the cost of nursing care is unknown.

In the past, it was assumed that the cost of nurses was a major part of hospital costs. When tough economic times came, the first cost reduction efforts were therefore aimed at nursing. Studies by the American Nurses Association Center for Nursing Research (McKibben, 1985) found that nursing accounted for only 20 to 28 percent of the costs of hospitalization for two-thirds of DRGs examined. Costing nursing services and developing standardized reimbursements based on cost will enhance the ability of nurse managers to control nursing resources and negotiate for a fair share of hospital financial resources.

There is some concern, however, that costing nursing services may not be beneficial to nursing. Costing strategies may make nursing more vulnerable to labor substitution efforts as hospital administrators experience increasing pressure to reduce costs. Isolating nursing costs might also lead to efforts to devalue nursing services by reducing wages or impeding salary increases (salary compression) (Buerhaus, 1995a).

Since 1983, many studies have been undertaken to determine the actual costs of nursing care. This fascinating research is expected to affect nursing practice profoundly in the future.

Impact of Cost Containment on Nursing Care

When the drive to provide high-quality nursing care meets the constraints of cost containment head-on, something has to give. What nurses hope, as both providers and consumers of health care, is that quality will not suffer because of the emphasis on "the bottom line." To many, this is a forlorn hope. Yet the financial realities that affect the institutions in which 68 percent of nurses practice—hospitals—cannot be ignored. To stay in business, hospitals must make at least enough money to pay personnel costs, maintain buildings and equipment, and pay suppliers of goods and services. One cost-reduction strategy has been to reorganize and restructure the delivery of hospital nursing services, reduce nursing personnel, and substitute unlicensed assistive personnel for registered nurses (Curtin, 1994). This strategy was explored in Chapter 13.

The financial vitality of a hospital depends in large measure on attracting physicians who will use that hospital's inpatient and outpatient services in providing medical care to their patients. A 1991 study done for the American College of Healthcare Executives by Arthur Andersen & Company examined the factors that influence physicians to seek affiliation with hospitals. When asked to rank factors, a panel of physicians ranked *quality of nursing staff* as the number-one factor affecting this choice (Arthur Andersen & Company and American

College of Healthcare Executives, 1991). If attracting physicians is essential to the financial stability of hospitals, and attracting physicians depends in large measure on the quality of the nursing staff, attaining or maintaining quality nursing care is of critical importance to the survival of hospitals.

The leadership of the American Nurses Association (ANA) has been outspoken in their assertion that overzealous cost-containment efforts have led to lower quality of hospital care. In 1996, the ANA president called on professional nurses to inform family members, friends, and acquaintances about the "eroding quality in acute care" (Betts, 1996, p. 4). ANA's "Every Patient Deserves A Nurse" campaign is a concrete step taken by the professional organization to educate the public about these concerns. News Note 16–3 elaborates on the effects of overemphasizing cost reductions in hospitals and other health care facilities.

Although hospital employment opportunities for nurses have leveled off or decreased, the dispersal of health care services into community settings is expected to continue to improve opportunities for community-based nursing services. Whether these new and expanded community settings will absorb all nursing personnel redirected from hospitals remains to be seen. Quality of care is expected to become a more important competitive feature among managed care and health network providers. To the extent that the nursing profession can link quality of care with nursing care, the demand for nursing services will continue to flourish (Buerhaus, 1995b).

COST CONTAINMENT AND QUALITY MANAGEMENT

Most people agree that there is potential for disaster if low cost is the only outcome that matters in the health care system. The challenge is to balance the cost-effectiveness and quality of patient care. Concern for maintaining high-quality services in the face of cost constraints has led to the development of a new health care initiative called **quality management.** As discussed in chapter 13, this field is growing and changing rapidly and creating change within hospitals. The interview in Box 16–4 with two nurses (Robertson, 1996, personal communication; Alexander, 1996, personal communication) involved in quality management gives insights into the complexities and satisfactions of participation in quality management initiatives.

HEALTH CARE REFORM AND NATIONAL HEALTH INSURANCE

In 1996, the United States and South Africa were the only two industrialized nations not providing universal access to health care to all citizens (Johnson, 1990). Despite the fact that 1994 health care expenditures averaged $3463 per person, infant mortality ranked twenty-second—lower than many countries with far fewer national resources. Two-thirds of inner-city children under 4 years of age did not have the full series of immunizations that could protect them from preventable childhood diseases (Burner and Waldo, 1995). There was no established minimum set of health services available to the entire population, and access to health care was not universal.

NEWS NOTE 16–3
Who's Taking Care of Mama?

The delivery of health care in America has changed a great deal. Unless you are very young, you probably remember doctors making house calls. We knew our doctors quite well and the nurses who worked with them. Those days are long gone, and with them, it's sad to say, is much of the trust that we reposed in our health care delivery system. Now, we must all ask who's taking care of mama when she goes to the hospital?

Nursing's Proud History
As a child, I dreamed of being a professional nurse. Caring for others who were not able to care for themselves was a calling for me as it has been for generations of nurses. There is simply no reward like that received for serving another human being who is depending upon you for their recovery or even their life.

Through the years, I have witnessed changes in our nursing profession that are both exciting for the professional nurse and essential for our patients. Nursing has made strides educationally and professionally that have brought it to the forefront of the national health care debate. Everyday, there is more evidence that the professional nurse is the key to successful and cost-effective health care delivery.

Research shows that when there are more nurses in a health facility, there will be lower mortality rates, shorter lengths of stay, lower costs and fewer complications. In addition to boosting health outcomes, professional nurse staffing levels are tied closely to a hospital's ability to provide care in the least costly, most highly effective means possible.

Opportunities Stifled
Despite this, changes in the health care community are stifling the opportunities that the professional nurse brings to health care delivery. Many external and internal forces, ranging from political and economic to social, are driving the health care industry to make sweeping but not yet fully evaluated changes in how, where and by whom health services are delivered.

These forces have been escalating rapidly over the past few years and include a heightened scrutiny by consumers and insurers about rising costs, pressure to move services to less expensive environments and embarrassing public health statistics. In addition, continually tightening federal reimbursement guidelines for Medicare and Medicaid have spawned a myriad of managed care networks that have resulted in even more changes.

I am disappointed to say that these forces have culminated in an institutional mentality in hospitals that is driven much more by the bottom line than by health outcomes. Health care facilities, in what they perceive as a scramble to survive, are borrowing cost-containment strategies utilized by other industries. These strategies include "downsizing" or "right-sizing" the work force to cut labor costs, and then crosstraining or "multi-skilling" remaining workers to maximize their productivity. Facilities are merging, closing and forming networks to better utilize existing services and resources—all in an effort to self-regulate and limit external controls and, perhaps, public accountability.

Dangers of Change
Professional nurses are greatly concerned about the implications of these changes in health care. Highest on the list of concerns is the impact on patient safety and quality of care and the current lack of data collection and sophisticated quality measurements to quantify these concerns. Nurses are concerned about the "de-skilling" of nursing, the fragmentation of comprehensive care into a series of tasks and the assignments of these tasks to unlicensed individuals. When a

(continued)

NEWS NOTE 16-3   *(Continued)*

hospital staff is diluted to a staff mix of as few as 50 percent registered nurses, the facility is risking increased mortality. When the hospital assigns more and more administrative functions to professional nurses, patient care also will suffer.

Hospitals have now reached the point that, in too many cases, the personnel tending its patients' needs are neither qualified nor trained adequately to perform the duties assigned to them. They are instead unlicensed employees who, while dressed appropriately, are not professional nurses at all. In some hospitals, professional nurses are told not to wear any identification indicating they are registered nurses (RNs) so that patients will not know the difference between the professional staff and the unlicensed, untrained staff. That is simply shocking!

Yet, these are exactly the kinds of changes that we are witnessing today, and it could not come at a more critical time in our history—a time when there is an increasing growth of an aging patient population that dictates an increased, rather than decreased, nursing service.

Consumer Education

As professional nurses, we feel obligated to tell our friends, families and the public that hospital care must be sought and procured with apprehension and diligence. No patient should be admitted to hospital care without an informed and active advocate, whether a relative or friend. Health care in America has changed dramatically and the public must change with it, or change it. Until then, America's professional nurse must educate consumers by issuing the warning that it is critical to ask: "Who's taking care of mama?"

(Reprinted with permission of Morris, E. A. (1996). Who's taking care of Mama? *The American Nurse*, 28(1), 4.)

Concerns about health care in the United States are not new. A 1991 *Time*/Cable News Network (CNN) poll of 1000 adults found that 91 percent believed that *fundamental change* in the health care system was needed, 75 percent believed costs were higher than necessary, and 83 percent advocated limiting physicians' fees. Two-thirds said health care is a right, and 70 percent expressed a willingness to pay more taxes to make sure all Americans have access to care (Castro, 1991, p. 36).

In the 1992 presidential campaign, candidates in both political parties advocated some type of health care reform. Nonpartisan groups also called for reform. These included nursing organizations, the American Association of Retired Persons, labor unions, the American College of Physicians, the National Leadership Coalition for Health Care Reform, and members of the U.S. Congress. Most of these groups put forward specific plans for reform, including "Nursing's Agenda for Health Care Reform," discussed in Chapter 4. Despite widespread public support for reform, as of 1996, federal reform efforts were stalled in Congress. Congressional inaction on controversial issues is common during election years. Lack of legislation on health care reform was aided by powerful interest groups such as the pharmaceutical, health insurance, and health equipment industries; the American Medical Association; and the American Hospital Association. These were the same groups that lobbied so vigorously against President Clinton's 1993 plan for health care reform.

JoAnn Alexander, MSN, RN, is Chief Operations Officer, and Charlene Robertson, MSN, RN, is Chief Nursing Officer, at a private not-for-profit hospital in a midsized city in the southeastern United States.

Q: *Tell me a little about the hospital—its size, services, and the number of nurses employed here.*

A: Robertson
This is a 365-bed hospital. We have all services including obstetrics, pediatrics, and behavioral health. There are 596 members on the nursing staff, which includes 464 RNs (registered nurses), 38 LPNs (licensed practical nurses), and 94 nursing assistants.

Q: *What specific cost-containment programs have been started here in the past few years that have influenced nursing care?*

A: Robertson
Specific cost containment programs began in 1992 with intensive education of physicians, nurses, and support staff on continuous quality improvement strategies, managed care strategies, and cost containment. The implementation of continuous quality improvement enhanced several multidisciplinary clinical groups to achieve good outcomes. For example:
- The Pneumonia Group reduced length of stay by 4 days and cost per discharge.
- A Multidisciplinary CareTrac (Clinical Pathway) tool was implemented housewide with physician support.
- A short-stay, one-stop unit for PTCA (percutaneous transluminal coronary angioplasty) patients was implemented. Patient care was also redesigned with a combination of an RN and Cardiac Tech who make up a "care pair." This approach has reduced cost by $1400 per case, with high patient and physician satisfaction.

Q: *What has been done to relieve nurses of nonnursing tasks?*

A: Robertson
Improvement in documentation comes immediately to mind, with charting by exception, bedside charting, computerized Kardexes and MAR, and the implementation of CareTracs, which has reduced redundant documentation. Other strategies include the formation of care pairs in the cardiac short stay unit, cross-training in the operative suite, and implementation of the Pyxis system.

Q: *What is the goal of quality management?*

A: Alexander
The focus of continuous quality improvement is to view our hospital system from our patient, physician, and family prospective. Multidisciplinary cross-functional teams identify barriers to service and systematically implement change using the PDCA (plan, do, check, and act) approach.

Q: *Who participates in quality management?*

A: Alexander
All members of the health care team, including physicians, nurses, and support and clinical services associates, participate in quality management. The cross-functional team allows all persons to have an active role. Customer service is everyone's responsibility.

(continued)

BOX 16–4 *(Continued)*

Q: *How are nurses involved in quality management?*

A: Robertson
About five years ago, we reorganized nursing and decentralized certain functions. The director of each unit has the responsibility of quality management and continuous quality improvement activities for that unit. When our hospitalwide and unit-specific quality monitoring programs reveal a problem, an action plan is developed either on the unit or by the nursing council. For example, the response on a hospitalwide patient satisfaction survey showed that patients felt that the call lights were not being responded to in a timely manner for pain medication or other needs.

The nursing staff was apprised of this concern and, as a means of addressing this concern, a nurse pager system was implemented. Patient care needs are communicated immediately. The pager dials in directly to the nurse who provides that care. This response is monitored internally by placing a phone call to the patient after discharge, and the unit secretary completes periodic monitoring of actual time frames of nurse response to patient call lights. By increasing the sensitivity of the patient's need for immediate call-light response and by implementing the new pager system, the patient satisfaction in this area has greatly increased.

The hospital is organized around a Service Line structure. The Chief Nursing Officer is accountable for nursing wherever nursing is practiced. Nursing leads some of the cross-functional teams and was involved with the development of the CareTracs. Most of the Care Managers are nurses who manage patients daily through the system and are starting to establish a method to manage across the continuum.

Q: *How does quality management affect the way nursing care is provided?*

A: Alexander
The CareTracs eliminate the need for nurses to be mind readers of other disciplines involved in the care of the patient. It allows better dialogue with the disciplines and the patient. It makes the truly collaborative model easier to live with on a daily basis. It also gives nurses more objective outcome data to measure the effectiveness of their care.

Q: *What would you say about cost containment and quality management to students of professional nursing around the United States?*

A: Alexander
It is important for nurses to adopt a philosophy of rather than finding *fault*, find a *remedy*. The public will not accept a continued escalation in cost, and nurses are in a good position to broaden their skills outside of the hospital and be primary care providers. I believe that the cross-functional team is the model that will provide productivity with time. Be a risk taker and have the initiative to try something different and remember that cost and quality can be measured.

(Courtesy of Charlene Robertson and JoAnn Alexander.)

In the present political climate, it seems unlikely that a systematic and comprehensive reform of the entire health care system is possible. Instead, we can expect to see piecemeal attempts to address specific issues of concern. Box 16–5 identifies some of the proposals under consideration in 1996. Most experts agree

---

BOX 16–5

Potential Health Care Reform Initiatives: Some Anticipated Changes to Health Insurance Laws and Regulations

Portable Health Insurance
Employees would be able to change employers without losing their health insurance benefits. (Eds. note: This legislation was signed into law in August 1996)

Universal Health Insurance
Every American would be covered by health insurance. Government would expand health insurance funding for all vulnerable populations, including those currently not covered. All employers might be expected to provide health insurance, or employees might be given an allowance and expected to purchase their own health insurance.

Catastrophic Limits Changed
Catastrophic coverage would be part of every health insurance plan, and lifetime limits on costs of care would be increased or limits eliminated altogether.

Medicare
Medicare payments for services would continue to decline. Co-pays or deductibles could rise. Increased pressure to enroll all Medicare recipients in managed care plans is likely.

Medicaid
Expansion of states requiring managed care enrollment for Medicaid recipients would occur. Changes in standard set of health services paid for by the program would occur, most likely reductions in services. Reduction in federal oversight would occur, freeing states to change eligibility standards for service. Some states might continue existing eligibility criteria; others might expand or reduce criteria. Minimal co-pays for services may be added.

Changes in Block Grants
Expect to see more federal funds distributed in block grants, less federal oversight of funded programs, and greater state autonomy in selection of services and populations served by federal funds.

Managed Care and Health Networks
The proportion of the population covered by managed care will continue to expand. Health care providers will continue to merge into large health networks.

Rationing
Current rationing of care is by ability to pay; insurance coverage ensures care for most. Because for-profit structures dominate the health market, there may be additional curtailments on such items as expensive therapies, disputes between providers and payors about what constitutes "experimental procedures," and shortening of allowable hospital recovery times. Legislation may be necessary to compel care. Unless a minimum standard of care is established at the federal level, each state may need to take action separately to address each inequity. For example, three states have already passed legislation that ensures a new mother's right to extend postdelivery hospital stays to 48 hours. Insurers had been willing to pay for 24 hours or less.

that reform efforts are doomed unless they are projected to reduce, or at least not increase, the cost of health care.

GUIDELINES FOR EVALUATING REFORM PROPOSALS

Despite wide-ranging differences of opinion about the specifics of health care reform proposals, there *are* areas of general agreement. Some general guidelines to look for in evaluating such proposals are:

1. Is there a uniform minimum set of benefits for all citizens, otherwise known as **universal care?**
2. Are coverage and benefits continuous and not dependent on where people live or work?
3. Are there mechanisms for controlling costs, especially administrative expenses?
4. Are provisions made for care to be provided by the most cost-effective personnel, taking quality issues and patient outcomes into consideration?
5. Are the issues of adequate facilities and personnel to ensure access for all addressed?
6. Is there an emphasis on quality care?
7. Are there incentives for healthy lifestyles and preventive care?

A point of particular interest to nurses is the issue of cost-effectiveness of personnel. If care is to be provided by the most cost-effective personnel, it should mean an expansion of the role of nurses as primary care providers. Studies have shown that nurses are cost-effective caregivers and are well accepted by the public (Holzemer 1990; Lampe 1987; Winslow 1990). Organized medicine, however, actively opposes moves to give clinical autonomy to almost all nonphysician providers (Winslow, 1990). This is a conflict that must be resolved for true reform to occur, and nurses themselves must be active in its resolution.

S U M M A R Y

How health care is financed in the United States has changed dramatically during the past 50 years from a system dominated by personal payment to one dominated by third-party payment. This change created basic economic disequilibrium in health care. People who do not pay directly for health care are not sensitive to the price of care. Medicare and Medicaid programs, begun in 1965, created a serious financial drain on federal and state budgets. In response, cost-containment efforts were begun by the federal government in the 1970s. Initial efforts were unsuccessful, so in 1982 more sweeping reforms were initiated. Retrospective payment was replaced by prospective payment. In the early 1990s, systemwide health reform efforts were supported by public opinion but failed to pass the U.S. Congress. Even without governmental action, many Americans have seen substantial changes in their health care plans, stimulated by business interests and employers. There has been a dramatic escalation in managed care plans and consolidation of health providers into larger health networks. The entire health care system, including nurses and nursing services, has been profoundly affected by these changes. Further changes are on the horizon. It remains to be seen whether these changes will improve access and maintain quality of health care for all Americans.

REVIEW AND DISCUSSION QUESTIONS

1. In your view, is access to health care a basic right? Be prepared to defend your opinion.
2. List the basic health care services that should be provided to all citizens. Compare your list with classmates' lists and discuss the reasons for your priorities.
3. Should there be a limit on the percentage of national resources expended on health care? If so, how should the limit be established?
4. What process should be used to determine how health care resources are allocated? List criteria you would suggest to determine whether or not a person should receive a kidney transplant.
5. Should people with healthy lifestyles pay the same for care or insurance as those whose habits result in a greater likelihood of illness? How could such a differentiation be determined?
6. Should there be rationing of extremely expensive procedures, such as heart transplants, even if the patient is able to pay? Give a rationale for your answer.

REFERENCES

AHA News. (1996). 39.7 million Americans uninsured in 1994. 31(50), 3.

Arthur Andersen & Company and American College of Healthcare Executives (1991). *The future of healthcare: Physician and hospital relationships*. Author.

Ashton, G. (1995). Getting tough on drive-through delivery. *AHA News*, 31(50), 3.

Berman, S. (1995). State block grants for Medicaid may increase number of poor children at risk. *JAMA*, 274(18), 1472–1473.

Betts, V. T. (1996). 1996—Speak out for quality care. *The American Nurse*, 28(1), 4.

Black, H. C. (1988). *Black's law dictionary*. St. Paul, MN: West Publishing.

Buerhaus, P. I. (1995a). Economics and reform: Forces affecting nurse staffing. *Nursing Policy Forum*, 1(2), 8–14.

Buerhaus, P. I. (1995b). Economic pressures building in the hospital employed RN labor market. *Nursing Economics*, 13(3), 137–141.

Burner, S. T., and Waldo, D. R. (1995). National health expenditure projections, 1994–2005. *Health Care Finance Review*, 16(4), 221–242.

Castro, J. (1991). Condition: Critical. *Time*, November 25, 1991, 34–42.

CPR (Current Population Reports). (1991). U.S. Bureau of the Census, Series P25No.1045. Washington, D.C.: U.S. Government Printing Office.

Cuniff, J. (1991). Soaring health costs need brake. *Chattanooga News—Free Press*, January 31, 1991, B5.

Curtin, L. (1994). Restructuring: What works—and what does not! *Nursing Management*, 25(10), 7–8.

Davis, K., and Schoen, C. (1994). Universal coverage building on Medicare and employer financing. *Health Affairs*, 13(1), 7–20.

DiVestea, N. (1985). The changing health care system: An overview. In F. A. Shaffer (Ed.), *Costing out nursing: Pricing our product*. New York: National League for Nursing.

Dougherty, C. J. (1989). Cost containment, DRGs, and the ethics of health care. *Hastings Center Report*, 19(1), 5–7.

Duston, D. (1996). Secret witness tells senators of Medicare fraud by hospitals. *Naples Daily News*, February 15, p. 2B.

Eason, F. R., Lee, B. T., and Spickerman, S. (1988). Analyzing cost: A learning module. *Nurse Educator*, 13(4), 9–10, 13.

Feldstein, P. J. (1993). *Health care economics* (4th ed). West Albany, NY: Delmar Publishers.

Fineman, H. (1995). Mediscare. *Newsweek*, CXXVI (12), 38–40.

Glieck, E. (1996). Picking a health plan: A how to guide. *Time*, 147(5), 60–61.

Gray, P. (1996). Gagging the doctors. *Time*, 147(2), 50.

Guidera, M. (1996). Care system to base in Columbia. *The Sun*, January 26, 1C, 3C.

Health care expenditures and other data: An international compendium from the Organization for Economic Cooperation and Development. (1989). *Health Care Financing Review*, annual supplement, 111–195.

Holzemer, W. L. (1990). Quality and cost of nursing care: Is anybody out there listening? *Nursing and Health Care*, 11(8), 412–415.

Horine, M. (1990). Assuring access to quality care. *Pension World*, 26(9), 26–28.

Jacobs, P. (1991). *The economics of health and medical care* (3rd ed.). Gaithersburg, MD: Aspen.

Johnson, P. A. (1990). A national health insurance program: A nursing perspective. *Nursing and Health Care*, 11(8), 416–429.

Kerr, P. (1991). Workers' comp fraud blamed for inflating cost of health care. *Chattanooga Times*, December 30, 1991, A1.

Khanna, V. (1995). Medicare HMOs: A bad deal for aged. *The Sun*, December 3, 6J.

Knox, R. (1989). Is a solution in sight for 1990? *Boston Globe*, April 17, A11, A14.

Lampe, S. (1987). *Costing hospital nursing services: A review of the literature*. Washington, D.C.: U.S. Department of Health and Human Services.

Larson, E. (1996). The soul of an HMO. *Time*, 147(4), 44–52.

Luciano, L. (1994). Get the health care you deserve. *Money*, October, 114–124.

Maurer, F. A. (1995a). Financing of health care: Context for community health nursing. In Smith, C., and Maurer, F. A. (Eds.), *Community Health Nursing: Theory and Practice*. Philadelphia: W.B. Saunders.

Maurer, F. A. (1995b). The United States health care system. In Smith, C., and Maurer, F. A. (Eds.), *Community Health Nursing: Theory and Practice*. Philadelphia: W. B. Saunders.

McKibben, R. C. (1985). *DRGs and nursing care*. Kansas City, MO: American Nurses Association Center for Research.

Medicare and Medicaid statistical supplement. (1995). Washington, D.C.: Health Care Finance Administration.

Morris, E. A. (1996). Who's taking care of Mama? *The American Nurse*, 28(1), 4.

Nornhold, P. (1995). What networks mean to you. *Nursing 95*, 25(1), 49–50.

Rowland, D., Lyons, B., Salganicoff, A., and Long, P. (1994). A profile of the uninsured in America. *Health Affairs*, 11(1), 283–287.

Sharpfstein, S. S. (1996). Psychiatry suffers under managed care. *The Sun*, February 4, 6J.

St. Anthony's DRG Guidebook 1995. (1994). Reston, VA: St. Anthony Publishing.

Statistical Abstract of the U.S. (1993). Washington, D.C.: U.S. Government Printing Office.

The Medicare Handbook. (1996). Washington, D.C.: U.S. Department of Health and Human Resources, Health Care Financing Administration.

Winslow, R. (1990). Nurses get public's vote as best bet to cut costs. *The Wall Street Journal*, September 21, B-1.

17

Carolyn Maynard

Illness and Its Impact on Patients and Families

OBJECTIVES

- Differentiate between acute and chronic illness.
- Describe the stages of illness.
- Describe behavioral responses to illness.
- Identify internal and external influences on illness behaviors.
- Discuss the influence of culture on illness behaviors.
- Characterize four levels of anxiety.
- Describe the physical, emotional, and cognitive effects of stress.
- Discuss how family functioning is altered during illness.

VOCABULARY

acute illness	dependency	learned resourcefulness
anxiety	disease	remission
chronic illness	exacerbation	stress
coping	hardiness	stressor
culture	illness	

Although prevention and health maintenance activities are primary functions of nurses, many nurse-patient interactions center on the management of illness. A unique characteristic of nursing is the emphasis on viewing patients holistically. Nurses recognize that human beings are complex organisms with physical, mental, emotional, spiritual, social, and cultural components, all of which affect how a person responds when ill. The effective nurse takes each of these dimensions into consideration when planning nursing care. This chapter explores the stages of illness, illness behaviors, internal and external influences on illness behaviors, and the impact of illness on patients and families.

ILLNESS

Kozier and associates (1994) described **illness** as a highly personal experience in which an individual feels unhealthy or ill. It involves the person's perceptions of disease. Illness is differentiated from **disease** in that **disease** is an alteration at the tissue or organ level causing reduced capacities or reduction of the normal life span. Illness is usually considered to be a subjective state. One may feel ill in the absence of a disease. Conversely, one may be unaware of a disease, such as high blood pressure, and not feel ill.

Ellis and Nowlis (1994) discuss the theory of "illness with evidence." This theory proposes that there must be demonstrable evidence of an organic nature for an illness to exist. According to this theory, health care professionals may define a state of illness, such as hypertension, even in the absence of subjective symptoms in the ill person.

People's perceptions of a change or loss play a major role in whether or not they see themselves as ill. People with mild arthritic changes who have no decrease in their activities and who need to use only over-the-counter analgesics such as aspirin may not consider themselves ill. To a radiologist looking at an x-ray, however, arthritic changes may be evident.

Whether the presence of illness is determined by the individual or by a health care provider, illness is experienced differently by different individuals and their families. The nurse's responses to patients must be defined in terms of each individual's reactions.

Acute Illness

Illnesses can be classified as either acute or chronic. **Acute illness** is characterized by severe symptoms that are relatively short-lived. Symptoms tend to appear suddenly, progress steadily, and subside quickly. Depending on the illness, the patient may or may not require medical attention. The common cold is an example of an acute illness that does not usually require a health care provider's attention. Others, such as appendicitis, may be fatal without rapid medical intervention. After treatment, people suffering from acute illness usually return rather quickly to their previous level of wellness.

Chronic Illness

Lupus erythematosus, coronary artery disease, arthritis, hypertension, emphysema, muscular dystrophy, and diabetes are examples of **chronic illness.** Chronic illnesses cannot normally be cured. They develop gradually, require ongoing medical attention, and may continue for the duration of the person's life.

It is increasingly important for nurses to understand chronic illnesses and their impact because they are one of the fastest-growing health problems in the United States (Thorne, 1993). It is estimated that one-third to one-half of the U.S. population has one or more chronic illnesses. Factors such as changing lifestyle trends and the aging of the population are expected to contribute to a continued increase in the number of chronically ill Americans.

Chronic illnesses are caused by permanent changes that leave residual disability. They vary in severity and outcomes, but there is generally not an end point at which normal health is regained. Some chronic illnesses are progressively debilitating and usually result in premature death, whereas others are as-

---

BOX 17–1
Comments of a Patient with Lupus Erythematosis

If there is one thing I want to say to nurses who work with patients with chronic disease it is, "Be patient and understand our problems and feelings." When I go to the doctor's office or to the hospital, I usually leave feeling guilty because I have been impatient with everyone I saw. Guilt and anger are the two feelings I seem to have had since I was diagnosed with this disease. I alternate between being angry that I got lupus and feeling that I should be grateful for the fact that I have something I can at least live with when others are not so fortunate.

I guess the thing that bothers me most is that the nurses keep telling me what changes I need to make to take better care of myself. They never seem to understand that I am doing the best I can do. I can't possibly get the amount of rest they seem to think I need, and I can't avoid as much stress as they seem to think I should avoid. Both my husband and I work hard at our jobs, and I hate asking him and my sons to take over my responsibilities at home when I am sick, so I wind up compromising. I ask them to help some and I do more than I should. When I get the lecture from the nurses on how I should take better care of myself, I usually just nod and say that I will even when I know that I probably won't be able to. (Anonymous)

---

sociated with a normal life span even though functioning is impaired. Chronic illnesses typically go through periods of **remission,** when symptoms subside, and **exacerbation,** when the symptoms reappear or worsen.

Chronic illnesses often lead to altered individual functioning and disruption of family life. Long-term medical management of chronic illness often creates financial hardship as well. Box 17–1 describes how one patient experiences her chronic illness.

Stages of Illness

Although the behaviors are different for each person, people who are ill tend to progress through certain recognizable stages. Ellis and Nowlis (1994) have identified five stages: disbelief and denial, irritability and anger, attempting to gain control, depression and despair, and acceptance and participation. Nurses encounter patients in each stage, so it is important to have some understanding of the types of behaviors that are associated with each.

STAGE I: DISBELIEF AND DENIAL

According to Ellis and Nowlis (1994), the first stage results from difficulty in believing that the signs and symptoms being experienced are caused by illness. Often, there is a belief that the symptoms will go away. Fear of illness often leads to the hope that the symptoms will subside without treatment.

Denial is a defense mechanism that people sometimes use to avoid the anxiety associated with illness. People who pride themselves on their vigor and health may downplay the significance of symptoms. If this occurs, they may avoid treatment or attempt inappropriate self-treatment. Extended denial can have serious results because some illnesses, left untreated, may become too advanced for effective treatment.

STAGE II: IRRITABILITY AND ANGER

As the ability to function is altered by illness, irritability results. Anger is directed toward the body because it is not performing as it should. With the current emphasis on wellness and prevention, anger may be directed inward, and guilt feelings may occur for failing to prevent the illness.

STAGE III: ATTEMPTING TO GAIN CONTROL

In this stage, people may try over-the-counter medications, folk medicine, or home remedies. They are aware that they are ill and usually experience some concern or even fear about the outcome. These fears usually stimulate treatment-seeking behavior as a way of gaining control over the illness.

STAGE IV: DEPRESSION

Depression is perhaps the most common mood that occurs with illness. The ability to work is altered, daily activities must be modified, and the sense of well-being and freedom from pain is lost. Illness results in many types of loss, and depression is a normal response to loss. The severity of the depression varies according to the severity and length of the illness as well as the individual's personality characteristics and coping abilities. Individuals with chronic illnesses often undergo cycles of depression as remissions and exacerbations occur. When depression is severe or prolonged, counseling is required.

STAGE V: ACCEPTANCE AND PARTICIPATION

By the time this stage occurs, the patient has acknowledged the reality of illness and is ready to participate in decisions about treatment. Active involvement and the hope attached to pursuing treatment usually lead to increased feelings of mastery and serve to decrease depression.

Not all individuals go through every stage, and they do not necessarily go through them at the same rate or in the same order. Individuals may become "stuck" in a stage before reaching the ideal stage of acceptance and participation. Those with acute illnesses may progress through stages in a different way than those with chronic illnesses. Nevertheless, these stages represent a useful model for nurses to keep in mind.

Illness Behavior and the Sick Role

Although illness is highly subjective and is experienced differently by each individual, a number of factors influence how a particular person will respond. One important factor is the societal expectation about how people *should* behave when ill.

Each society generally requires that certain criteria be met before people can qualify as "sick." Talcott Parsons (1951), a sociologist, identified five attributes and expectations of the sick role that guided the view of illness in mainstream U.S. society for decades. According to Parsons, the sick person:

1. Is exempt from social responsibilities.
2. Cannot be expected to care for himself or herself.
3. Should want to get well.
4. Should seek medical advice.
5. Should cooperate with the medical experts.

Although the current expectation is that people should accept responsibility for their own care rather than turn themselves completely over to health care providers, there continues to be some presumption that ill people should want to get well and should behave in a way that leads to wellness. The individual who does not do so will probably not be seen as legitimately ill. In addition, there must be an inability to get well just by choosing to do so. Those who call themselves sick and who refuse to accept treatment may be seen as malingering, or faking illness, to avoid responsibilities.

Illness carries both privileges and obligations. The ill person is often allowed to evade some troubling situations or to escape the necessity of having to live up to others' expectations. Frequently the ill person is entitled to be taken care of for some period and to give up some or all of the usual duties. The degree of exemption from responsibilities usually depends on the extent and severity of the illness.

Although there are benefits from being ill, there are also obligations. One obligation is to seek and accept competent help. People who are ill generally must accept help with the duties they are unable to perform. For instance, the housewife who prides herself on doing everything for her family must accept help with cooking the meals and cleaning the house while she is restricted to bed.

The expectation that ill persons should want to get well and return to their normal duties as quickly as possible usually means that they should cooperate in the treatment process and, to a great extent, become submissive and compliant, placing themselves in the hands of the caretakers. Persons who refuse to take medications as ordered or who refuse to perform prescribed activities, such as adhering to an exercise program or therapeutic diet, are viewed in a negative light. Their friends and family members may become irritated at their lack of participation in getting well again.

In caring for patients with acute and chronic illnesses, it is important for nurses to refrain from making judgments about patients' lifestyle choices. Emphasis should be on encouraging and reinforcing healthy behaviors. Education and support are important role functions for the nurse, especially in the management of chronic disorders.

Working with patients with chronic illnesses can be particularly challenging for nurses. The inability of modern medicine to effect a cure sometimes leads caregivers to feel hopeless and powerless. They may also feel overwhelmed and inadequate at times. Self-aware nurses recognize these feelings and do not allow them to interfere with the nurse-patient relationship.

Influences on Illness Behavior

Although there are some behaviors expected of sick people, there is also a wide variation of responses. Each person who is newly diagnosed with diabetes behaves somewhat differently from other people with the same condition. Both internal and external variables affect how an individual acts when ill. An ill individual's personality has a great deal of influence on his or her response to illness. Past experiences with illness and cultural background also influence illness behaviors.

INTERNAL INFLUENCES

The personality structure of an individual is an internal variable that determines, to a large extent, how one manages illness. Personality characteristics the nurse should consider when assessing the ill person are dependence/independence, coping ability, hardiness and learned resourcefulness, and spirituality.

Dependence and Independence.   Patients have greater or lesser needs to be dependent that are unrelated to the severity of their illnesses. Some patients who are ill adopt a passive attitude and rely completely on others to take care of them. Others may deny that they are ill or have problems with being dependent and try to continue to do what they did before becoming sick.

We have all known sick people who have said something like, "I don't ask any questions—I know that my doctor and nurses know what is best for me, and I do what they tell me." Perhaps you also know someone who reacted to illness by saying, "They don't know what they are talking about. I don't need to be in bed, and I don't need to take that medicine." These two sentiments are at the opposite ends of the **dependency** continuum.

People who perceive themselves as helpless may be more willing to turn themselves over to health care personnel and do what they are told. Those who are used to being in charge and see themselves as being independent may resent the enforced dependency of hospitalization and illness. These two different attitudes are illustrated in the following clinical vignettes.

Clinical Vignette: Dependency
Mrs. Johnson has been in the hospital for several days following abdominal surgery. Even after she progressed to the point that she could feed herself, turn over in bed, and get up to go to the bathroom unaided, she continued to call for assistance when she needed to turn or to get out of bed. She now calls the nurse every few minutes, making some small request that she is quite capable of performing for herself. She is communi-

cating to the nurse that she needs a great deal of assistance and is demonstrating overly dependent behavior.

Clinical Vignette: Independence

Mr. Thomas is just back to his room from surgery. The nurse found him trying to get out of bed by himself. He does not call to ask for medication. He says that he is used to doing things for himself and feels uncomfortable asking the nurses for help. Mr. Thomas is demonstrating behavior that is too independent for his current physical status.

Both overly dependent and overly independent behavior can be frustrating to nurses. They sometimes become angry with patients who request help with activities they are capable of doing for themselves. The patient who is too dependent requires assistance to assume more responsibility for self gradually. The patient who needs to be "in charge" may have problems turning enough control over to caregivers and is often too independent. This patient needs assistance in recognizing limitations and using available resources to get needs met.

Because nurses most often focus on independence, they may react negatively to patients who are exhibiting dependent behavior. It is important for the nurse to be aware of personal feelings about dependent behaviors and to keep in mind that dependent behaviors may be the patient's way of signaling that he or she has an increased need for security or support. Sometimes independence may not be the desired outcome. For patients with chronic illnesses who must rely on others for assistance in meeting their needs, independence may actually be dysfunctional (Whiting, 1994).

Coping Ability. An individual copes with disease or illness in a variety of ways. **Coping** is the method a person uses to assess and manage demands. With an acute illness, coping is generally of short duration and leads to a return to the preillness state. With chronic disorders, the length and complexity of the coping required is greatly magnified.

Sick people use coping methods to deal with the negative consequences of the disorder, such as pain or physical limitations. Each individual has a unique coping repertoire that is called into play to achieve a sense of control. With chronic health problems, there is a continuous need for adjustments to maintain well-being and prevent the feelings of despair that can result from high stress conditions (Bowsher and Keep, 1995).

Hardiness and Learned Resourcefulness. **Hardiness** and **learned resourcefulness** are two concepts that have received attention as personal characteristics related to coping. Hardiness, as described by Kobasa, is viewed as a function of resistance to stressful life events (Bowsher and Keep, 1995). The tendency to believe that one can influence the course of events, viewing change as a challenge, and feeling commitment to values or goals are seen as the interrelated dimensions of hardiness.

The person with greater hardiness is believed to be better able to manage the changes associated with illness and to have less physical illness resulting from stress. Hardy people are likely to perceive themselves as having some control over what happens to them, even when ill. The feeling of being able to exert some control over the situation can affect a person's sense of well-being and adaptation to chronic health problems.

Zauszniewski (1995) has described the concept of learned resourcefulness as a characteristic useful in promoting adaptive, healthy lifestyles. Throughout life, individuals acquire a number of skills that enable them to cope effectively with stressful situations. The resulting attitude of self-control can be particularly helpful in reducing the feelings of depression and helplessness that often accompany the numerous stressors of chronic illness.

The nurse can enhance both hardiness and resourcefulness by teaching new coping skills. Stress inoculation, self-regulation skills, problem-solving skills, conflict resolution skills, and emotion-control skills are examples of the types of educational interventions the nurse may implement.

Spirituality. The role of spiritual beliefs in health and illness has only recently been formally investigated. A growing number of scholars and health professionals think that spiritual beliefs have psychological, medical, and financial benefits that can and have been proven scientifically.

One of the leading proponents of the spirituality and healing movement in American medicine is Doctor Herbert Benson, a Harvard Medical School cardiologist. He originated the relaxation-response therapy to reduce stress in patients with hypertension, chronic pain, and other stress-related illnesses. According to Benson, many people use prayer as part of the relaxation response. His Mind/Body Medical Institute of Pathway Health Network in Boston has studied the effects of the relaxation response and claims the following benefits (Larson, 1996):

- A 36 percent reduction in physician visits by chronic pain patients.
- Significantly fewer postoperative complications in open heart surgery patients.
- Lowered blood pressure and decreased use of medications in 80 percent of hypertensive patients.
- A 50 percent reduction in Health Maintenance Organization (HMO) visits by relaxation response users.

Other indications that meeting patients' spiritual needs is becoming a priority in health care settings is evidenced by an increase in chaplain presence in some inpatient and outpatient settings. More than 90 percent of the patients surveyed believed that having a chaplain available was helpful, and 60 percent were more likely to return to a hospital with a pastoral presence in an otherwise frightening and confusing environment (Larson, 1996).

Nurses are participating in the use of spirituality in healing. St. Francis Hospital's Congregational Nurse Program in Evanston, Illinois, for example, is reaching 15,000 local families in an interfaith health project. Following training as congregational nurses, nurses spend approximately 20 hours weekly at churches and other places of worship providing classes, counseling, and referrals. They dovetail their efforts with the spiritual beliefs and customs of each congregation. The congregational nurse concept is being implemented in numerous communities around the United States. By respecting and treating the whole person, these practitioners are affirming that a key dimension of health and healing is spiritual.

EXTERNAL INFLUENCES

External factors that bear on illness behaviors include past experiences and cultural group. Both directly influence how one perceives and responds to illness. The values that guide one's feelings about illness and steer one toward particular methods of treatment are acquired primarily in the family of origin and in the culture.

Past Experiences.   Adults who were pampered during childhood illnesses may accept being ill fairly easily. Relying on others to care for them may not concern them, and they may settle into the sick role easily. Adults who received childhood messages such as "It is weak to be ill" or "One must keep going even when not feeling well" may have difficulty accepting illness and the restrictions that accompany it. Still other adults who were hospitalized as small children or threatened with injections for misbehaving may see hospitals and nurses as threatening. Clearly these adults behave differently when ill.

Nurses should determine the patient's past experiences with illness and the health care system during a careful admission assessment. They can then use these findings to individualize care.

Culture.   One's **culture** is a pattern of learned behavior and values, reinforced through social interactions, shared by members of a particular group, and transmitted from one generation to the next. Culture exerts considerable influence over most of an individual's life experiences, including illness. Meanings attached to illness and perceptions of treatment are affected to a large degree by one's culture. Culture determines when one seeks help and the type of practitioner consulted. It also prescribes customs of responding to the sick. Culture determines whether illness is seen as a punishment for misdeeds or as the result of inadequate personal health practices. It influences whether one goes to an acupuncturist, an herbalist, or a physician.

Knowledge of the patient's culture assists the nurse in understanding behaviors and provides direction for appropriate approaches to patient problems. Because culture may guide the patient's response to health care providers and to the care provided, it is necessary for the nurse to be knowledgeable about cultural influences. Understanding a patient's cultural background can facilitate communication and assist in establishing an effective nurse-patient relationship.

The shared values and beliefs in a culture enable its members to predict each other's actions. They also influence how members react to each other's behavior. When nurses work with patients from cultures about which little is known, they lack familiar guidelines for predicting behavior. This can cause anxiety and feelings of distrust for both patient and nurse.

In an effort to predict behavior, the nurse may resort to stereotyping patients from different cultures. It is important that nurses refrain from overgeneralizing and stereotyping members of cultures or ethnic groups that are different from their own. Individual assessment is always the best basis for care, whatever the patient's culture or ethnic group.

The nurse should keep in mind that patterns of communication are strongly influenced by culture. The Asian patient who smiles and nods may be communicating politeness and respect rather than agreeing or indicating understanding. Americans tend to value a direct approach to problems, but in other cultures, subtlety and indirectness may be valued. Although Western culture values direct eye contact, some cultures view this as impolite, particularly direct eye contact between men and women.

The amount of personal space needed is another factor that varies depending on cultural experience. Some cultures use touch as a major form of communication; in others, touching between persons who are not considered family is disrespectful.

Culture also has a primary influence on the type of stress its members experience at various points in their lives. Every society places stress on its members at one or more stages of development. For instance, American adolescents are typically under great stress as they struggle with independence issues. Amish adolescents tend to experience less stress because their behavior during this period is more rigidly prescribed by their culture.

Values held by the nurse may come into conflict with patients' cultural values. In the Navajo culture, for example, great value is placed on keeping pain and discomfort to oneself. Letting others know how you feel is seen as weak. The nurse who expects patients to complain and ask for medication when in pain may assume that the Navajo patient is comfortable when he or she is not. A nurse who values suffering in silence may underrate the discomfort of a patient who comes from a culture that proclaims pain loudly and uses dramatic physical gestures to communicate discomfort.

The role expectations of nurses also vary from culture to culture. A common white, middle-class American view of nurses is that they treat people as equals, are passive, and take direction from physicians. These patients feel free to ask questions of their nurses. Asians, however, may expect nurses to be authoritative, to provide directives, and to be expert practitioners who take charge. Out of respect for authority, they may not speak until spoken to and may verbally agree with anything nurses propose. The following patient vignette illustrates a culture difference between patient and nurse in regard to expressing pain.

Clinical Vignette: Cultural Expression of Pain

Mrs. L., a 42-year-old Asian woman, became ill and required surgery while visiting her daughter in the United States. Following surgery, she was placed on a patient-controlled analgesia pump (PCA). The nurse explained how she should self-administer medication when she felt pain. Mrs. L. smiled and nodded her head when asked if she understood the instructions. Much later the nurse noticed that this patient appeared to be in great pain. On talking with her daughter, the nurse realized that Mrs. L. had not understood how to use the equipment but felt that she should not ask for additional instructions or complain of pain.

Nurses respond to sick people based not only on their formal education, but also on the socialization and culture in their own background. The nurse who

---

BOX 17-2
Sociocultural Self-Assessment

Directions: Use your answers to these questions to understand your own social and cultural beliefs and expectations better.

1. To what groups do I belong? What is my cultural heritage? My socioeconomic status? My age group? My religious affiliation?
2. How do I describe myself? What parts of the description come from the groups I belong to?
3. What kinds of contact have I had with persons from different groups?

4. What about my different groups do I feel proud of? What would I change if I could?
5. Have I ever experienced the feeling of being rejected by another group?
6. When I was growing up, what messages did I get from parents and friends about people from groups different from mine?
7. What are the major stereotypes I hold about people from different groups?
8. To work effectively with people from different groups, what do I need to change about myself?

---

identifies personal beliefs and expectations and how they influence care is more able to recognize and deal with any factors that may impede patient care. Cultural assessment, therefore, begins with self-assessment.

To begin a cultural self-assessment, ask what your own values are. What behavior do you expect from people who are ill? Toward what groups do you have prejudices or biases? The nurse who is frustrated at the difficulty of caring for a patient from a different culture may benefit from taking a few minutes to imagine what it would be like to be hospitalized in a foreign country. Candidly answering the questions in Box 17–2 will help you begin the important process of self-assessment.

The nurse who does not take cultural differences into consideration may misinterpret patient behavior and fail to recognize problems that need to be managed. Cultural norms must be included in the care plan to achieve the desired goals. Being knowledgeable about other cultures can promote feelings of respect and enhance understanding of attitudes, behaviors, and the impact of illness.

IMPACT OF ILLNESS ON PATIENTS AND FAMILIES

Illness results in a number of changes for both patients and families. Common experiences include behavioral and emotional changes, changes in roles, and disturbed family dynamics. Illness creates stress and other emotional responses.

Severe illnesses that profoundly affect physical appearance and functioning are more likely to result in high levels of anxiety and extensive behavioral changes than are short-term, non–life-threatening illnesses. The impact of a chronic illness is significant and continues for the lifetime of the patient. When planning care, the nurse must take into consideration how the family both influences and is influenced by the illness of a member.

Impact of Illness on Patients

Illness creates a variety of emotional responses. The most common responses are guilt, anger, anxiety, and stress.

GUILT

Individuals may experience guilt about becoming ill, particularly if the illness is related to lifestyle choices, such as smoking. Guilt may also be associated with the inability to perform usual activities because of illness. A mother who is unable to perform child care tasks or a father who has to take a lower-paying job because of illness may experience considerable guilt. Nurses who identify and encourage patients to discuss guilt feelings may help prevent the depression that can be a consequence of illness-induced alterations in lifestyle.

ANGER

Anger is another common emotional response to illness. When patients must make sacrifices to manage their illnesses, such as giving up favorite foods or activities, they may experience anger about the changes. At times, they may feel that their bodies have betrayed them, which results in self-directed anger. Anger may also be directed toward caregivers for their inability to produce a cure, reduce pain, or prevent negative consequences of the illness. Nurses must be prepared to accept such angry feelings, to refrain from rejecting or avoiding patients who express their fears through anger, and to encourage the adaptive expression of angry feelings.

ANXIETY

Anxiety is a common and universal experience. It is also a common emotional response to illness and hospitalization. Anxiety is an ill-defined, diffuse feeling of apprehension and uncertainty (Ellis and Nowlis, 1994). Anxiety occurs as a result of some threat to an individual's selfhood, self-esteem, or identity.

A number of threats are associated with illness. Illness may alter the way people view themselves. Some illnesses result in a change in physical appearance. Often, there is some change in the ability to function, creating alterations in relationships, work performance, and abilities to meet others' expectations. In addition to potential changes caused by illness, there may be concern about pain and discomfort associated with illness or treatment. Because of real and potential threats and changes arising from illness, nurses must develop skills that enable them to help patients recognize and manage anxiety.

Although the responses are similar, there is general agreement that anxiety and fear are different. Fear results from specific, known causes, whereas with anxiety the cause of the feelings is unknown (Ellis and Nowlis, 1994). For example, if you are home alone at night and you hear an unusual noise outside, your heartbeat and respirations increase, your stomach tightens, and you perspire. The emotion in this situation is fear. If you begin to have the same feelings but have heard no noises and cannot identify a source of fear, you are experiencing anxiety. Both emotions may be present at the same time. The patient who is in the hospital for an operation may experience anxiety about the unknown consequences of the surgery and fear of the procedure itself.

Symptoms of Anxiety. Nurses should be familiar with the numerous symptoms of anxiety. They are classified as physiological, emotional, and cognitive. Physiological symptoms include increased heart rate, respirations, and blood pressure; insomnia; nausea and vomiting; fatigue; sweaty palms; and tremors. Emotional responses include restlessness, irritability, feelings of helplessness, crying, and depression. Cognitive symptoms include inability to concentrate, forgetfulness, inattention to surroundings, and preoccupation.

Responses to Anxiety. Responses to anxiety occur on a continuum. Peplau (1963) described four levels: mild, moderate, severe, and panic. In the mild level, there is increased alertness and ability to focus attention and concentrate. There is an expanded capacity for learning at this stage.

At the moderate level, the person is able to concentrate on only one thing at a time. Frequently, there is increased body movement and more rapid speech. There is subjective awareness of discomfort.

At the severe level, thoughts become scattered. The severely anxious person may not be able to communicate verbally, and there is considerable discomfort accompanied by purposeless movements such as handwringing and pacing.

At the panic level, the person becomes completely disorganized and loses the ability to differentiate reality and unreality. There are constant random and purposeless movements. The individual experiencing the panic level of anxiety is unable to function without assistance. Panic levels of anxiety cannot be continued indefinitely because the body will become exhausted, and death may occur if anxiety is not reduced. Box 17–3 lists the characteristics of each level of anxiety.

Because anxiety is such a common response to illness and hospitalization, nurses often encounter patients who are experiencing mild or moderate anxiety.

B O X 1 7 – 3
Levels of Anxiety

Mild Anxiety
Increased alertness, increased ability to focus, improved concentration, expanded capacity for learning

Moderate Anxiety
Concentration limited to one thing, increased body movement, rapid speech, subjective awareness of discomfort

Severe Anxiety
Scattered thoughts, difficulty with verbal communication, considerable discomfort, purposeless movements

Panic
Complete disorganization, difficulty differentiating reality from unreality, constant random movements, unable to function without assistance

Occasionally, patients who are severely anxious are seen. When interacting with an anxious patient, the nurse should carefully assess the level of anxiety before attempting to develop the plan of care.

According to Peplau (1963), anxiety is communicated interpersonally. In other words, it is "contagious." For this reason, it is crucial that the nurse be aware of and manage personal anxiety so that it is not inadvertently transferred to patients. Self-awareness is also essential to prevent absorbing patients' anxiety.

STRESS

Stress is another internal variable that affects patients. Stress is both a response to illness and an important factor in the development of illness. Because illness and hospitalization involve so many alterations in lifestyle, they tend to cause a great deal of stress.

Stress is a part of life that is unavoidable and essential. To survive and grow, individuals must cope adaptively with constantly changing demands. The stress related to examinations, for example, motivates most students to grow by studying and learning. Although stress is unavoidable, and even sometimes desirable, some control can be exerted over the number and types of **stressors** encountered, and responses to the stressors can often be managed.

Hospitalized patients are removed from their usual support systems. They lose much of their control because nurses and other care providers make decisions for them. Being ill often means that they are no longer able to perform activities as they did before the illness occurred. Stress is a common response to all these changes.

Differentiating Between Stress and Anxiety.
Stress and anxiety have some characteristics in common. The physiological responses are similar. Anxiety is a response to some real or perceived threat to the individual, whereas stress is an interaction between the individual and the environment. Stress includes all the responses the body makes while striving to maintain equilibrium and deal with demands.

Clinical Vignette: Stress and Anxiety

Mary S. is a 32-year-old single mother and a lawyer who was recently hired as the first woman in an established law firm. One morning as she prepares to take her 2-year-old daughter to the child care center, she receives a call saying that the woman who has provided child care was in an accident and will be closing the center indefinitely. Ms. S. experiences both stress and anxiety in this situation. She has a number of demands placed on her from her workplace and from her family that lead to stress. The additional demands caused by the sudden change in her plans results in even higher levels of stress. In addition, even though none of the male lawyers have responsibility for child care, Ms. S. has placed the expectation on herself that she will perform her job exactly like the men in the firm do. Being late or missing work because of having to make new arrangements for child care conflicts with her self-expectations and poses a threat to her self-esteem. This threat leads to feelings of anxiety.

Internal, External, and Interpersonal Stressors. Selye (1956) defined stress as the nonspecific response of the body to any demand made upon it. He named it the *general adaptation syndrome* and identified three stages through which the body progresses while responding to stress.

Stressors trigger the body's stress response. Stressors are agents, or stimuli, that an individual perceives as posing a threat to homeostasis (Ellis and Nowlis, 1994). Stressors may come from external, interpersonal, or internal sources. External stressors include such things as noise, heat, cold, malfunctioning equipment (such as a car that will not run), or organizational rules and expectations. Interpersonal sources of stress include the demands made by others and conflicts with others. Placing unrealistic expectations on oneself is an example of an internal stressor. In the example of Mary S., an internal stressor is her expectation that her child care responsibilities will not affect the hours she works. It is an unrealistic expectation for any single parent of a small child to expect that the child's needs will never interfere with work.

Responses to Stress. Outward responses to stress are determined by the individual's perception of the stressor. Cognitive appraisal, or the way one thinks about a specific situation, determines whether that situation is stressful for that particular individual. For example, loud music at a rock concert may be perceived as considerably less stressful by an adolescent than by his or her parents.

Another factor related to the assessment of threat is whether the individual feels capable of handling the threat, that is, whether the person exhibits hardiness. The person who feels capable of dealing with whatever problem arises can be expected to feel less stress than the person who does not generally feel competent.

Stress affects the physical, emotional, and cognitive areas of functioning just as anxiety does. Physically, there is a feeling of fatigue; muscles feel tight and tense. There is an increase in heart rate and respiration. The person who is under prolonged stress may be unable to sleep or eat, or there may be excessive sleeping or eating in an attempt to avoid or cope with the stress.

Emotionally, stressed people feel drained and unable to care for themselves or others. This can result in social isolation and distancing from others. There is difficulty with enjoying life. There may be feelings of hopelessness and of being out of control. Irritability and impatience often occur.

Cognitively, stress causes decreased mental capacity, and problem-solving skills are reduced. Therefore, there is a tendency to have difficulty making decisions.

Stress and Illness. It has been known for some time that stress plays a major role in the development of illness. More recent research has provided better understanding of the links between prolonged stress and body functioning.

The person who is under stress for long periods of time is at risk for a number of physical problems. The exhaustion that results from excessive, unmanaged stress leads to physiological breakdowns and predisposition to a number of problems. Disorders such as peptic ulcers, hypertension, and rheumatoid arthritis are called *stress-related* diseases because they frequently occur in individuals who have been severely stressed.

Stress has been found to be related to a reduction in the immune response,

which can delay healing and result in greater susceptibility to infectious disorders such as colds and flu. Holmes and Rahe (1967) conducted long-term studies of persons with medical illness and found that the more stress people experienced in a given year, the more likely they were to develop physical illness. See Chapter 10 for Holmes and Rahe's Social Readjustment Rating Scale.

Coping with Stress. Nurses have a role in helping patients modify their stressors. Nurses should assess patients' abilities to recognize symptoms of stress and their usual methods of coping.

Coping with stress can be direct or indirect. In using direct action, nurses assist patients to identify those situations that can be changed and take responsibility for changing them. The focus is on using problem-solving skills and planning to eliminate or avoid as many stressors as possible. It is important to realize that completely eliminating stress from one's life is neither possible nor desirable.

In helping patients use indirect coping, nurses' actions are aimed at reducing the affective (feelings) and physiological (bodily) disturbances resulting from stress. Patients are taught techniques such as deep breathing, muscle relaxation, and imagery, which help them cope more effectively with stress (Boxes 17–4 and 17–5).

To assist patients to manage stress, it is important that nurses be skilled in assessing and managing their own personal stress. Nurses who are feeling stressed themselves have difficulty assisting patients to deal with similar problems. Identifying your own sources of stress is an important first step. The questions in Box 17-6 can help you begin the process of becoming self-aware and thereby effective in helping patients deal with stress.

Teaching and Learning. Patient education is a major part of nursing practice, and nurses have a professional responsibility to ensure that their patients' learning needs are met. When patients are competent in the knowledge and skills they need to manage their illnesses, they tend to feel more masterful and less stressed.

BOX 17–4
Breathing Exercises

1. Sit comfortably with feet on the floor and eyes closed.
2. Inhale slowly and deeply through the nose and fill the lungs completely. As you breathe in, imagine the oxygen flowing to all your cells. Hold your breath while slowly counting to 4.
3. Slowly release all the air while thinking the word *calm*. As you breathe out, imagine the air taking all the tension out with it.
4. Repeat the cycle four times. Try to banish all thoughts except those related to your breathing, but don't fight them if other thoughts creep in.
5. When you have completed the exercise, open your eyes slowly and sit for a moment before resuming your regular activities.

BOX 17–5
Relaxation Exercises

Get into a comfortable position in a place where you will not be interrupted. First focus on slow, deep breathing. Close your eyes and begin to think about the muscle sensations in your body. Identify where you are feeling tense now. Slowly inhale as you stretch like a cat, then exhale and allow the tension to flow out.

Neck and Shoulders
Slowly bend your head forward and backward, then side to side three times. Bring your shoulders up as if you were trying to touch them to your ears. Slowly relax and feel the difference in tension.

Arms and Hands
Make a tight fist in one hand and tighten the muscles throughout your arm. Slowly release the muscles from the shoulder to the hand. Repeat with the other arm and hand.

Head
Make a wide smile and hold for a count of 5. Slowly relax your face muscles and let your jaw go loose. Tightly close your eyes and feel the tension. Slowly give up the tension and allow your eyes to remain gently closed.

Stomach
Make your stomach muscles tight by pushing them out as far as possible. Make your stomach hard and feel the tension. Slowly relax your muscles and notice the difference.

Legs and Feet
Holding your leg still, curl your toes down to point to the floor. Do first one leg and then the other. As you tighten your muscles, feel the tension. Then slowly relax.

Sit quietly for a few moments and feel the relaxation in your body before you resume your activities.

BOX 17–6
Personal Stress Inventory

	Very Often	Sometimes	Rarely or Never
1. I feel tense, anxious, and have some nervous indigestion.			
2. People at home, school, or work make me feel tense.			
3. I eat, drink, and/or smoke in response to tension.			
4. I have tension or pain in my neck or shoulders.			

(continued)

B O X   1 7 – 6   *(Continued)*

	Very Often	Sometimes	Rarely or Never
5. I have headaches or insomnia.			
6. I have trouble turning off my thoughts long enough to feel relaxed.			
7. I find it difficult to concentrate on what I am doing for worrying about other things.			
8. I take tranquilizers or other medications to relax or sleep.			
9. I feel a lot of pressure at work or school.			
10. I do not feel that my work is appreciated.			
11. My family does not appreciate what I do for them.			
12. I feel I do not have enough time for myself.			
13. I have difficulty saying "no."			
14. I wish I had more friends to share with.			
15. I do not have enough time for physical exercise.			

Scoring: Give yourself 2 points for every check in the *Very Often* column, 1 point for every check in the *Sometimes* column, and 0 points for every check in the *Rarely or Never* column.

Total the number of points.

A score of 20 to 30 represents a high level of stress. If you scored in this range, you should take steps to reduce your stress level.

A score from 10 to 19 means that you are experiencing midlevel stress. You should monitor your stress and begin relaxation exercises.

A score of 9 or under means that you are experiencing relatively low stress at the present time.

Nurses can assist patients in acquiring new methods of coping with stressors through learning, but first they must identify factors that can create barriers to learning. One factor is anxiety.

Mild anxiety improves learning by increasing the ability to focus on the task. As anxiety increases, however, the ability to listen, pay attention, and concentrate decreases. Information is not retained, and the patient is unable to make the cognitive connections that are required for learning to take place.

Physiological factors may also impede learning. Visual or hearing deficits must be overcome. Unmet physiological needs, such as fatigue, shortness of breath, hunger, or thirst, decrease the patient's attention to learning. Pain dramatically impairs the ability to learn. Nurses who ensure that patients' physiological needs are met enhance their readiness to learn.

Culture also influences learning. This is especially true when patient and nurse have different languages and patterns of learning. When the nurse works toward an educational goal that is not seen as desirable by a patient of a different culture, their cultural values may be in conflict. Understanding the meaning of illness in the patient's culture is necessary. Using language the patient can understand and handouts written in the patient's native language and reading level are important. Using an interpreter also shows sensitivity to cultural differences.

Lack of motivation and readiness are often significant barriers to education. The patient may not be motivated to learn what the nurse plans to teach. Often, nurses believe that simply pointing out what they need to know is sufficient to motivate patients. It is usually more effective to assist patients to make their own decisions about what knowledge is needed. This may require greater effort initially, but it is more efficient in the long run to assess patient motivation and readiness before engaging in patient teaching.

The nurse who is preparing to teach should also assess and manage the environment. A setting that is private, comfortable, and free of distractions is beneficial to the learning process. Boxes 17–7 and 17–8 review several principles of adult learning and teaching-learning concepts that are useful in working with patients.

Impact of Illness on Families

Families are best understood as systems, which means that change in one member changes the functioning of the total family. It is important to remember that

---

BOX 17–7
Principles of Adult Learning

- Prior experiences are resources for learning.
- Readiness to learn is usually related to a social role or developmental task.
- Motivation to learn is greater when the material is seen as immediately useful.

BOX 17–8
Teaching and Learning Concepts

- The learner learns best when there is active involvement.
- Feedback should include both positive and negative comments.
- The presentation should proceed from simple to complex concepts.

- Practice, or frequent repetition, reinforces skill acquisition.
- Learning is enhanced when multiple senses are used: Seeing, hearing, telling, and doing make the best combination.

---

the entire family system is affected by a member's illness. Illness and hospitalization are situations that can drastically increase stress in a family and cause disruptions in how the family functions.

Stress is one of the greatest threats to the healthy functioning of a family. The most important factor in how a family tolerates stress is the coping abilities of the members as individuals and as a group. Families already experiencing difficulties may find that their problems are intensified to the point of disruption when acute or chronic illness occurs in a family member.

When a member of a family becomes ill, the sick member has to give up responsibility to other family members. The family must continue to fulfill its usual functions while dealing with the alterations imposed by the illness or absence of a member. Flexible family members who are able to shift and assume different roles, who can share their feelings, and who seek assistance as needed can be expected to adjust to changes better.

Both acute and chronic illness cause changes in family functioning. Chronic illness can be particularly difficult because it is never completely cured. Families experience emotional highs and lows as the patient has remissions and exacerbations.

Resentment may be experienced in families with a sick member. Those family members who must take over the sick person's responsibilities may be angry and then feel guilty about the anger. Family members who are unable to deal with feelings of anger may displace them onto nurses by becoming critical and demanding. Similarly, patients may feel guilty about creating hardships for loved ones. They may become convinced that they are no longer essential because others are capably taking over their roles.

Family members sometimes withdraw from each other because they fear that their negative feelings may not be understood and accepted. This mutual withdrawal leads to feelings of isolation for both patients and family members.

Families are often confused or uncertain about how to treat the sick member. They may have problems accepting and responding appropriately to the patients' dependency needs. As discussed earlier, patients may react to illness with either overly dependent or overly independent behaviors. Nurses need to monitor whether family members foster dependence, thereby keeping the patient from becoming more independent. Nurses should also be aware that some families are uncomfortable with the ill person being in a dependent role and do not allow the necessary dependency for recovery. For example, if a man who is very much in control in a family has a heart attack and is in the coronary care unit, family members may have difficulty seeing the usually strong father in a helpless position. They may continue to bring family problems to him. Other families may find it difficult to shift responsibilities back to the formerly ill member as he or she becomes able to resume role functions, thereby fostering dependence.

The accompanying Research Note concerns how illness affects family roles.

The nurse needs to recognize the anxiety in the family and take steps to reduce it. Talking with members, explaining what is happening and what to expect, and teaching them how to participate in their loved one's care can help the family considerably.

The nurse should assess the family functioning and the ability of the family to provide support for the patient. Observe for feelings of anger, resentment, and guilt and assist the family in identifying adaptive methods of expressing these feelings. The nurse needs to determine the level of knowledge of the family members and assist them to identify concerns and make realistic plans. Providing information and including the family in the planning can result in increased support for the patient and more effective care.

Nurses must be prepared to accept the anger and distrust that often is directed toward care providers who are unable to cure disease or relieve the negative consequences of illness. Understanding that anger expressed by patients and families is not personally directed can enable nurses to assess patients objectively and respond to feelings expressed in a nondefensive manner.

Despite the numerous stresses and adjustments necessitated by illness of a family member, many families find that there are also positive experiences. Find-

RESEARCH NOTE

Research on how illness affects family roles increases the knowledge base needed to develop effective nursing interventions to meet family needs. Johnson and colleagues undertook a study designed to identify the changes in family roles and responsibilities resulting from the hospitalization of a family member in a critical care unit. They also studied how these changes were affected by the passage of time.

The study involved 52 family members who visited patients in critical care units in a large midwestern medical center. The subjects completed the Iowa ICU Family Scale each day during the first week and weekly thereafter as long as the patient remained in the unit. Family members were asked to describe changes in family roles and responsibilities. Approximately 59 percent reported that they experienced changes in family roles or responsibilities as a result of the hospitalization. Qualitative analysis of their responses identified seven themes: (1) pulling together, (2) fragmentation, (3) increased dependence, (4) increased independence, (5) increased responsibilities, (6) change in routine, and (7) change in feelings. The researchers recommended that further research be conducted to examine how family roles vary within family systems.

(Adapted with permission of Johnson, S., Craft, M., Titler, M., Halm, M., Kleiber, C., Montgomery, K., Nicholson, A., and Burkwalter, K. (1995). Perceived changes in adult family members' roles and responsibilities during critical illness. *IMAGE: Journal of Nursing Scholarship*, 27(3), 238–243. Copyright 1995 by Sigma Theta Tau International.)

ing new activities to share and working together to meet the challenges can lead to feelings of closeness that were not present before. Previously unrecognized individual strengths may be identified as new roles and responsibilities are assumed. New meanings for the entire family may emerge as values are reassessed and shifted.

SUMMARY

Illness involves a perception of loss. Sick people tend to progress through stages of disbelief and denial, irritability and anger, attempting to gain control, depression, and acceptance and participation. Societal expectations of sick people are that they want to get well, will seek appropriate care, and will cooperate in treatment. In return, they are exempted from some of their usual responsibilities during their illnesses.

Although society has expectations about how sick people should behave, there are several factors that influence actual behavior. Previous experience and personality characteristics are factors that affect individuals' responses to illness.

Because of the stress and anxiety involved with illness, it is important for the individual to have methods of handling them. Coping ability is enhanced in people who exhibit personality characteristics of hardiness and learned resourcefulness. Spiritual beliefs may also play a role in stress reduction.

Providing holistic care means that nurses must consider their patients' families. The family is a system in which a change in one member affects all the other members. Illness causes alterations in usual family functioning that can result in feelings of anger and guilt. The nurse needs to assess both how the family is influencing the patient and how they are being influenced by the member who is ill.

An understanding of the factors that affect behaviors associated with illness can provide a better framework for the delivery of nursing care that is satisfying to patients, families, and nurses. As nurses view responses to illness in the context of the person's total life, they are better able to understand and accept the unique ways in which individuals and families react to illness.

REVIEW AND DISCUSSION QUESTIONS

1. Think of your most recent illness. Can you identify any benefits you gained from being ill?
2. If you or someone close to you has been hospitalized, how did the nurses encourage or discourage dependent behaviors?
3. How much do you value your independence? Would it be easy or hard to allow yourself to be bathed and have other intimate needs met by nurses?
4. Identify your own cultural group's response to illness. What are your family's characteristic responses to illness of a member?
5. Interview someone from another cultural background to learn how he or she perceives illness.
6. Speculate about the potential changes in the family of a husband and father of four small children who has experienced a severe illness and will be unable to work for an extended period. What stresses is this family likely to

encounter? How would these stresses change if the wife and mother were the sick family member?

REFERENCES

Bowsher, J., and Keep, D. (1995). Toward an understanding of three control constructs: Personal control, self-efficacy, and hardiness. *Issues in Mental Health*, 16, 33–50.

Ellis, J., and Nowlis, E. (1994). *Nursing: A human needs approach* (5th ed.). Philadelphia: J. B. Lippincott.

Johnson, S., Craft, M., Titler, M., Halm, M., Kleiber, C., Montgomery, K., Nicholson, A., and Burkwalter, K. (1995). Perceived changes in adult family members' roles and responsibilities during critical illness. *IMAGE: Journal of Nursing Scholarship*, 27(3), 238–243.

Kozier, B., Erb, G., Blais, K., and Wilkinson, J. (1994). *Fundamentals of nursing* (5th ed.). New York: Addison-Wesley.

Larson, L. (1996). Heaven and hospitals: The role of spirituality in healing. *AHA News*, 32(1), 7.

Miller, J. F. (1992). *Coping with chronic illness* (2nd ed.). Philadelphia: F. A. Davis.

Parsons, T. (1951). *The social system*. New York: Free Press.

Peplau, H. (1963). A working definition of anxiety. In S. F. Burd and M. A. Marshall (Eds.), *Some clinical approaches to psychiatric nursing*. New York: Macmillan.

Selye, H. (1956). *The stress of life*. New York: McGraw-Hill.

Thorne, S. E. (1993). *Negotiating health care: The social context of chronic illness*. Newbury Park, CA: Sage Publications.

Whiting, S. A. (1994). A Delphi study to determine defining characteristics of interdependence and dysfunctional independence as potential nursing diagnoses. *Issues in Mental Health Nursing*, 15, 37–47.

Zauszniewski, J. A. (1995). Learned resourcefulness: A conceptual analysis. *Issues in Mental Health Nursing*, 16, 13–31.

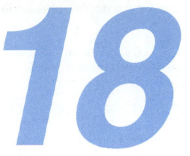

Kay K. Chitty

Communication and Collaboration in Nursing

OBJECTIVES

- Describe "therapeutic use of self."
- Explore the role self-awareness plays in the ability to use nonjudgmental acceptance as a helping technique.
- Discuss factors creating successful or unsuccessful communication.
- Evaluate interactions according to criteria for successful communication: feedback, appropriateness, efficiency, and flexibility.
- Differentiate between therapeutic and social relationships.
- Recognize own helpful and unhelpful communication patterns.
- Identify key prerequisites of collaboration.
- Explain the impact of gender culture on nurse-physician relationships.

VOCABULARY

acceptance	feedback	open posture
action language	flexibility	perception
active listening	incongruent	receiver
appropriateness	irrational belief	self-awareness
clarification	message	sender
communication	nonjudgmental	somatic language
congruent	acceptance	stereotypes
context	nonverbal	transmission
efficiency	communication	ventilation
evaluation	nurse-patient	verbal communication
false reassurance	relationship	

Interpersonal skills are important to professional nurses. Regardless of the settings in which they work and the roles they assume within those settings, most nurses interact with numerous other people every day. The way they relate to patients, families, colleagues, and other professionals and nonprofessionals determines the level of comfort and trust others feel and, ultimately, how successful their interactions are. This chapter includes information that enhances the development of self-awareness, nonjudgmental acceptance of others, communication skills, and collaboration skills, all of which are essential components of effective interpersonal relationships in nursing.

THERAPEUTIC USE OF SELF

As mentioned in Chapter 11, Hildegard Peplau first focused on the importance of the nurse-patient relationship in her 1952 book *Interpersonal Relations in Nursing*. She called using one's personality and communication skills to help patients improve their health status "therapeutic use of self."

The ability to use oneself therapeutically can be developed. Nurses develop this ability by acquiring certain knowledge, attitudes, and skills that assist them in relating effectively to patients, patients' families, co-workers, and other health care professionals.

Developing Self-Awareness

Awareness of oneself, called **self-awareness,** is basic to effective interpersonal relationships. Robert Burns, the eighteenth-century Scottish poet, described the desire for self-awareness in his poem *To a Louse:* "Oh wad some Power the giftie gie us/To see oursels as ithers see us!" (Barke, 1955).

Few people have the innate capacity to recognize their own emotional needs, biases, and blind spots as well as their impact on others. With practice, however, most can become more effective in doing so, thus improving self-awareness.

An important guideline in professional nursing is that nurses should get their own emotional needs met outside of the **nurse-patient relationship.** When nurses' strong unmet needs for **acceptance,** approval, friendship, or even love enter into their relationships with patients, professionalism is lost, and relationships become social in nature. Becoming aware of one's needs and making conscious efforts to meet those needs in one's private life make professional, therapeutic relationships with patients possible. Table 18–1 outlines several differences in social and professional relationships.

Nurses care for a widely diverse array of patients whose values, beliefs, and lifestyles may challenge the nurses' own. Patients sometimes are attractive or re-

---

TABLE 18–1
Differences in Social and Professional Relationships

Social	Professional
Not time limited	Limited in time
Not necessarily goal directed	Goal directed
Centered on meeting both parties' needs	Centered on meeting patient needs
No obligation to problem solve	Obligation to problem solve
May or may not include nonjudgmental acceptance	Includes nonjudgmental acceptance
Aim is pleasure for both parties	Aim is improved health for one party
Spontaneous interactions	Planned and purposeful interactions

pellant to nurses. Sometimes nurses find themselves meeting their own needs to be liked or needed through relationships with patients. Nurses who have emotional reactions to patients, positive or negative, sometimes feel disturbed or guilty about these feelings. Part of self-awareness is recognizing one's feelings and understanding that although feelings cannot be controlled, behaviors can. Effective nurses control their behaviors to prevent their own prejudices, beliefs, and needs from intruding into nurse-patient relationships.

Developing Trust

A reality of contemporary nursing practice is that an interaction with a patient may be brief, sometimes lasting only minutes. Even in the briefest contacts, nurses must orient patients and help them feel comfortable and as trusting as possible.

Certain nursing behaviors help patients develop the feeling that the nurse can be trusted. A straightforward, nondefensive manner is important. Answering all questions as fully as possible and admitting not knowing everything also facilitate trust. Promise to find out the answer and report the information to the patient as soon as possible. Be there at the designated time or make arrangements to let the patient know of a change in plans. Use active listening behaviors and accept the patient's thoughts and feelings without judgment.

Congruence between verbal and nonverbal communication is a key factor in the development of trust. Communicating in a congruent manner requires that nurses be aware of their own thoughts and feelings and be able to share those with others in a nonthreatening manner. The communication patterns self-assessment in Box 18–1 is the type of activity that can help improve self-awareness.

BOX 18–1
Communication Patterns Self-Assessment

Directions: Answer the following true/false questions as honestly as possible. Then review your answers and draw at least two conclusions about your habitual communication patterns. Check your conclusions for accuracy with a friend who knows your style of communicating well.

1. I usually listen about as much as I talk.
2. I rarely interrupt others.
3. I pay close attention to what others say.
4. I usually make eye contact with the person I am talking with.
5. I can usually tell if someone is angry or upset.
6. I would hesitate to interrupt someone to ask for clarification.
7. People often tell me personal things about themselves.
8. I find it is best to change the subject if someone gets too emotional.
9. If I can't "make things better" for a friend with a problem, I feel uncomfortable.
10. I am comfortable talking with people much older or much younger than myself.

Avoiding Stereotypes

Stereotypes and prejudices are attitudes developed through interactions with family, friends, and others in each individual's social and cultural system. It is not uncommon for even well-educated professionals to have stereotyped expectations about groups of people different from themselves. These stereotypes are established through childhood experiences and affect relationships with people in the stereotyped group. Because stereotypes and prejudices tend to persist despite contrary experiences, they are **irrational,** or illogical, **beliefs.**

The subtle intrusion of stereotyped expectations into the nurse-patient relationship can cause disturbed patterns of relating. For example, the expectation that all elderly people are irritable and demanding may cause the nurse to avoid all elderly patients or treat their complaints as unimportant.

Professional nurses deliver high-quality care to all patients regardless of ethnicity, age, gender, religion, lifestyle, or diagnosis. The *Code for Nurses* (see Box 4–1) calls upon nurses to do this. Nurses are not without stereotypes and prejudices, however, and must strive to be aware of their own irrational feeling responses toward patients. Every professional nurse's goal is to accept patients as individuals of dignity and worth who all deserve the best nursing care possible.

Becoming Nonjudgmental

Acceptance is not always easy because prejudices are strong, and judging others as "good" or "bad" is often automatic. It is important to remember that acceptance conveys neither approval nor disapproval of patients, their personal beliefs, habits, expressions of feelings, or chosen lifestyles. **Nonjudgmental acceptance** means that nurses acknowledge all patients' rights to be different and to express their "differentness."

Therapeutic use of self begins with the ability to convey acceptance to patients and requires self-awareness and nonjudgmental attitudes on the part of nurses. Ongoing examination of attitudes toward others is both a lifelong process and an essential part of self-awareness and interpersonal growth.

COMMUNICATION THEORY

Communication is the exchange of thoughts, ideas, or information and is at the heart of all relationships. Communication is a dynamic process that is the primary instrument through which change is effected in nursing situations. Nurses use their communication skills in all phases of the nursing process. These skills are vital to effective nursing care and to effective interaction with others in health care.

Jurgen Ruesch (1972, p. 16), a pioneer communications theorist, defined communication as "all the modes of behavior that one individual employs, conscious or unconscious, to affect another: not only the spoken and written word, but also gestures, body movements, somatic signals, and symbolism in the arts."

Communication begins the moment two people become aware of one another's presence. It is impossible *not* to communicate when in the presence of another person, even if no words are spoken. Even when alone, people routinely engage in "self-talk," which is an internal form of communication.

Levels of Communication

Communication exists on at least two levels: verbal and nonverbal. **Verbal communication** consists of all speech and represents only a small part of communication. The majority of communication is **nonverbal communication,** which consists of grooming, clothing, gestures, posture, facial expressions, tone and volume of voice, and actions, among other things (Fig. 18–1). Because individuals tend to exercise less conscious control over their nonverbal communication than the verbal, nonverbal is considered a more reliable expression of feeling.

Consider, for example, a young woman who is angry with her boyfriend. She may "clam up," pout, or otherwise show her displeasure nonverbally but when asked, "What's wrong?" may reply, "Nothing. Nothing at all!" The wise suitor would pay more attention to her nonverbal communication than to the spoken word. If he pays attention only to her words, she may become even more annoyed at his lack of perceptiveness. His job in evaluating her intent is made more difficult by the incongruence between her verbal and nonverbal messages.

F I G U R E   1 8 – 1
Nonverbal communication consists of grooming, clothing, gestures, posture, facial expressions, tone and volume of voice, and actions. (Courtesy of the University of Akron.)

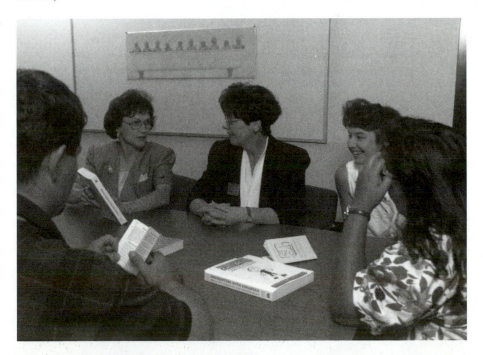

When **congruent** communication occurs, the verbal and nonverbal aspects match and reinforce each other. For example, the words "I'm glad to see you!" spoken in a pleasant tone and accompanied by a smile and a proffered hand represent congruence between verbal and nonverbal behavior. The same words spoken listlessly, in a monotone, and without eye contact convey **incongruent** communication. Incongruent communication creates confusion in receivers, who are unsure to which level of communication they should respond.

Elements of the Communication Process

Ruesch identified five major elements that must be present for communication to take place: a sender, a message, a receiver, feedback, and context. The **sender,** is the person sending the message, the **message** is what is actually said plus accompanying nonverbal communication, and the **receiver** is the person receiving the message. A response to a message is termed **feedback.** The setting in which an interaction occurs—the mood, relationship between sender and receiver, and other factors—is known as the **context.** All of these elements are necessary for communication to occur.

Consider the classroom situation. During a lecture, the professor is the sender, the lecture is the message, and students are the receivers. The professor (sender) receives feedback from the students (receivers) through their facial expressions, alertness, posture, and attentiveness. The atmosphere in the classroom is the context. If the atmosphere is a relaxed one of give-and-take between students and professor, the feedback is quite different from feedback in a more formal context. Figure 18–2 shows the relationships among the five elements of communication.

FIGURE   18 – 2
Elements of the communication process.

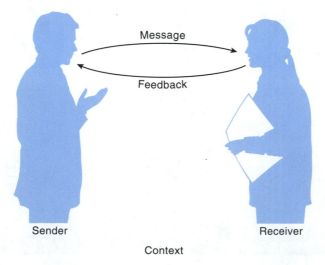

Sender

Receiver

Context

Operations in the Communication Process

In addition to the five elements of communication, Ruesch also identified three major operations in communication. They are perception, evaluation, and transmission.

PERCEPTION

Perception is the selection, organization, and interpretation of incoming signals into meaningful messages. In the classroom situation just given, students select, organize, and interpret various pieces of the professor's message or lecture. Different students perceive the information differently, based on factors such as personal experience, previous knowledge, alertness, sensitivity to subtleties of meaning, and sociocultural background.

EVALUATION

Evaluation is the analysis of information received. Is the content of the professor's lecture useful? Is it important or relevant to the students' needs? Is it likely to be on the next test? Each student evaluates the message in a different manner.

TRANSMISSION

Transmission refers to the expression of information, verbally or nonverbally. While the professor is transmitting his verbal message to the students, his nonverbal behavior of excitement about his subject matter also transmits a message to the class.

INFLUENCES ON PERCEPTION, EVALUATION, AND TRANSMISSION

Perception, evaluation, and transmission are influenced by many factors. The gender and culture of the sender and receiver; the interest and mood of both parties; the value, clarity, and length of the message; the presence or absence of feedback; and the atmosphere of the context all are powerful influences. Also involved are individuals' needs, values, self-concepts, sensory and intellectual abilities or deficits, and sociocultural conditioning. Given the variety of factors involved, it is clear that communication is a complex human activity worthy of nurses' attention.

HOW COMMUNICATION DEVELOPS

People learn to use language (and therefore to communicate verbally) through a certain developmental sequence, which begins in infancy. Infants use **somatic**

language to signal their needs to caretakers. Somatic language consists of crying; reddening of the skin; fast, shallow breathing; facial expressions; and jerking of the limbs. The sequence progresses to **action language** in older infants. Action language consists of reaching out for or crawling toward a desired object, or closing the lips and turning the head when an undesired food is offered. Last to develop is verbal language, beginning with repetitive noises and sounds and progressing to words, phrases, and complete sentences.

If a child's development is normal, any one or combination of these forms of communication can be used. Somatic language usually decreases with maturity, but because it is not under conscious control, some somatic language may persist past childhood. A familiar example is facial blushing when embarrassed or angry.

The development of communication is determined by inborn and environmental factors. The amount of verbal stimulation an infant receives can enhance or retard the development of language skills. The extent of a caretaker's vocabulary and verbal ability is therefore influential. Some families engage in lengthy discussions on a variety of issues, thereby providing intense verbal stimulation, whereas others are less verbal.

Nonverbal communication development is similarly influenced by environment. Some families communicate through nonverbal gestures such as touch or facial expressions, which children learn to "read" at young ages. Other families ascribe to the adage, "Children should be seen and not heard," thus discouraging verbal expression and increasing dependence on nonverbal cues for communicating.

The ability to communicate effectively is dependent on a number of factors. Primary among these are the quantity and quality of verbal and nonverbal stimulation received during early developmental periods.

CRITERIA FOR SUCCESSFUL COMMUNICATION

Everyone has had the experience of being the sender or receiver of unsuccessful communication. An example is arriving for an appointment with a friend at the wrong time or wrong place because of a communication mix-up. Unsuccessful communication creates little harm when done under social circumstances. In nursing situations, however, accurate, complete communication is vitally important. Nurses can achieve successful communication on most occasions if they plan their communication to meet four major criteria: feedback, appropriateness, efficiency, and flexibility. Each of these criteria is examined.

Feedback

When a receiver relays back to a sender the effect that the sender's message has had, feedback has occurred. Feedback was identified as one of Ruesch's five elements necessary for communication (see Fig. 18–2). It is also a criterion for successful communication. In making the social appointment mentioned previously, if the receiver of the message had said, "Let's make sure I understand you.

We'll meet at 12:30 on Tuesday at Cafe Al Fresco," that feedback could have led to successful communication.

In a nurse-patient interaction, a nurse can give feedback to a patient by saying, "If I understand you correctly, you have pain in your lower abdomen every time you stand up." The patient can then either agree or correct what the nurse has said: "No, the pain is there only when I arise in the morning." Effective nurses do not assume that they fully understand what their patients are telling them until they feed the statement back to the patient and receive confirmation.

Appropriateness

When a reply fits the circumstances and matches the message, and the amount is neither too great nor too little, **appropriateness** has been achieved. In day-to-day conversation among acquaintances passing on the street, most people recognize the question, "How are you?" as a social nicety, not a genuine question. The individual who launches into a detailed description of how his morning has gone has communicated inappropriately. The reply does not fit the circumstances, and the quantity is too great. An appropriate response is, "Fine, and how are you?"

If a patient asks, "When is my lunch coming?" the nurse, knowing that the patient has already eaten lunch, will be alert to other inappropriate messages by this patient that may signal a variety of problems. In this instance, the inappropriate message does not match the context.

Efficiency

Using simple, clear words that are timed at a pace suitable to participants meets the criterion of **efficiency.** Explaining to an adult that she will have "an angioplasty" tomorrow morning probably will not create successful communication. Telling her she will have "a procedure where a small balloon is threaded into an artery and inflated to open up the vessel so more blood can flow through" will more likely ensure her understanding. This message would not be an efficient one for a small child, however. Messages must be adapted to each patient's age, verbal level, and level of understanding.

Some examples of patients who require special assistance in evaluating and responding to messages are young children, depressed people, some people with neurological deficits, and those recovering from anesthesia. For efficient communication to occur, nurses must recognize patients' needs and adjust messages accordingly.

Flexibility

The fourth criterion for successful communication is **flexibility.** The flexible communicator bases messages on the immediate situation rather than preconceived expectations. When a student nurse who plans to teach a patient about diabetic diets enters the patient's room and finds her crying, the nurse must be flexible enough to change gears and deal with the feelings the patient is expressing. Pressing on with the lesson plan in the face of the patient's distress shows a lack of compassion as well as inflexibility in communicating.

Nurses can learn to use these four measures of successful communication to enhance their effectiveness with patients. The continuing absence or malfunction of any of these four criteria can create disturbed communication and hamper the implementation of the nursing process.

BECOMING A BETTER COMMUNICATOR

People are not born being good communicators. Communication skills can be developed if you are willing to put forth a moderate amount of time and energy. Becoming a better listener, learning a few basic helpful responding styles, and avoiding common causes of communication breakdown can put you on the path to becoming a better communicator.

Listening

A requirement of successful verbal communication in any setting is listening. **Active listening** is a method of communicating interest and attention. Using such signals as good eye contact, nodding, use of "mumbles" (mmhmm), and encouraging the speaker ("Go on" or "Tell me more about this") all help to communicate interest. Facing the speaker squarely and using an **open posture** (arms uncrossed) also communicate interest.

Having someone listen to concerns, even if no problem solving takes place, is considered therapeutic. **Ventilation** is the term used to describe the verbal "letting off steam" that occurs when talking about concerns or frustrations. The experience of feeling "listened to" is becoming so rare in contemporary American society that a columnist in the *Christian Science Monitor* was prompted to write about it (News Note).

Nurses may have difficulty listening for a variety of reasons. They may be intent on accomplishing a task and be frustrated by the time it takes to be a good listener. They may be planning their own next response and not hear what the patient is saying. Similar to other people, nurses have their own personal and professional problems that sometimes preoccupy them and interfere with effective listening. Nurses must remember that no verbal message can be received if the receiver (the nurse) is not listening.

Three common listening faults include interrupting, finishing sentences for others, and lack of interest. It is important for nurses to remember that what the patient is saying is just as important as what the nurse wishes to say.

Being listened to meets the patient's emotional need to be respected and valued by the nurse. Listening can help avert problems by letting people ventilate about the pressures they feel. Hospitalized patients particularly may feel that their lives are out of control and may need to discuss those feelings with someone who will listen without becoming defensive (Fig. 18–3).

Nurses at all levels find listening a useful skill. Nurse managers often use lis-

NEWS NOTE
Where Did All the Listeners Go?

When everybody learned how to tune out their machines—blabbing-off radio and television ads, hanging up on computer phone calls, and so on—they also learned how to tune out other people.

During the talkiest era ever, nobody listens. Or so it is assumed. In his new novel, "A Tenured Professor," Harvard economist John Kenneth Galbraith puts it nicely:

"By long custom, social discourse in Cambridge is intended to impart and only rarely to obtain information. People talk; it is not expected that anyone will listen. A respectful show of attention is all that is required until the listener takes over in his or her turn."

But wait. Just as it seems that the glazed-over eye and the numbed ear typify the Age of the Non-Listener, there is heartening news.

In Milwaukee, the Roman Catholic Archdiocese is sponsoring six "listening sessions" to give Catholic women a chance to express their feelings about abortion.

The first session, held last month in a college gymnasium in Fond du Lac, Wis., drew 100 women. While participants gathered in small groups to discuss the volatile issue, Archbishop Rembert Weakland, who organized the event, moved from table to table, listening and reportedly saying little.

Archbishop Weakland, considered one of the more liberal Catholic leaders, has been criticized within his church for his gesture. But as he explained to a reporter, "The polarization about this issue has become so great that I had to admit we needed dialogue about it within the Catholic community."

It is one thing for equals to listen to equals, or for subordinates to listen to those in authority. But it is a high tribute when individuals in power listen to those below them.

Once upon a time, being a "good lis-tener" was considered a social grace. At least 51 percent of the world were "good listeners." They were also called women. A young woman learned by example that her gender role was to listen to what others—especially men—were saying. Her mouth was primarily for smiling at what she heard, with an occasional rhythmic "uh-huh."

Today that "uh-huh" is increasingly likely to come from a stranger. Lending an ear has become a paid profession. As if to signify a national hunger for "listening sessions," an entire industry has sprung up.

Eight-year-olds phone latchkey hotlines for after-school comfort and conversation while Mom—the original "good listener"—is off at work. Bereaved dog and cat owners call on pet grief counselors for animal-loving shoulders to cry on. Even technology offers an ear, this one electronic, as answering machines and voice mailboxes do more and more of the listening.

Then of course there is the biggest listening post of all, the talk show. What does it say about the desperate yearning for an audience, any audience, that guests are willing to bare their souls and share their most intimate secrets not with close friends but with Oprah, Phil, Geraldo—and millions of TV viewers?

Is this what it takes to get a word in edgewise in the late 20th century?

Outside the TV studio, other cameras reveal that finding a "good listener"—or any listener at all—can be a tricky business in classrooms as well, especially for women.

Catherine Krupnick, a researcher at the Harvard Graduate School of Education, videotaped thousands of hours of college classes. She discovered that even when male students made up just one-tenth of a class, the men would do one-quarter of the talking. Other studies over

(continued)

NEWS NOTE *(Continued)*
Where Did All the Listeners Go?

the past two decades confirm Ms. Krup-nick's findings, showing that professors are more likely to call on men.

The philosopher Mortimer Adler has called listening "the untaught skill." Those like Archbishop Weakland may be thought of as pioneers in retraining. But the changeover from mouth to ear won't come easily. The thing about listening is that it takes more time and, in fact, more thought than merely talking.

When a reporter, after one of the "listening sessions" in Wisconsin, asked the Archbishop what he thought, he gave the right answer: "I'm still listening."
—Marilyn Gardner

tening as a tool for dealing with staff members' problems and concerns and find that no other intervention is required. Listening is a talent that can be developed; properly used, it can be an important part of a nurse's communication repertoire.

FIGURE   18–3

Being an active listener is an important part of communication. (Courtesy Memorial Hospital, Chattanooga, Tennessee.)

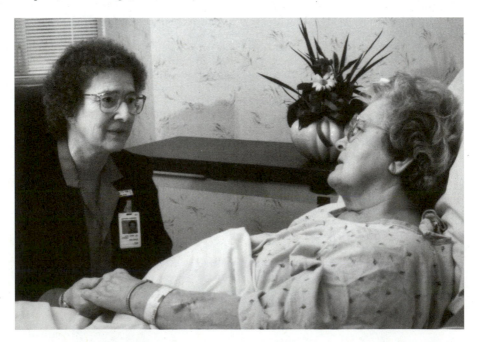

Using Helpful Responding Techniques

There are many helpful responding techniques nurses can use to demonstrate respect and encourage patients to communicate openly. Helpful responses that have already been discussed in this chapter include being nonjudgmental, observing body language, and active listening. Other useful responses include empathy, open-ended questions, giving information, reflection, and silence. These communication-enhancing techniques are covered fully in psychosocial nursing courses.

Avoiding Common Causes of Communication Breakdown

Just as there are many factors influencing successful communication, unsuccessful communication can occur for many reasons. A sender may send an incomplete or confusing message. A message may not be received, or it may be misunderstood or distorted by the receiver. Incongruent messages may cause confusion in the receiver. In nursing situations, there are several common causes of communication breakdown. They include failing to see each individual as unique, failing to recognize levels of meaning, using value statements, using false reassurance, and failing to clarify unclear messages.

FAILING TO SEE THE UNIQUENESS OF THE INDIVIDUAL

Failing to see the uniqueness of each individual is a frequent cause of communication breakdown. This failure is caused by preconceived ideas, prejudices, and stereotypes. This problem is illustrated by the following interchange between a patient and a nurse:

P: My back is really hurting today. I can hardly turn over in bed.

N: I guess we have to expect these little problems when we get older.

 This nurse has pigeonholed her patient in her mental group "old people" and therefore does not react to the patient as an individual. The nurse could have promoted continued communication by responding to the patient as an individual:

N: Tell me exactly how your back hurts, Mrs. Jameson.

FAILING TO RECOGNIZE LEVELS OF MEANING

When nurses recognize no level of meaning other than the obvious ones, communication breakdown can occur. Patients often give verbal cues to meanings that lie under the surface content of their verbalizations:

P: It's getting awfully warm in here.

N: (*Responding only to surface meaning*) I'll adjust the air conditioning for you.

This response does not help the patient express himself fully. A different type of response focuses on the symbolic level of meaning.

N: Perhaps the questions I am asking are making you uncomfortable.

Although it takes a lot of experience to know when and how to respond to symbolic communication, nurses should be aware of its existence.

USING VALUE STATEMENTS AND CLICHÉS

Using value statements and clichés is another communication problem. The use of clichés, which are trite, stereotyped expressions, is common in social conversation. Consider the prevalence of the cliché "Have a good day." This statement has come to have little real meaning.

This common error can cut off communication by showing the patient that the nurse does not understand the patient's true feelings.

P: My mother is coming to see me today.

N: How nice. Do you want to put on a fresh gown?

This nurse has failed to verify that the patient actually wishes to see her mother. In fact, the patient and her mother may have a difficult relationship, and the patient may dread the impending visit. By assuming otherwise, the nurse has contributed to communication breakdown. This patient probably will not attempt to discuss her relationship with her mother any further with this nurse. A more helpful response would be:

N: How do you feel about her visit?

This allows the patient to ventilate her feelings about her mother's visit, whether positive or negative. The nurse has conveyed a genuine interest in the patient's true feelings.

GIVING FALSE REASSURANCE

Using **false reassurance** is another communication pitfall. It may help the nurse feel better but does not facilitate communication and help the patient.

P: I'm so afraid the biopsy will be cancer.

N: Don't worry. You have the best doctor in town. Besides, cancer treatment is really good these days.

For a fearful patient, this type of glib reassurance does not help. This nurse has no way of knowing that the patient's concerns are not legitimate. She may indeed *have* cancer. A more sensitive response would be:

N: Why don't we talk about your concerns?

This kind of response keeps the lines of communication open between patient and nurse.

FAILING TO CLARIFY

Failing to clarify the patient's unclear statements is a fifth common communication pitfall.

P: I've got to get out of the hospital. They have found out I'm here and may come after me.

N: No one will harm you here.

This nurse has responded as if the patient's meaning was clear. A more clarifying response might be:

N: Who are "they," Mrs. Johnson?

Confused patients or those with psychiatric illnesses often communicate in ways that are difficult to understand. It is reassuring to patients to know that nurses are trying to understand them, even if they are not always successful. Communication is facilitated by **clarification** responses.

Practicing Helpful Responses

Nurses can practice using helpful responses and avoiding common communication pitfalls with family members, friends, and co-workers as well as in patient contacts. Being a good communicator takes practice and usually feels unnatural at first. Any new behavior takes time to integrate into habitual patterns. By continuing to practice, nurses soon find themselves feeling more natural. They find that these newly acquired skills are beneficial both professionally and personally. Box 18–2 compares different responses in a nurse-patient interaction.

COMMUNICATION WITH PROFESSIONAL COLLEAGUES

This chapter has focused on nurse-patient communication as the core of the nursing process and foundation of the therapeutic use of self. In addition to patients and their families, however, nurses must also communicate effectively with a variety of professional and unlicensed personnel such as physicians, other nurses, and nursing assistants. Health care delivery suffers when the members of the health care team experience communication breakdown.

As a general rule, nurses can use the same communication skills with colleagues that have been discussed as part of nurse-patient communication. The attitude of respect for others, regardless of position, is essential. Active listening, acceptance, and nonjudgmentalism are key elements, as are the conscious use of feedback, appropriateness, efficiency, and flexibility.

Wise nurses do not leave their communication skills at the patient's bedside

BOX 18–2
Case Study: Helpful and Unhelpful Responding Techniques

Directions: Critique both interactions, identifying the helpful and unhelpful responses used by the nurse. Describe how you imagine the patient might feel at the close of each interaction. Itemize what the nurse has accomplished in each instance.

Mr. Goodman has been admitted to the hospital for coronary bypass surgery. During the admission process, the following interactions might take place.

Interaction #1
N: Mr. Goodman, I am Mrs. Scott. Can I get some information about you now?

P: Okay.

N: You're here for bypass surgery?

P: Yes, that's what they tell me.

N: (*Taking blood pressure*) Do you have any allergies to foods or medications?

P: Not that I know of. I've never been in a hospital before.

N: Well, your blood pressure looks good. (*Silence while patient has thermometer in mouth*) This is a really nice room—just remodeled. I know you'll be comfortable here. Will your wife be coming to see you tonight? (*Removes thermometer*)

P: My wife is sick. She hasn't been able to leave home for two years. I don't know what will happen to her while I am here.

N: Gosh, I'm so sorry to hear that. I guess having you back home healthy is what she wants though, isn't it? And you've got a great surgeon. Well, I've got to run now. Check on you later.

Interaction #2
N: Good afternoon, Mr. Goodman. I'm Mrs. Scott, and I'll be your nurse this evening. If this is a good time, I'd like to ask you some questions and complete your admission process.

P: Okay.

N: First, I'll get your temperature and blood pressure, and then we'll talk. (*Silence while nurse takes vital signs*) Everything looks good. Do you have any allergies to foods or medications?

P: Not that I know of. I've never been in a hospital before.

N: Hospitals can be a little overwhelming, especially when you've never been a patient before. Now, would you please tell me in your own words why you are here?

P: Well, the doc tells me I have a clogged artery, and I need a bypass. I guess they'll open up my heart.

N: What exactly do you know about the surgery?

P: Not too much, really. He told me yesterday that I need it right away—and here I am.

N: It sounds like you need some more information about what will happen. Later this evening I will come back, and we'll talk some more. Are you expecting to have visitors tonight?

P: No, my wife can't leave home. I don't know what she will do without me while I'm here. This came up so suddenly.

N: I can see that this is a serious concern for you. We can explore some possibilities when I come back this evening. I'll plan to come around 7:15, if that suits you.

P: Sure, I can use all the help I can get.

but use them throughout their personal and professional lives. Using clear, simple messages and clarifying the intent of others constitute a positive goal in all personal and professional communication. As with patients, trust must exist before communication with co-workers can be effective.

COLLABORATION SKILLS

Collaboration is a complex process that is related to communication. An often misunderstood concept, collaboration in health care settings is far more than simply cooperation or compromise. Henneman and colleagues analyzed collaboration to understand its complexities better. They asserted that collaboration implies working jointly with other professionals, all of whom are respected for their unique knowledge and abilities, to benefit a patient's wellness or illness needs or to solve an organizational problem. It involves sharing knowledge and authority and is nonhierarchical. For collaboration to occur, a variety of human and organizational factors must be in place (Henneman, Lee, and Cohen, 1995).

Human Factors in Collaboration

Although it may seem obvious, all collaborating parties must be willing to work together if the collaboration is to be successful. They must have attained a level of readiness to collaborate through education, maturity, and prior experience (Henneman, Lee, and Cohen, 1995). They must know what knowledge and expertise they bring to the table and have confidence in the worth of their contributions. They must understand their own limits and their discipline's boundaries while respecting what other professions and professionals can contribute. Above all, they must communicate effectively, trust one another, and be committed to working together (Henneman, Lee, and Cohen, 1995).

Organizational Factors in Collaboration

Just as the people involved must have certain attributes that facilitate collaboration, the organization in which the collaboration takes place also must be supportive. According to Henneman and colleagues, factors supporting collaboration include a flat, as opposed to a multitiered, organizational structure; encouragement and support of individuals to act autonomously; recognition of team accomplishments, as opposed to individual accomplishments; cooperation as opposed to competition; and valuing of knowledge and expertise rather than titles or roles. Collaborative organizations have values that support equality and interdependence rather than status and pecking orders. Creativity and shared vision are also valued (Henneman, Lee, and Cohen, 1995).

Outcomes of Collaboration

Collaboration is a positive process that benefits the people involved, as individuals and as a group; the organization in which they work; and health care consumers. Henneman and colleagues identified increased feelings of self-worth; a sense of accomplishment; *esprit de corps*; enhanced collegiality and respect; and increased productivity, retention, and employee satisfaction as positive benefits of collaboration. They suggested that patient outcomes are also improved by collaboration among health care professionals (Henneman, Lee, and Cohen, 1995).

Nurse-Physician Collaboration

Among the most problematic relationships that nurses encounter during practice are those with physicians. Despite rising male enrollments in nursing schools and even more dramatic female enrollments in medical schools, practicing physicians are predominantly male and practicing nurses overwhelmingly female. This leads to differences in styles of communicating and behaving that can cause difficulty in collaborative relationships.

During female-dominated nursing school experiences, most nurses are encouraged to view physicians as teammates and to collaborate with them whenever possible. Male-dominated medical schools, however, tend to instill in their graduates a hierarchical model of teamwork with the physician at the top of the hierarchy. These two divergent cultures, when combined with gender differences in communication and teamwork patterns, further complicate the relationship between the two professions. Too often, gender differences are interpreted as professional differences, leading to further misunderstanding.

People realize that there are differences in communication styles and behavior among individuals of different cultures. What too few people recognize is that gender is a culture because men and women grow up learning different lessons about what is appropriate adult behaviors. From birth, boy babies and girl babies are dressed differently, given different toys, praised for different types of behavior, and socialized to gender-appropriate behavior in dozens of more subtle ways. Teachers treat boys and girls differently; authors of children's books and television scripts depict men and women differently. Team games and being "coached" are predominantly male experiences (Heim, 1995). Is it any wonder that as adults, men and women have different expectations of professional relationships?

Women tend to treat other people as equal, regardless of their position in the organizational hierarchy. They spend time chatting with others, building and maintaining relationships, and frequently make friends at work. Even when in management roles, they tend to tell people what to do indirectly. They come to meetings expecting to discuss the issues and make decisions depending on the outcome of the discussion. They value the process aspects of decision making as much as the outcome (Heim, 1995).

Men tend to see other workers as above, below, or parallel to them in the organizational structure and to treat them accordingly. They chat less, are friendly but tend not to become friends with co-workers, and are likely to tell subordinates what to do directly. They come to meetings already having discussed the issues, make decisions beforehand, and line up the votes they need to get their decisions approved. They are more goal-oriented and pay less attention to process than to outcome (Heim, 1995).

Differences in gender cultures create problems in all aspects of personal and professional life if they are not understood. For insight into how gender culture may affect your working relationships, take the self-awareness exercise in Box 18–3 and discuss it in a small group composed of both genders.

BOX 18–3
Gender Culture Self-Assessment

Directions: For each of the paired statements, select the one that most accurately expresses your experiences or feelings.

Column One

I prefer to compete to win.

I like work where I know the hierarchy so I know what is expected of me.

When I lead a meeting, I prefer to sit in front of the group or at the head of the table.

In arriving at a decision, I study the options, select one, and move ahead with it.

I define a "team player" as someone who follows orders, supports the leader unquestioningly, and does what is needed no matter how he or she feels.

I can disagree or even argue with my friends and not allow it to affect the friendship.

In the workplace, competent people don't worry about being nice.

I spend little time in getting to know my co-workers personally.

Column Two

I prefer to find win-win solutions.

I like to work in situations where power is equally shared.

When I lead a meeting, I prefer to sit with the group or in a circle.

In arriving at a decision, I usually ask several other people for their opinions.

I define a "team player" as someone who shares ideas, listens even when they disagree, and works collaboratively.

I expect my friends to side with me in disagreements and tend to take it personally if they don't.

In the workplace it is possible to be both competent and nice.

It is worthwhile to spend time getting to know my co-workers on a personal level.

Scoring instructions: If most of your checks were in Column One, you have a predominantly male gender style. When you work with women, you can anticipate some difficulties because of differences in behavior and conversational patterns.

If most of your checks were in Column Two, you have a predominantly female gender style. When you work with men, you can anticipate some difficulties because of differences in behavior and conversational patterns.

If your checks were about equally balanced between Column One and Column Two, you have a combination of male and female gender styles. You should be able to work successfully with both men and women.

Collaboration with Assistive Personnel

Relationships between registered nurses and unlicensed assistive personnel, formerly known as nurse's aides or nursing assistants, affect the quality of care given to hospitalized patients. All too often, mutual respect and cooperation are missing in these important relationships, and both groups feel frustrated and unappreciated.

In many areas, ethnic and cultural differences complicate the relationship between nurses and unlicensed personnel. Language is often a barrier as well as nonverbal and other culturally determined behaviors, such as the value placed on being punctual. Differences in beliefs, values, perceptions, and priorities create conflict, poor teamwork, and reduced job satisfaction and ultimately have a negative impact on patient care (Grossman and Taylor, 1995).

Hayes (1994) reported on team building sessions with registered nurses and unlicensed personnel on three general hospital units. The purpose was to identify and align work-related relationship needs of both groups with the needs of the nursing unit. This is a key step in team building, which was the model chosen to encourage collaboration between the two groups.

Teams were defined as groups of workers that were fairly stable in composition. They worked interdependently and "shared a common purpose" (Hayes, 1994, p. 52). To emphasize that the nurses and unlicensed personnel needed to work cooperatively, each group was asked questions such as, "What do you need from each other to make your day go better?" "What is important for you to have in the way of working relationships on this nursing unit?" "What do you need from the registered nurses?" "What do you need from the nursing assistants?" (Hayes, 1994, p. 52).

Unlicensed personnel reported needing to feel welcome, appreciated, and respected but instead reported feeling unwelcome, unrecognized, and unappreciated. They did not realize that registered nurses were expected to plan, supervise, and evaluate the unlicensed personnels' work. The registered nurses expressed the need to feel competent as managers and to have unlicensed personnel comply with requests and give feedback about assigned activities. Some registered nurses reported that they preferred to complete work themselves rather than experience embarrassment when unlicensed personnel failed to comply with their requests.

Team-building sessions centered around identifying problematic feelings and misperceptions and correcting them. For example, in response to the unlicensed personnel's belief that their contributions to patient welfare were unappreciated, the registered nurses replied, "We could not run the unit without you" and "What you do makes the difference in how comfortable the patients feel" (Hayes, 1994, p. 53).

During team building with these groups, Hayes reported that misperceptions were aired and discussed, and expectations were clarified. Registered nurses' legitimate authority and responsibility for unlicensed personnel were clarified. The result was an increase in mutual respect and understanding.

To stress the importance of positive working relationships, Diann B. Uustal, clinical ethicist and consultant, adapted the familiar poem, "Children Learn What They Live" (Box 18–4). It reminds us that professional co-workers deserve respectful concern as much as do patients.

BOX 18–4
Colleagues Learn What They Live

If a colleague lives with criticism,
s/he learns to condemn.
If a colleague lives with hostility,
s/he learns to fight.
If a colleague lives with ridicule,
s/he learns to be shy.
If a colleague lives with shame,
s/he learns to feel guilty.
If a colleague lives with tolerance,
s/he learns to be patient.
If a colleague lives with encouragement,
s/he learns confidence.
If a colleague lives with praise,
s/he learns to appreciate.

If a colleague lives with fairness,
s/he learns justice.
If a colleague lives with security,
s/he learns to have faith.
If a colleague lives with approval,
s/he learns to like her/himself.
If a colleague lives with acceptance and friendship, s/he learns to find satisfaction in professional nursing.

Adapted with permission of Uustal, D. B. (1985).

SUMMARY

The "therapeutic use of self" means using one's personality and communication skills effectively while implementing the nursing process to help patients improve their health status. Communication is the core of all relationships and is the primary instrument through which desired change is effected in others.

Acceptance of others' values, beliefs, and lifestyles is important in nursing. Developing awareness of biases can help nurses to prevent the intrusion of these biases into nurse-patient relationships.

Communication is both verbal and nonverbal and consists of a sender, a receiver, a message, feedback, and context. Perception, evaluation, and transmission are the three major operations in communication.

Communication develops sequentially. It may be successful or unsuccessful. Successful communication meets four major criteria: feedback, appropriateness, efficiency, and flexibility. Active listening is a key factor in successful communication. Unsuccessful communication is caused by a variety of factors that can be identified and eliminated.

In addition to communicating well with patients, nurses use communication skills to collaborate effectively with physicians, other nurses, unlicensed personnel, and other members of the health care delivery team. Professional nurses must be sensitive to sociocultural factors such as ethnicity and gender that can affect communication and collaboration.

REVIEW AND DISCUSSION QUESTIONS

1. Explain why nonverbal communication may be more revealing than verbal communication.

2. List as many factors as you can that influence the communication process.
3. Identify a recent interaction you have had in which communication was incongruent. Analyze what effect the incongruence had on the communication. When are you most likely to use incongruent communication?
4. Think of a person with whom you have experienced difficult communication. Identify which of the barriers to successful communication are functioning in that person's communication with you and analyze your responses to that person.
5. Describe a collaborative experience you have had. What factors differentiated it from cooperation or compromise?

REFERENCES

Barke, J. (Ed.). (1955). *Burns' poems and songs*. London: Collins.

Gardner, M. (1990). Where did all the listeners go? *Christian Science Monitor*, April 27, 1990, 14.

Grossman, D., and Taylor, R. (1995). Cultural diversity on the unit. *American Journal of Nursing*, 95(2), 64–66.

Hayes, P. M. (1994). Team building: Bringing RNs and NAs together. *Nursing Management*, 25(5), 52–55.

Heim, P. (1995). Getting beyond "she said, he said." *Nursing Administration Quarterly*, 19(2), 6–18.

Henneman, E. A., Lee, J. L., and Cohen, J. I. (1995). Collaboration: A concept analysis. *Journal of Advanced Nursing*, 21(1), 103–109.

Peplau, H. (1952). *Interpersonal relations in nursing*. New York: G. P. Putnam's Sons.

Ruesch, J. (1972). *Disturbed communication: The clinical assessment of normal and pathological communicative behavior*. New York: W. W. Norton.

CHAPTER 19

Pamela S. Chally

Nursing Ethics

OBJECTIVES

- Differentiate between morals and ethics.
- Discuss the importance to nursing of having a code of ethics.
- Identify basic theories and principles central to ethical dilemmas and moral development.
- Describe ethical dilemmas resulting from conflicts between patients, health care professionals, and institutions.
- Describe a model for ethical decision making.
- Discuss the impact of ethical issues on nurses and other health care professionals.

VOCABULARY

advance directives	ethical decision making	patients' rights
autonomy	ethics	personal value system
beneficence	justice	utilitarianism
bioethics	moral development	veracity
code of ethics	morals	
deontology	nonmaleficence	

To understand ethics and its relationship to health care, the terms *morals*, *ethics*, and *bioethics* must first be clarified. It is important to realize that there are conflicting viewpoints by philosophers and scholars on how to define these terms. **Morals** are established rules in situations in which a decision about right and wrong must be made. Morals provide standards of behavior. These standards guide the behavior of an individual or social group. Morals reflect the *is* or reality of how individuals or groups behave. An example of a moral standard is "Good people do not lie."

Morals reflect the *is* of human behavior, whereas **ethics** is a term used to reflect the *should* of human behavior. Ethics identify what should be done for individuals to live with one another. Ethics are process oriented and involve critical analysis of actions. If ethicists, people who study ethics, reflected on the moral statement "One should not lie," they would clarify definitions of lying and

explore whether or not there are circumstances under which lying might be acceptable.

Despite the fact that differences between ethics and morals are noted by several authors (Davis and Aroskar, 1991; Silva, 1990; Thompson and Thompson, 1990), in everyday usage the terms are often used interchangeably.

When ethical theories and principles are applied to problems in health care, the field of study is called **bioethics.** Bioethics as an area of ethical inquiry came into existence around 1970, when health care began to shift its focus from curing disease toward concern for the total patient (Husted and Husted, 1995). A new term, *clinical ethics,* is increasingly being used.

Advances in medicine, science, and technology sometimes create ethical dilemmas. For example, people can now be kept "alive" even when brain dead. Should they be kept alive under these circumstances just because we now have the technology to do so? This kind of issue mandates that nurses be concerned with what *should* be done for patients they care for. It is important that actions be critically analyzed for their appropriateness because health care professionals possess a good deal of power over those in their care.

Within this context, nurses need to study codes of ethics, ethical theories and principles, moral development, ethical dilemmas, and ethical decision-making models. Such knowledge increases nurses' ability to participate in the resolution of ethical dilemmas. The accompanying *Letter to Nursing Students from a Critical Care Nurse* highlights some of the reasons why professional nurses need ethical decision-making skills.

NURSING CODES OF ETHICS

As discussed in Chapter 6, an essential characteristic of professions is that they have a **code of ethics.** A code of ethics is an implied contract through which the profession informs society of the principles and rules by which it functions.

Ethical codes help with professional self-regulation. They serve as guidelines to the members of the profession, who then can meet the societal need for trustworthy, qualified, and accountable caregivers. It is important to remember that codes are useful only if they are upheld by the members of the profession.

American Nurses Association Code for Nurses

The *Code for Nurses with Interpretive Statements* (American Nurses Association, 1985) is the nursing profession's expression to the public of its ethical values and duties (Fowler, 1992). The need for a code of ethics was expressed by the Nurses' Associated Alumnae (forerunner of the American Nurses Association [ANA]) as early as 1897 (Veins, 1989). A written code was actually adopted in 1950. During that 53-year time span, nursing was emerging as a profession in its own right.

The 1950 *Code* consisted of 17 short, succinct statements depicting the nurse in action (*e.g.*, "The nurse accepts . . . ," "The nurse sustains . . . ") (Veins, 1989). Even in 1950, the broad spectrum role of the nurse—in illness, prevention, and health promotion—was stressed. In addition, this code encouraged

Letter to Nursing Students From a Critical Care Nurse

Dear Nursing Student,

As you begin your nursing education, you may be focused on correctly performing manual clinical skills, i.e., fixed routines requiring psychomotor dexterity. The need to be continually aware of potential ethical dilemmas and knowledgeable of ethical decision-making strategies may seem to be near the end of a long list of overwhelming responsibilities. However, a solid ethical decision-making foundation will long outlast the anxiety associated with acquiring new psychomotor skills.

In your nursing career, you will be challenged routinely with opportunities to develop your ethical decision-making skills. What are some points to consider when developing these skills? First, take a critical look at yourself. Identify your values and beliefs. Are these values and beliefs firmly entrenched, or are you easily swayed toward change by outside pressure? Are you willing to take a firm advocacy stance on an issue you believe is correct? Are you just as willing to admit if you are wrong and learn from your experiences? Are you comfortable with sensitive or confidential information placed in your possession? Can you comfortably accept both personal praise and criticism from associates? When necessary, can you take a neutral stance and avoid the temptation to give advice?

Like many of these questions, ethical dilemmas cannot always be answered by a simple "yes" or "no." Ethical dilemmas are challenging, with some situations more dramatic than others. You may encounter such situations as supporting a patient or family through a "do not resuscitate" decision, the decision to terminate life support systems in a nonviable patient, or organ donation decisions. You may encounter the suicidal patient who confides in no one else. You may encounter chemically impaired or incompetent physicians, nurses, or other health care providers. Most of you will come up against ethical dilemmas almost on a daily basis.

As you mature in your nursing experience, encountering and resolving ethical dilemmas can prove to be a personally rewarding experience for both you and those who benefit from your abilities. Do not avoid ethical dilemmas. Instead, meet these challenges with confidence and professionalism using principles of moral decision making.

Best wishes as you continue your nursing studies,

Sandra H. Carr, CCRN, BSN

(Courtesy of Sandra H. Carr.)

---

nurses to participate in lifelong learning activities. Minor revisions to the first *Code* were agreed upon by delegates to the ANA's conventions throughout the 1950s.

In 1958, the ANA's Committee on Ethical Standards began reviewing the entire *Code*, and in 1960, major revisions were suggested (Veins, 1989). The 1960 *Code* also contained 17 statements, but new statements were added and some were deleted. The new statements addressed nurses' responsibilities to participate in the professional organization and the necessity of identifying and upholding professional standards. Another new statement addressed nurses' participation in negotiating terms of employment. This opened the way, in later years, for the ANA to function as a collective-bargaining agent for nurses. An earlier statement, describing nurses' obligations to physicians, was eliminated from the 1960 *Code* (Veins, 1989).

The next major revision of the *Code*, completed in 1976, resulted in 11 statements. The emphasis of the 1976 *Code* was the nurse's relationship to the client. No longer was the word *patient* used. *Client* was adopted in the belief that it was a more inclusive term than *patient*. All gender-related language was eliminated. A paragraph dealing with consequences of breaking the *Code* was also added. Accordingly the nurse who violated the *Code* could be censured, suspended, or expelled from the ANA. Any violations of civil law would subject the nurse to legal action as well (American Nurses Association, 1976). Clarifying statements were added to each point in the *Code* in the 1976 revision. These interpretations provided definitions of key terms and elaborated on the meaning of each statement.

In 1985, the *Code* was again reviewed. All 11 statements remained the same, but the interpretations were updated. In particular, more emphasis was placed on clients' rights. The 1985 *Code for Nurses* is the latest version of nursing's ethical code. See Box 4–1 for the *Code for Nurses* (American Nurses Association, 1985).

International Council of Nurses Code for Nurses

The International Council of Nurses (ICN) (1973) also has published a code of ethics for the profession. This document discusses the rights and responsibilities of nurses related to people, practice, society, co-workers, and the profession. The ICN first adopted a code of ethics in 1953. Its last revision in 1973 represents agreement by more than 80 national nursing associations that participate in the international association. Inherent in the *International Council of Nurses Code for Nurses* is nursing's respect for the life, dignity, and integrity of all people unmindful of nationality, race, creed, color, age, sex, political affiliation, or social status (Mitchell and Grippando, 1993). Box 19–1 contains this code.

ETHICAL THEORIES

There is no single ethical theory ascribed to by all philosophers or ethicists. Numerous theories have been developed. We discuss two of the primary ethical theories that nurse ethicists have identified as useful.

Utilitarianism

Utilitarianism theory was first described by David Hume (1711–1776) and was developed further by many notable philosophers, including Jeremy Bentham (1748–1826) and John Stuart Mill (1806–1873). Mill had a significant influence on utilitarian ethics as we know it today.

According to Mill (1985; originally published in 1863), a "right action" conforms to the "greatest happiness principle." In other words, it is right to maximize the greatest good for the happiness or pleasure of the greatest number of

---

BOX 19–1
International Code for Nurses

The fundamental responsibility of the nurse is fourfold: to promote health, to prevent illness, to restore health, and to alleviate suffering.

The need for nursing is universal. Inherent in nursing is respect for life, dignity, and rights of man. It is unrestricted by considerations of nationality, race, creed, color, age, sex, politics or social status.

Nurses render health services to the individual, the family and the community and coordinate their services with those of related groups.

Nurses and People
The nurse's primary responsibility is to those people who require nursing care.

The nurse, in providing care, promotes an environment in which the values, customs and spiritual beliefs of the individual are respected.

The nurse holds in confidence personal information and uses judgment in sharing this information.

Nurses and Practice
The nurse carries personal responsibility for nursing practice and for maintaining competence by continual learning. The nurse maintains the highest standards of nursing care possible within the reality of a specific situation.

The nurse uses judgment in relation to individual competence when accepting and delegating responsibilities.

The nurse when acting in a professional capacity should at all times maintain standards of personal conduct which reflect credit upon the profession.

Nurses and Society
The nurse shares with other citizens the responsibility for initiating and supporting action to meet the health and social needs of the public.

Nurses and Co-Workers
The nurse sustains a cooperative relationship with co-workers in nursing and other fields. The nurse takes appropriate action to safeguard the individual when his care is endangered by a co-worker or any other person.

Nurses and the Profession
The nurse plays the major role in determining and implementing desirable standards of nursing practice and nursing education.

The nurse is active in developing a core of professional knowledge.

The nurse, acting through the professional organization, participates in establishing and maintaining equitable social and economic working conditions in nursing.

(Reprinted with permission of International Council of Nurses. (1973). *International Council of Nurses Code for Nurses*. Geneva, Switzerland: Author.)

---

people. Utilitarian ethics calculates the effect of all alternative actions on the general welfare of present and future generations. Thus, this position is also referred to as "calculus morality" (Davis and Aroskar, 1991).

The utilitarian approach to ethics assumes that it is possible to balance good and evil. The goal is that most people experience good rather than evil. Benefits are to be maximized for the greatest number of people possible. In this approach, each individual counts as one.

Professional health care personnel employ utilitarian theory in many situations. The concept of triage, in which the sick or injured are classified by the severity of their condition to determine priority of treatment, is an example of utilitarianism. In triage, those who are so gravely ill or injured that they cannot possibly recover are not treated at all. Although this seems cruel, when there are many more sick and wounded than available facilities to care for them, triage is accepted worldwide as an ethical basis for determining treatment.

Frequently, utilitarianism is the basis for deciding how health care dollars should be spent. Money is more likely to be spent on research for diseases that affect large numbers of people than for research on diseases that affect only a few. A difficulty of this approach is that although the appeal is made to the happiness of the majority, the individual or minority, who also deserves help, may be overlooked.

Deontology

The major proponent of **deontology** was Immanuel Kant (1724–1804). Kant (1985; originally translated in 1959) believed that the rightness or wrongness of an action depended on the inherent moral significance of the action. He believed that an act was moral if it originated from good will. Ethical action consisted in doing one's duty. To do one's duty was right; not to do one's duty was wrong.

Deontology can be further divided into either act or rule deontology. Act deontologists determine the right thing to do by gathering all the facts and then making a decision. Much time and energy are needed to judge each situation carefully in and of itself. Once a decision is made, there is commitment to universalizing it. In other words, if one makes a moral judgment in one situation, the same judgment will be made in any similar situation.

Rule deontologists emphasize that principles guide our actions. Examples of rules might be "Always keep a promise" or "Never tell a lie." In all situations, the rule is to be followed. Deontologists are not concerned with the consequences of always following certain rules or actions. If the principle believed in is "Always keep a promise," the deontologist will keep promises, even if circumstances have changed. For example, if a father has promised that he will take his son to a baseball game and then a close family member becomes critically ill, the baseball game promise will be kept regardless of the changed circumstances.

In nursing, there are many rules and duties that nurses follow. One such rule is "Do no harm" (**beneficence**). Another justifiable rule is "The patient should be allowed to make his or her own decisions" (**autonomy**). Consider the situation of a severely depressed young man who wishes to end his life by committing suicide and asks the nurse's assistance. Clearly the rule about doing no harm conflicts with allowing the young man to make his own decisions. You can see that dilemmas cannot always be resolved using theoretical approaches alone.

ETHICAL PRINCIPLES

Respect for persons is the most fundamental human right (Aroskar, 1995). It requires that each person be respected as a unique individual that is equal to all others. This means valuing every aspect of a person's life, not just the parts that are easy to value because they are congruent with your own values. Respect for persons is the foundation for all ethical principles.

Justice

The principle of **justice** states that equals should be treated the same and that unequals should be treated differently (Beauchamp and Childless, 1989). In other words, patients with the same diagnosis and health care needs should receive the same care. Those with greater or lesser needs should receive different care.

In health care, the most common concern about justice relates to allocation of resources. How much of our national resources should be appropriated to health care? Which health care problems should receive the most financial resources? Which clients should have access to health care services? According to the principle of justice, the answer to these questions is based on treating all individuals equally.

Numerous models have been developed for distributing health care resources. These models include:

1. To each equally.
2. To each according to merit. (They may include past or future contributions to society.)
3. To each according to what can be acquired in the marketplace.
4. To each according to need (Jameton, 1984).

All of these suggestions for distribution have merit and make it difficult to decide who should be treated for what. It would be ideal if all patients could receive all available treatment for their health needs. Unfortunately, this is not possible because of the cost involved.

Justice as a principle often leaves us with more questions than answers. It raises our consciousness about making ethical decisions but certainly does not determine what the answer should be.

Autonomy

The principle of autonomy is the claim that individuals have the right to determine their own actions. Freedom to make one's own decisions is respected under the principle of autonomy. The principle refers to the control individuals have over their own lives. Respect for the individual is the cornerstone of this principle.

Autonomy applies to both decisions and actions. Autonomous decisions have several characteristics. They

1. Are based on individuals' values.
2. Use adequate information.
3. Are free from coercion.
4. Are based on reason and deliberation.

Autonomous actions result from autonomous decisions.

The concept of autonomy has featured prominently in ethics and philosophy since the time of the ancient Greeks. Philosophers and lawyers agree that people have a right to make decisions for themselves. It was established in health care settings more than 75 years ago that professionals should not act against the wishes of an adult human being of sound mind (*Schoendorf v. Society of New York Hospital*, 1914).

It is almost impossible to disagree with autonomy. Autonomy is a basic principle of the U.S. Constitution. Throughout the history of the United States, people have fought and died for the right of individual autonomy. Disregard for autonomy, however, is glaringly evident in the health care system.

Health care professionals often take actions that profoundly affect patients' lives without adequate consultation with the patients. Incorporating the principle of autonomy in all health care situations is difficult, if not impossible. Patients cannot always make their own choices. Examples of those unable to participate in decisions include infants or small children, mentally incompetent patients, and unconscious patients. Other patients may be unable to participate in decision making because of external constraints, such as financial limitations, lack of necessary information, or the norms of their culture.

Beneficence

Beneficence is commonly defined as "the doing of good." According to Frankena (1988), there are several duties involved with this principle. They include:

1. Not to inflict harm or evil (**nonmaleficence**).
2. To prevent harm or evil.
3. To remove harm or evil.
4. To promote or do good.

The first duty, not to inflict harm, takes priority over the three following duties. Even so, all four duties are obligations that must be taken into account. Additional considerations may take precedence when there is conflict about the appropriate course of action. For example, a surgical procedure inflicts harm on the body but potentially has long-term benefits. The procedure may be lifesaving, or it may diminish pain or increase mobility. In this sense, even though it inflicts harm in the short-term, it is justified because of the long-term good that results.

Virtually everyone would agree that causing good and avoiding harm are important to all human beings—and certainly to health care professionals. It is therefore surprising how often conflicts center around this principle. In addition to consideration of both short-term and long-term benefits, the principle of beneficence conflicts with other ethical principles. Consider the elderly patient who has just broken her hip for the second time and refuses to eat. Should she be allowed to decide autonomously not to eat even though it will harm her? The principles of autonomy and beneficence are in conflict in this example.

Veracity

Veracity is defined as "telling the truth." Truth telling has long been identified as fundamental to the development and continuance of trust among human beings. Telling the truth is expected. It is necessary to basic communication, and societal relationships are built on the individual's right to know the truth.

All communication between individuals has the potential to be misleading. It is easy for information to be misunderstood, misinterpreted, or not comprehended. Usually these misunderstandings are unintentional. *Intentional* deception, however, is considered morally wrong.

Despite that well-established fact, much intended deception occurs between health professionals and people seeking health care. Persons seeking health care often are not truthful when giving their health histories. An example that commonly occurs relates to truthfulness concerning use of drugs and alcohol.

At the same time, health care professionals are not always truthful in responding to patients' questions. The nurse may choose to answer only part of a question, rather than giving all the known facts. A long tradition of a double standard in truth telling exists in health care (Tschudin, 1993). Health care professionals are not responsible for false information given to them by their patients. They *are* responsible for information that they give *to* patients, however.

A number of reasons have been proposed to justify deception by health care professionals. For the most part, the justifications are related to the idea that patients would be better off not knowing certain information or that they are not capable of understanding the information. Based on these justifications, health care professionals often believe they have the right to decide what people should know and should not know about their illnesses. If both patient and health care provider are respectful of one another as individuals, it is difficult to accept that deception between two human beings is ever justified.

THEORIES OF MORAL DEVELOPMENT

How does a person become moral or able to make decisions about right and wrong? Answering this question moves us into the realm of **moral development.** Moral development describes how a person learns to deal with moral dilemmas from childhood through adulthood. Two major theorists who have worked at understanding this area of human development are Lawrence Kohlberg (1973, 1986) and Carol Gilligan (1982, 1987).

Kohlberg's Levels of Moral Development

Kohlberg (1976, 1986) proposed three levels of moral development:

1. Preconventional.
2. Conventional.
3. Postconventional.

In the preconventional level, the individual is inattentive to the norms of society when responding to moral problems. Instead the individual's perspective is self-centered. At the preconventional level, what the individual wants or needs takes precedence over right or wrong. Kohlberg saw this level of moral development in most children under nine years of age as well as in some adolescents and adult criminal offenders.

The conventional level is characterized by making moral decisions that conform to the expectations of one's family, group, or society. When confronted with a moral choice, people functioning at the conventional level follow family or cultural group norms. According to Kohlberg, most adolescents and adults generally function at this level.

The postconventional level involves more independent modes of thinking than previous stages, so that the individual is able to define his or her own moral values. People at the postconventional level may ignore both self-interest and group norms in making moral choices. They create their own morality, which may differ from society's norms. Kohlberg believed that only a minority of adults achieve this level.

Each of Kohlberg's levels is subdivided into two stages. Progression through the stages occurs over varying lengths of time, but each stage is sequential and is characterized by higher capacity for logical reasoning than the preceding stage.

Kohlberg (1976) suggested that certain conditions may stimulate higher levels of moral development. Intellectual development is one necessary characteristic. Individuals at higher levels intellectually are generally more advanced in moral development than those operating at lower levels of intelligence.

An environment that offers people opportunities for group participation, shared decision-making processes, and responsibility for the consequences of their actions also promotes higher levels of moral reasoning. Further moral development is stimulated by the creation of conflict in settings in which the individual recognizes the limitations of present modes of thinking. Students have been stimulated to higher levels of moral reasoning through participating in courses on moral discussion and ethics (Kohlberg, 1973).

The Research Note discusses moral dilemmas further.

Gilligan's Levels of Moral Development

Gilligan (1982) was a student of Kohlberg who was concerned that Kohlberg did not give adequate acknowledgment to the experiences of women in moral development. She recognized that Kohlberg's theories had largely been generated from research with men and boys. When women were tested using Kohlberg's levels of moral development, they scored lower than men.

Gilligan believed that this was due not to inadequate moral development in women but to the fact that women's identities are largely dependent on relationships with others. Because of the basic difference in the way men and women feel about relationships, Gilligan believed that Kohlberg's theory was inadequate to explain women's moral development.

She suggested that women view moral dilemmas in terms of conflicting responsibilities. The sequence she described included three levels and two transitions, with each level representing a more complex understanding of the relationship of self and others and each transition resulting in a crucial re-evaluation of the conflict between selfishness and responsibility. Gilligan's levels of moral development are:

1. Orientation to individual survival.
2. A focus on goodness as self-sacrifice.
3. The morality of nonviolence.

RESEARCH NOTE

The purpose of this study was to determine if the theoretical perspective described by Kohlberg or Gilligan exemplifies the approach critical care nurses use when confronted with a moral dilemma. More specifically, the research project determined if either theoretical perspective described by Kohlberg or Gilligan exemplified the perspective used by nurses when confronted with a moral dilemma.

Fifty-five experienced intensive care nurses were interviewed concerning moral dilemmas they have experienced in professional practice. Subjects also completed Rest's Defining Issues Test (DIT) and a demographic questionnaire. Interpretive analysis sought to understand how nurses make moral decisions by listening for specific approaches in audiotaped interviews. The principled thinking scores on the DIT were analyzed among the groups identified by interpretive analysis.

The results indicated that nurses used more than one perspective as they deliberated moral dilemmas. The predominant number of nurses, 42 percent, used a perspective of justice. The care perspective was the basis for moral decisions for 24 percent of the nurses. The remaining nurses, 34 percent, combined the care/justice perspective when deliberating moral dilemmas. There was no evidence that justice, care, or care/justice groups differed in their principled thinking as measured by the DIT. The researchers concluded that both care and justice are important to understanding moral decision making among nurses. The mature moral reasoning of all human beings must be developed and supported no matter what their gender or moral perspective.

(Adapted from Miller, S. E., Hamilton, J., Chally, P. S., Jacobs, M. and Dunnagan, S. (1995). *Moral decision making in critical care nursing*. Unpublished research.)

The moral person is one who responds to need and demonstrates a consideration of care and responsibility in relationships. Gilligan described a moral development perspective focused on care. This perspective differed from the orientation toward justice described by Kohlberg (1973, 1976).

More recent work by Gilligan and Attanucci (1988) has attempted to define the relationship between the two moral orientations of justice and care. They determined that both perspectives were present when people faced real-life moral dilemmas, but people generally tended to focus on one set of concerns and paid only minimal attention to the other perspective. As expected, the care focus was more often exhibited by women, and the justice focus was more often exemplified by men.

The justice and care perspectives in themselves are not competing theories but are two separate moral perspectives that organize thinking in different ways (Chally, 1990). The justice perspective strives to treat others fairly, whereas the care perspective is strongly based on relationships with others.

Gilligan, Brown, and Rogers (1988) described a combined care/justice perspective that incorporates both viewpoints as moral deliberations are made. Moral development theory must incorporate all perspectives, some of which may not yet be identified. Analysis of interviews of nurses suggest that nurses at times combine the care/justice perspective when forced to make ethical decisions (Chally, 1995).

UNDERSTANDING ETHICAL DILEMMAS IN NURSING

Ethical dilemmas occur frequently in nursing practice. This is to be expected because nurses focus on life and death issues involving human beings. Many ethical dilemmas arise in nursing because of conflicts between patients, health care professionals, and institutions. To understand these conflicts, the following areas are explored:

1. Personal value systems.
2. Peers' and other professionals' behaviors.
3. Patients' rights.
4. Institutional and societal issues.

Role of Personal Value Systems

Values are important preferences that influence the behavior of individuals. Value systems are learned beliefs that help people choose among difficult alternatives.

As discussed in Chapter 9, each person has a value system. This value system has a beginning foundation in beliefs, purposes, attitudes, qualities, and objects that are important to a child's early caregivers. In time, individuals develop their own value systems. A **personal value system** is a rank ordering of values with respect to their importance to one another.

Value systems vary from individual to individual. Something important to one individual may hold greater or lesser significance to someone else. For example, a clean, neat home means more to some individuals than others.

Variations in value systems become highly significant when dealing with critical issues such as health and illness or life and death. Value systems enable people to resolve conflicts and decide on a course of action based on a priority of importance. In professional nursing, it is not enough to recognize and act on one's values. In addition, one must determine if the value system is ethical. Only after careful reflection can nurses take action based on their personal or professional values.

Identifying your personal value system and its influence on decision making helps you understand your behavior more clearly. In addition, it gives you clues as to why other people's choices are different from your own. The "Childhood Value Messages" exercise in Box 19–2 can help you identify values learned as a child that may still influence you today.

To see how value conflicts can affect health care delivery, consider the following patient vignette:

Mrs. Hamid has recently relocated to the United States from Iran. It is important in her religious faith that men not be present during labor and delivery or at anytime when a woman's body is exposed. A female obstetrician is delivering Mrs. Hamid, but complications develop. Her baby's heart rate drops abruptly, and a cesarean delivery is indicated. The only anesthesiologist available in the hospital for this emergency surgery is a man. What action should the nurse take?

BOX 19-2
Childhood Value Messages

By the time we are about 10 years old, most of our values have already been "programmed." Values are taught to us by family members and friends, through the media, in churches and schools, and by watching other people. What are the value messages you learned as a child?

Recall as many values as you can remember hearing as a child and write them in the space provided. Here are a few examples to get you thinking:

"Nothing worthwhile ever comes easy."

"Life is fatal—you're eternal."

"You can accomplish almost anything you want to if you persevere."

"Clean your plate, there are starving children in China!"

"You are your brother's keeper—reach out to others."

"Tell me the truth and I won't punish you!"

"Get your work done first, then you can play."

Now it's your turn to write some of your childhood values.

How many of these values still influence the way you think and act today? Which ones influence you professionally?

If you want to explore further:

1. Next to each value on your list, write the person's name who taught or modeled that value.
2. Put a star next to those messages that are still your values today.
3. Put a check next to those messages that you need to alter.
4. How are some of these values still influencing you today? Is this a positive or negative influence?

(Reprinted with permission of Uustal, D. B. (1993). *Clinical ethics and values: Issues and insights in a changing healthcare environment.* East Greenwich, RI: Educational Resources in HealthCare, Inc.)

1. _____
2. _____
3. _____
4. _____
5. _____
6. _____
7. _____
8. _____

Dilemmas Involving Peers' and Other Professionals' Behavior

All practicing nurses participate as members of the health care team. This involves cooperation and collaboration with other professionals. As is true in all situations involving human beings, conflicts can easily develop, particularly in stressful circumstances. These conflicts may be between two nurses, the nurse and physician, the nurse and hospital administration, or the nurse and any other health care professional.

As discussed in the section on personal value systems, conflicts can evolve because of differing value systems. A nurse may believe that assisting with abortions is wrong, whereas the institution performs many abortions daily. Some conflicts develop because individuals are not respectful of the human rights of other individuals.

Conflicts in human rights often center around one of the ethical principles discussed earlier: justice, autonomy, beneficence, or veracity. In some circumstances, the ethical dilemma may result from a violation of even more basic human rights, those guaranteed by the U.S. Constitution.

A serious issue today is the large number of nurses and other health care professionals impaired by drug dependence or other addictions. Deciding how and when to confront a suspected drug user may result in an ethical dilemma. Fortunately, some employers and state nurses associations have developed plans to assist impaired nurses in getting the help they need and make provisions for them to return to the profession once they are far enough along in their recovery process. Your state nurses association can provide information on specific programs for impaired nurses in your state.

To understand the ethical dilemmas that can result from conflict between peers, consider the following vignette:

> Miss Corbin, RN, works on a surgical floor. She has just assisted in the transfer of Mr. Hudson to his room from the postanesthesia unit after surgery and noticed that he was resting comfortably. Miss Corbin sees a nurse colleague drawing up a pain medication. The nurse colleague returns to the medicine room 10 minutes later with an empty syringe. Miss Corbin asks, "Who needed pain medication?" "Mr. Hudson," the colleague replies. "He was in pain after surgery." Confused, Miss Corbin checks Mr. Hudson's room and learns from his wife that he has not asked for or received pain medication. What should Miss Corbin do now?

Conflicts Regarding Patients' Rights

Years ago, health professionals, particularly physicians, were considered "all-knowing" experts. Few patients questioned the physician, let alone demanded their basic human rights. Now consumers of health care are increasingly demanding to have a say in matters affecting their health care. *A Patient's Bill of Rights* (American Hospital Association, 1992) outlines currently accepted **patients' rights** (see Box 3–4). The patient's relationship with the physician as well as the relationship between the patient and hospital are discussed.

Many other specialty groups have developed published lists of rights. Examples include *Declaration of the Rights of Mentally Retarded Persons, Dying Person's Bill of Rights, Pregnant Patient's Bill of Rights, Rights of Senior Citizens,* and the *United Nations Declarations of the Rights of the Child.* As consumers have become more aware of their rights, conflicts between patients, health care professionals, and institutions have developed. Many of the rights demanded by consumers are their legal as well as moral rights and have been upheld by the judicial system.

It is beyond the scope of this chapter to discuss all rights due patients. Many have been identified, however, including informed consent, the right to die, privacy, confidentiality, respectful care, and information concerning medical condition and treatment. In addition, patients have the right to be informed if any aspect of treatment is experimental. Based on that knowledge, they can refuse to participate in research projects.

PATIENT SELF DETERMINATION ACT

Another safeguard for patients, the Patient Self Determination Act, gives patients the legal right to determine how vigorously they wish to be treated in life or death situations. The Patient Self Determination Act forces individuals to think about the type of medical and nursing treatment they want if they become critically injured or ill. When questions arise, the patient is often unconscious or too sick to make decisions or communicate personal wishes.

This act, which went into effect in December 1991, calls for hospitals to abide by patients' **advance directives.** Advance directives are legal documents that indicate the wishes of individuals in regard to end-of-life issues. The Patient Self Determination Act specifies that any organization receiving Medicare or Medicaid funds must inform patients of state laws regarding directives, document the existence of directives in the patient's medical record, and educate the community about directives.

Advance directives were designed to ensure individuals the rights of autonomy, refusal of medical intervention, and death with dignity (Norman and Pinkham, 1994). Critically ill individuals can remain in charge of their own end-of-life decisions if their advance directives are carried out.

Families should talk about how each member wishes critical situations to be handled. Individual preferences can then be understood, and family members, caregivers, and courts should not need to be involved. Often the first time a patient learns about advance directives is upon admission to a health care facility. The question then arises as to who is responsible for discussing this sensitive issue with the patient. The ideal time for patients to make difficult end-of-life decisions is well in advance of the need (Fig. 19–1).

Advance directives have not been without controversy. One problem is that states have passed different legislation, and there is no guarantee that one state will honor another's advanced directives. Another problem sometimes arises when a person is designated as the proxy to decide about medical treatment if the patient cannot do so. In some situations, persons have been named as proxies without their knowledge. Conflict still arises among caregivers in honoring certain advance directives (News Note).

The following case illustrated a conflict related to patients' rights:

A 28-year-old quadriplegic man is admitted to the hospital with pneumonia and severe pressure ulcers. He asks not to be given antibiotics and to be allowed to die with dignity. At the insistence of the hospital administration, the physician orders intravenous antibiotics. What is the nurse's responsibility?

More information about patient rights and the Patient Self Determination Act is found in Chapter 20.

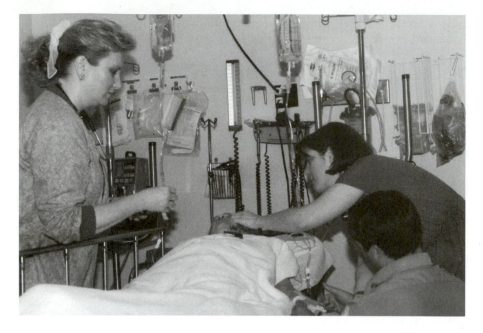

FIGURE 19–1
Patients must make end-of-life decisions early and discuss them with family members and caregivers to avoid unwanted, life-prolonging interventions. (Courtesy of Memorial Hospital, Chattanooga, TN.)

Conflicts Created by Institutional and Societal Issues

Nurses experience ethical dilemmas when conflicts develop between policies of their employing institution and themselves. Controversial health care policies at the local, state, or national level can also interfere with the nurse's ability to implement care safely and effectively.

Grave concerns over health care have centered around the cost of care. The rising cost of health care over the past 25 years is a matter that has prompted worry for individuals, groups, and communities as well as governmental officials. All health care agencies are stressing cost-containment measures to survive. At times, cost-containment policies conflict with the value system of the nurse, whose goal is to provide high-quality, individualized patient care.

Other institutional and societal concerns can result in ethical dilemmas for the nurse whose personal value system does not support the policies set forth by those in authority. Examples include policies concerning access to health care for the elderly, children, and persons with acquired immunodeficiency syndrome (AIDS).

Nurses today work in many settings. The scope and complexity of these settings vary significantly from large multiservice medical complexes to small clinics or offices. All organizations, however, that receive governmental funds are subject to public scrutiny and accountability. Ethical dilemmas may develop be-

A Troubling Death: Wishes of Terminally Ill Patients Are Often Ignored, New Study Says

Perry Elfmont knew he had heart problems. And, as a physician, he knew the questionable future he could face should he suffer a heart attack.

So, like many Americans, he wrote a "living will" saying that he didn't wish to be resuscitated when the inevitable time arrived that his heart would stop.

That time came in May 1994, when he was 88. After he awoke one morning seeming disoriented, his wife, Sabrina, took him to the hospital. She went home 14 hours later to rest—but not before reminding a doctor and nurse about her husband's living will.

Yet she returned the next morning to a horrifying sight. Her husband, whose heart had stopped during the night, had been revived despite his wishes. He was connected to numerous tubes and his hands were restrained "because, the nurses said, he wanted to pull them out," she recalls.

Now her husband, who once spoke five languages, no longer can read, speak or recognize anyone. He lies in bed or sits listlessly, not reacting to anything. His wife is bitter. "No one has the right to change a person's living will," she says.

A quarter century after the living will movement began, many people like Elfmont are unable to achieve their goal of dying with dignity.

A new study, financed by the Robert Wood Johnson Foundation and published in the *Journal of the American Medical Association*, found that almost half of all seriously ill hospital patients who asked their doctors to issue do-not-resuscitate orders for them did not get their wish—at least initially.

The result, in many cases, is a now familiar litany of lives senselessly prolonged by futile treatment of seriously ill patients who spend their final days in pain or twilight existences.

The study found that even an organized effort to improve in-hospital communications about patients' wishes—by using nurses as liaisons between patients and doctors—had little effect.

What's a person to do? While improved long-range answers are being thought out, experts say, most individuals could make better use of the tools we already have. These include writing out your wishes before a medical emergency arises, aggressively informing family members, doctors and religious counselors about these wishes and—most important—naming at least one trusted surrogate to vigorously represent you should you become incapacitated.

Fewer than one-third of Americans have even prepared advance directives spelling out their wishes. "There is a tremendous amount of denial, discomfort and fear on the part of the public and doctors," says Robert Butler, M.D., professor of geriatrics at Mt. Sinai School of Medicine in New York.

Denial leads many people to wait until the last minute—often, when they're sick or unable to think clearly—to fill out advance directives.

Preparing the required forms can be relatively easy: the AARP, American Bar Association and American Medical Association have jointly prepared a patient guide that includes a model living will and health-care power of attorney. Instructions and forms also can be obtained from Choice in Dying, a New York-based non-profit group.

These organizations also can help you make sure your documents are consistent with the laws of the state (or states) in which you reside. That's important because state laws vary on some significant issues.

Once you've written an advance directive, insist it be in a prominent spot in your medical records.

Arthur Caplan, director of the Center for Bioethics at the University of Pennsylvania, recommends updating your directive every couple of years. "People will not trust a document you filled out 10

(continued)

A Troubling Death: Wishes of Terminally Ill Patients Are Often Ignored, New Study Says

years ago as much as one you just signed," he notes.

Caplan has another bit of advice: "Never fill out an advance directive alone." The reason: Your loved ones should know your wishes so that they can become forceful advocates for you when you're facing death. Moreover, doctors are more comfortable stopping aggressive treatment when families are united behind the decision.

Besides lining up your family members, try to gauge whether your physician or health maintenance organization would honor your wishes to accept death rather than fight it beyond a point you consider appropriate.

If your doctor won't discuss the issue, he or she may also have trouble letting you die when the time comes.

To assess a caregiver's familiarity and comfort with letting people die with dignity, "ask whether they know the nuts and bolts of how do you die at home," suggests Joanne Lynn, M.D., director of the Center to Improve the Care of the Dying at George Washington University and co-director of the study.

Lynn suggests asking "if people who are dying sometimes have to be in pain." A doctor knowledgeable about pain management and comfortable with it, she explains, should confidently answer "no," while one who focuses only on fighting death might give a less definite response.

Having a personal physician who supports your views can enhance your chances of dying with dignity. Even if the attending physician isn't your own doctor, he or she is more likely to act as you wish if that action is backed by a doctor who knows you, according to William Prip, program associate for Choice in Dying.

You should also discuss your wishes with your religious counselor, who may be present when you are seriously ill. And warn your attorney, suggests Robert Veatch, director of the Kennedy Institute of Ethics at Georgetown University. The mere act of involving your lawyer puts a physician on no-

tice that you are serious about having your wishes honored, he argues.

And experts increasingly emphasize the importance of appointing representatives, with properly executed powers of attorney, to make sure your wishes are carried out.

"A living will may be too vague to guide practitioners," argues Robert Harootyan, a senior research associate at AARP who formerly headed a study by the congressional Office of Technology Assessment on "Life-Sustaining Technologies and the Elderly." "Having a health-care proxy who is legally appointed removes a lot of ambiguity and vagueness." he says.

But be careful whom you appoint to be your representative. Make sure he or she appreciates your values—whether you'd sacrifice extra months of life in order to die at home, for instance. And make sure that he or she is physically able to represent you forcefully.

Still, even if you have taken all these steps, you can't be sure that your wishes will be fulfilled.

Many authorities say the ultimate solution will be to fundamentally change the American way of dying—among other things, by making it easier for people to die at home or in hospices rather than in hospitals.

"We're a victim of our own success," says William Knaus, M.D., chairman of the Department of Health Evaluation Sciences at the University of Virginia School of Medicine, and a study co-director. "A lot of this technology is very useful, and we have wanted to make sure it is widely available.

"Now we have to make it just as easy," he adds, "to get pain relief, comfort and dignity at the end of life as it is to get high-technology care."

(Reprinted with permission of Conte, C. (1996). A troubling death: Wishes of terminally ill patients are often ignored, new study says. *AARP Bulletin*, 37(1), 4–5.)

tween nurses and the organizations that employ them concerning policies dictated by the organizations or mandated by governmental agencies.

Ethics committees were created to assist with ethical dilemmas in institutional settings. Ethics committees are multidisciplinary groups charged with the responsibility of providing consultation and emotional support in situations in which difficult ethical choices are necessary. Cases needing consideration are referred to the committee by those desiring help, usually clinical caregivers such as physicians and nurses.

The following vignette illustrates an ethical conflict between a nurse and the employing institution:

> Dina Cook is a nurse working in a critical care unit. All beds in the unit are full. For the past two days, Miss Cook has been assigned to care for a 92-year-old woman critically ill with heart failure. The patient has no financial resources of her own, and no family member has seen her since she was admitted from a nursing home. She remains in very critical condition. Suddenly, orders come for the elderly woman to be transferred to a bed on a regular nursing unit. As she is being moved out of the intensive care unit, a state senator's son in a diabetic coma is admitted to her recently vacated bed. What is the nurse's responsibility?

ETHICAL DECISION MAKING

Nurses encounter situations daily that require them to make professional judgments and act on those judgments. The judgments or decisions are often made in conjunction with other persons involved in the situation: patients, families, and other health care professionals. When an ethical decision is made, everyone must respect and value the perspective held by others. Through respectful collaboration, the best decision can be reached in even the most difficult dilemma. Notice that it is suggested that the best decision will be made. In an ethical dilemma, there is not a right or wrong answer. Instead, we search for the best answer.

Ethical Decision-Making Model

Whether involved in a collective or individual decision, nurses need to be knowledgeable about the steps in **ethical decision making** (Table 19–1). Various mod-

TABLE 19–1
Comparison of Nursing Process and Ethical Decision-Making Model

Nursing Process	Ethical Decision-Making Model
Assess	Clarify the ethical dilemma
	Gather additional data
Analyze	Identify options
Plan	Make a decision
Implement	Act
Evaluate	Evaluate

els of ethical decision making have been developed. Each model is unique to some degree, but the models do share commonalities. Although the models all have steps, they are not intended to be rigid processes for decision making. Instead, ethical decision making is a process in which ideas are thoroughly examined to determine the best solution to a difficult situation.

The following steps can be used in ethical decision making.

1. CLARIFY THE ETHICAL DILEMMA

What is the specific issue in question? Who owns the problem and should actually make the decision? Who is affected by the dilemma? Determine the ethical principle or theory related to the dilemma. Are there value conflicts? What is the time frame for the dilemma?

2. GATHER ADDITIONAL DATA

After clarifying the ethical dilemma, in most instances more information needs to be gathered. It is important to have as many facts about the situation as possible. Make sure you are up-to-date on any legal cases related to the situation because ethical and legal issues often overlap.

3. IDENTIFY OPTIONS

Most ethical dilemmas have multiple solutions, some of which are more feasible than others. The more options that are identified, the more likely it is that an acceptable solution can be identified. Brainstorm with others and consider every possible alternative.

4. MAKE A DECISION

To make a decision, think through the options that are identified and determine each options' impact. Ethical principles and theories may help determine the significance of each option. When confronted with an ethical dilemma, a decision should be made. Refusing to make a decision is not a responsible professional behavior.

5. ACT

Once a course of action has been determined, the decision must be carried out. Implementing the decision usually involves working collaboratively with others.

6. EVALUATE

Unexpected outcomes are common in crisis situations that result in ethical dilemmas. It is important for decision makers to determine the impact this decision may have on future ones. It is also important to consider if a different course of action might have resulted in a better outcome. If the action accomplished its purpose, the ethical dilemma should be resolved. If the dilemma has not been resolved, additional deliberation is needed.

Case Study

Eleanor Gift, age 68 years, is scheduled for triple bypass surgery. Martha Blake, RN, is the nurse doing her preoperative teaching the evening before the procedure is scheduled. It is apparent to Miss Blake that Mrs. Gift does not want to have surgery. She expresses great apprehension about the procedure and generally feels quite negative about the outcome. The surgeon, however, has convinced Mrs. Gift and her family that she must undergo the surgery to survive. Although far from comfortable with the situation, Mrs. Gift is resigned to undergo the impending surgery in the morning. What is the nurse's responsibility in this situation?

1. CLARIFY THE ETHICAL DILEMMA

Many questions are not answered in this case study. Clearly the decision regarding having surgery should be made by the one most affected (i.e., Mrs. Gift). Others are affected by her decision, however. There is no information given about her family or how involved they are in her health care. Other caregivers also may play a significant role. The ethical principle of autonomy is important in this scenario. Unfortunately, time is quite short because Mrs. Gift's surgery is scheduled in the morning.

2. GATHER ADDITIONAL DATA

The nurse needs to know information from Mrs. Gift's medical history related to the extent of her cardiovascular disease. It is also important to know what she has been told about the surgery and her need for it. Has she been given the necessary information to allow her to make an informed decision?

3. IDENTIFY OPTIONS

The following nursing actions are options for the nurse in this situation:

- Continue preoperative teaching under the assumption that surgery will take place as scheduled.
- Continue preoperative teaching and let the increased knowledge be used as an additional tool to assist Mrs. Gift in decision making.
- Inform the surgeon about Mrs. Gift's concerns.
- Inform the supervisor about Mrs. Gift's concerns.
- Advise the patient to refuse to have surgery tomorrow.

- Encourage Mrs. Gift to include her family in the decision.
- Explore Mrs. Gift's concerns thoroughly and help her deal with her apprehension and fears.
- Determine insofar as possible if Mrs. Gift has autonomously consented or been coerced to have surgery.
- Encourage Mrs. Gift to make her own decision based on the information she has already been given. Continue preoperative teaching if she agrees to the surgery.

4. MAKE A DECISION

Choose one of the options. In this situation, it seems most appropriate to explore Mrs. Gift's concerns and feelings about the surgery. It is important to determine if Mrs. Gift truly feels the surgery is in her best interest and if she has made an autonomous decision.

5. ACT

Once a decision is made, it is important to implement the action. In this situation, the nurse decides to explore Mrs. Gift's concerns and determine if an autonomous decision was made by the patient.

6. EVALUATE

This step is important, even though it may seem obvious. It is necessary to evaluate the implications of the decision that was made. The nurse must determine if the action implemented accomplished what was intended. Evidence that the intervention was successful would include a decrease in Mrs. Gift's anxiety level and negative feelings about the probable outcome of the surgery.

S U M M A R Y

The terms *morals* and *ethics* are often used interchangeably. Technically, however, morals reflect what is done in a situation, whereas ethics are concerned with what should be done. It is important that nurses are familiar with ethical theories and principles, moral development, and decision-making models to participate actively in resolving ethical dilemmas. Codes of ethics, developed by the profession's members, are important to the development of professional status. The ANA *Code for Nurses* (1985) serves as a guideline for nurses regarding ethical behavior. The history of the *Code for Nurses* is reflective of nursing's history as a profession. Ethical dilemmas occur in all areas of nursing practice. Often dilemmas are present because of conflicts between personal value systems, patients, health care professionals, institutions, and societal issues. Ethical decision-making models are helpful in determining the best action to take concerning an ethical dilemma.

REVIEW AND DISCUSSION QUESTIONS

1. What is the difference between morals and ethics? Give an example of each from your own value system.
2. How can the American Nurses Association's *Code for Nurses* be used by the bedside nurse?
3. Compare the American Nurses Association's *Code for Nurses* with the *International Council of Nurses Code for Nurses*. How are they similar, and how are they different?
4. Select an ethical theory or principle that is most congruent with your approach to ethical dilemmas. Use it as a basis for resolving the ethical dilemmas in this chapter. How well does it hold up under these test conditions?
5. Discuss your reactions to the following questions in a small group:
   A. Mrs. Otto has recently undergone extensive surgery for gynecological cancer. The day after surgery, she is asking for more pain medication than the physician has prescribed. You have called once and have an order to increase the pain medication dosage, but she still is complaining every two hours that she cannot tolerate the pain. What should be done?
   B. Mrs. Perton suffers from severe chronic pain, the cause of which has not been definitely diagnosed. Her husband has brought her into the emergency department for the fifth time this month asking for narcotic relief from the pain. In tears she states, "A shot of Demerol is the only thing that takes the edge off." She threatens suicide if she is sent home without some help. The physician has ordered a placebo. What is the nurse's responsibility?
   C. You are caring for a neonate in intensive care who needs a minor emergency operative procedure. The resident on call immediately begins the procedure in the unit without any anesthesia. The infant is intubated and makes no sound, but she becomes very restless and her pulse rises significantly. You believe that she is experiencing pain. What should you do?

REFERENCES

American Hospital Association (1992). *A patient's bill of rights*. Chicago: Author.

American Nurses Association (1991). *Position statement on promotion of comfort and relief of pain in dying patients*. Kansas City, MO: Author.

American Nurses Association (1985). *Code for nurses with interpretive statements*. Kansas City, MO: Author.

American Nurses Association (1976). *Code for nurses with interpretive statements*. Kansas City, MO: Author.

Aroskar, M. A. (1995). Envisioning nursing as a moral community. *Nursing Outlook*, 43(3), 134–138.

Beauchamp, T. L., and Childless, J. F. (1989). *Principles of biomedical ethics* (3rd ed.). New York: Oxford University Press.

Chally, P. S. (1995). Nursing research: Moral decision making by nurses in intensive care. *Plastic Surgical Nursing*, 15(2), 120–124.

Chally, P. S. (1990). Theory derivation in moral development. *Nursing and Health Care*, 11(6), 302–306.

Conte, C. (1996). A troubling death: Wishes of terminally ill patients are often ignored, new study says. *AARP Bulletin*, 37(1), 4–5.

Davis, A. J., and Aroskar, M. A. (1991). *Ethical dilemmas and nursing practice* (3rd ed.). Norwalk, CT: Appleton & Lange.

Fowler, M. D. (1992). A chronicle of the evolution of the code for nurses. In G. B. White (Ed.), *Ethical dilemmas in contemporary nursing practice* (pp. 149–154). Washington, D.C.: American Nurses Publishing.

Frankena, W. K. (1988). *Ethics* (2nd ed.). Englewood Cliffs, NJ: Prentice-Hall.

Gilligan, C. (1987). Moral orientation and moral development. In E. Kittay and D. Meyers (Eds.), *Women and moral theory* (pp. 19–33). Totowa, NJ: Rowman & Littlefield.

Gilligan, C. (1982). *In a different voice: Psychological theory and women's development.* Cambridge, MA: Harvard University Press.

Gilligan, C., and Attanucci, J. (1988). Two moral orientations: Gender differences and similarities. *Merrill-Palmer Quarterly,* 34(3), 223–231.

Gilligan, C., Brown, L., and Rogers, A. (1988). *Psyche embedded: A place for body, relationships, and culture in personality theory* (Monogr. No. 4). Cambridge, MA: Harvard University, Laboratory of Human Development.

Husted, G. L., and Husted, J. H. (1995). *Ethical decision making in nursing* (2nd ed.). St. Louis: C. V. Mosby.

International Council of Nurses. (1973). *International Council of Nurses code for nurses.* Geneva, Switzerland: Author.

Jameton, A. (1984). *Nursing practice: The ethical issues.* Englewood Cliffs, NJ: Prentice-Hall.

Kant, I. (1985). The categorical imperative. In J. Feinburg (Ed.), *Reason and responsibility: Readings in some basic problems of philosophy* (6th ed.) (pp. 540–547). Belmont, CA: Wadsworth. (Reprinted from Kant, I. [1959]. *Foundations of the metaphysics of morals,* trans. L. W. Beck. Indianapolis: Bobbs-Merrill, pp. 31–49.)

Kohlberg, L. (1986). A current statement on some theoretical issues. In S. Modgil and C. Modgil (Eds.), *Lawrence Kohlberg: Consensus and controversy* (pp. 485–546). Philadelphia: Falmer Press.

Kohlberg, L. (1976). Moral stages and moralization: The cognitive developmental approach. In T. Lickona (Ed.), *Moral development and behavior* (pp. 31–53). New York: Holt, Rinehart & Winston.

Kohlberg, L. (1973). Continuities and discontinuities in childhood and adult moral development revisited. In L. Kohlberg (Ed.), *Collected papers on moral development and moral education.* Cambridge, MA: Moral Education Research Foundation.

Mill, J. S. (1985). Utilitarianism. In J. Feinburg (Ed.), *Reason and responsibility: Readings in some basic problems of philosophy* (6th ed.) (pp. 503–515). Belmont, CA: Wadsworth. (Original work published 1863.)

Mitchell, P. R., and Grippando, G. M. (1993). *Nursing perspectives and issues* (5th ed.). Albany, NY: Delmar.

Norman, E. M., and Pinkham, D. B. (1994). Advance directives: Understanding their impact on care. In O. L. Strickland and D. J. Fishman (Eds.), *Nursing issues in the 1990s* (pp. 267–279). Albany, NY: Delmar.

Schoendorf v. Society of New York Hospital, 105 N.E. 92 (N.Y. 1914).

Silva, M. C. (1990). *Ethical decision making in nursing administration.* Norwalk, CT: Appleton & Lange.

Thompson, J. B., and Thompson, H. O. (1990). *Professional ethics in nursing.* Malabar, FL: Robert E. Krieger.

Tschudin, V. (Ed.). (1993). *Ethics: Nurses and patients.* London: Scutari Press.

Uustal, D. B. (1993). *Clinical ethics and values: Issues and insights in a changing healthcare environment.* East Greenwich, RI: Educational Resources in HealthCare, Inc.

Veins, D. C. (1989). A history of nursing's code of ethics. *Nursing Outlook,* 37(1), 45–49.

Virginia Trotter Betts
Frances I. Waddle

Legal Aspects of Nursing

OBJECTIVES

- Describe the components of a model nursing practice act.
- Discuss the authority of state boards of nursing.
- Explain the conditions that must be present for malpractice to occur.
- Identify nursing concerns related to delegation, assault and battery, informed consent, and confidentiality.
- Describe strategies nurses can use to protect themselves from legal actions.

VOCABULARY

administrative law	duty to report	Patient Self-
advance directives	expert witness	Determination Act
assault	informed consent	prescriptive authority
battery	law	privileged
"captain of the ship"	legal authority	communication
doctrine	licensure	proximate cause
civil law	licensure by	respondeat superior
common law	endorsement	risk management
competency	malpractice	standard of care
confidentiality	managed care	standard of nursing
criminal law	National Practitioner	practice
delegation	Data Bank	statutory law
documentation	negligence	tort
duty of care		

Professional nurses have many complex and interesting relationships with the law that are important to identify and understand. This is an area that is both extremely important and constantly changing. Therefore, nursing education programs sometimes offer required or elective courses in law as applied to nursing. "Nursing and the law" is also one of the most popular continuing education topics for nurses. This chapter highlights key issues in the law for professional nurses to develop interest in further study, which is essential to maintain a working knowledge of the law as it relates to professional nursing practice.

AMERICAN LEGAL SYSTEM

The purpose of the law in the United States is found in the Preamble to the U.S. Constitution: to assure order, protect the individual person, resolve disputes, and promote the general welfare. To achieve these broad objectives, the law concerns itself with the legal relationships between persons and the government.

U.S. law evolved from centuries-old English **common law.** Common law is decisional or judge-made law. Every time a judge makes a legal decision, the body of common law expands.

In addition to common law, there are **statutory laws,** which are laws established through formal legislative processes. Every time the U.S. Congress or a state legislature passes legislation, the body of statutory law expands.

An important distinction to understand is the difference between civil and criminal law. **Civil law** involves issues between individuals, whereas **criminal law** involves public concerns against unlawful behavior that threatens society.

All law in the United States flows from the U.S. Constitution and must conform to its principles. The Constitution provides for division of powers through the establishment of three branches of government—the judicial, executive, and legislative branches. The chief functions of the judicial branch are to resolve legal disputes, interpret statutory laws, and amend the common law. The executive branch implements laws through governmental agencies. The legislative branch may delegate authority to governmental agencies to create **administrative law** to meet the intent of a statute. Both federal and state administrative laws have the force and effect of statutory law. The legislative branch makes statutory laws and speaks most directly for the people.

The word **law** is defined as the sum total of man-made rules and regulations by which society is governed in a formal and binding manner (Hemelt and Mackert, 1982). It encompasses the actions of the legislative branch in enacting statutes, the executive branch in administering the statutes through rules, and the judicial branch in interpreting statutes and rules.

Professional nurses need to be aware of a wide array of legal issues. Nurses must be particularly aware of the statutory authority governing nursing practice, executive authority of state boards of nursing, the civil law areas of torts, privacy rights, and the evolving common law related to health care. The remainder of this chapter focuses on these key areas.

NURSING AS A PRACTICE DISCIPLINE

Disciplines such as nursing, medicine, dentistry, law, and many others are regulated by the individual states. The practitioners of these disciplines cannot legally practice without a license. The purpose of licensing certain professions is to protect the public safety. The statute that defines and controls nursing is called a nursing practice act. All 50 states and several U.S. territories have nursing practice acts.

Statutory Authority of State Nursing Practice Acts

Nurses, as health care providers, have certain rights, responsibilities, and recognitions through various state laws, or statutes. The nursing practice act in each state does at least four things:

1. Defines the practice of professional nursing.
2. Sets the educational qualifications and other requirements for licensure.
3. Determines the legal titles and abbreviations nurses may use.
4. Provides for disciplinary action of licensees for certain causes.

In many states, nursing practice acts also define the responsibilities and authorities of the state board of nursing. Thus, the nursing practice act of each state is the most important statutory law affecting nurses (Fig. 20–1).

Once the law regarding nursing practice is established, the legislative branch delegates authority to an executive agency, usually the state board of nursing. State boards of nursing are responsible for enforcing the nursing practice acts in the various states. The state board of nursing promulgates rules and regulations that flesh out the law. The statutory law plus the rules and regulations promulgated by the state board of nursing give full meaning to the nursing practice act in each state.

FIGURE   20–1
The nursing practice act and other state rules and regulations are vital documents that affect the legal practice of nursing. (Photo by Fielding Freed.)

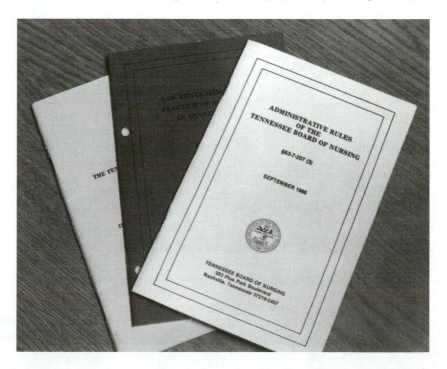

Nursing practice acts are revised from time to time to keep up with new developments in health care and changes in nursing practice. State nurses associations are usually instrumental in lobbying for appropriate updating in nursing practice acts.

Because of the importance of practice acts to professional nurses, the American Nurses Association (ANA) has developed suggested language for the content of state nursing practice acts. The document *Model Practice Act* was published in 1996 to guide state nurses associations seeking revisions in their nursing practice acts (American Nurses Association, 1996). The guidelines encourage consideration of the many issues inherent in a nursing practice act and the political realities of each state's legislative and regulatory processes. Through this document, the ANA recognizes the great importance of the nursing practice act and urges that the following content be included:

1. A clear differentiation between advanced and generalist nursing practice.
2. Authority for boards of nursing to regulate advanced nursing practice, including authority for prescription writing.
3. Authority for boards of nursing to oversee unlicensed assistive personnel.
4. Clarification of the nurse's responsibility for delegation to and supervision of other personnel.
5. Support for mandatory licensure for nurses while retaining sufficient flexibility to accommodate the changing nature of nursing practice.

The ANA document provides a broad definition of the practice of professional nursing and appropriate professional practice activities. It incorporates aspects of technical nursing practice and identifies technical activities (American Nurses Association, 1996).

The guidelines recognize the baccalaureate degree with a major in nursing (BSN) as the minimum educational credential for the professional nurse.

There has been extensive debate about the need to change the minimum educational qualifications for professional nursing practice. In the early 1980s and again in 1995, the ANA reaffirmed its long-standing position that the baccalaureate should be the minimum educational qualification for professional nursing practice and the associate degree the minimum educational qualification for technical nursing practice.

To date, only North Dakota has fully implemented these changes in the minimum educational qualifications for nurses. Many state nurses associations, however, consider such changes a priority for future nursing practice act modifications.

Executive Authority of State Boards of Nursing

Both federal and state laws provide for the executive branch of government to administer and implement laws. The state executive, or governor, generally delegates the responsibility for administering the nursing practice act to an executive agency, the state board of nursing. In most states, the state board of nursing consists of registered nurses (RNs), licensed practical nurses (LPNs), and consumers, all of whom are generally appointed by the governor.

The state board of nursing's authority is limited. It can adopt rules that clarify general provisions of the nursing practice act, but it does not have the authority to enlarge the law.

State boards of nursing usually have three functions:

1. Quasiexecutive—authority to administer the nursing practice act.
2. Quasilegislative—authority to adopt rules necessary to implement the act.
3. Quasijudicial—authority to deny, suspend, or revoke a license or to otherwise discipline a licensee or to deny an application for licensure.

Each of these functions is as broad or as limited as the state legislature specifies in the nursing practice act and related laws.

Establishing Rules Regulating Nursing Practice

The federal government and each state have an administrative procedures act (APA) that specifies the process executive branch agencies such as the state board of nursing must use in promulgating rules to implement a specific law. Although one state's APA may differ in certain areas from others', there are recommended principles for all APAs. The principles for promulgation of rules include:

1. Written notice and publication of the proposed rules.
2. Opportunity for oral and written comments about the proposed rules.
3. A public hearing or forum for response to the proposed rules.
4. Identification of options the executive agency may exercise to withdraw, modify, or adopt the proposed rules.
5. Review of the adopted rules by a legislative committee or legal review, such as by the office of the state attorney general.
6. Publication of the final rules in an official governmental document.
7. Codification of the adopted rules in an official publication such as the federal *Code of Federal Regulations (CFR)* or a state administrative code.

In some states, rules may be proposed through a petition to the executive agency.

The APA also specifies a process that executive agencies such as state boards of nursing must follow when considering action on a specific professional or occupational license or permit. This process is consistent with an individual's constitutional right to due process. An executive agency may have the authority to suspend a license or a permit to practice if there is evidence of a threat to the public health and welfare if the license or permit remains in effect while the action is pending. The APA-specified process usually includes:

1. Notice of a complaint or cause of the proposed action.
2. Notice of the date, time, and place of a hearing on such complaint.
3. Right of the applicant or licensee to legal counsel.
4. Right of the applicant or licensee and the agency to subpoena witnesses and records and to examine and cross-examine such witnesses.

5. The agency's authority in such matters.
6. Right of either party to appeal the decision.
7. Final decision and notice to applicant or licensee.

State boards of nursing may be independent agencies in the executive branch of state government or part of a department or bureau such as a department of licensure and regulation. Some state boards have authority to carry out the nursing practice act without review of their actions by other state officials. Others must recommend action to another department or bureau and receive approval of the recommendation before the decision is finalized.

LICENSING POWERS

The legal regulation of nursing practice is accomplished primarily through state licensure of nurses. The *Report of the National Advisory Commission on Health Manpower* concluded: "The first requirement for assuring that health care approaches its potential quality is to make licensure effective to the limit of its capabilities" (U.S. Department of Health, Education and Welfare, 1968).

The accepted definition of individual **licensure** is: "The process by which an agency of government grants permission to persons to engage in a given profession or occupation by certifying that those licensed have attained the minimal degree of competency necessary to ensure that the public health, safety and welfare will be reasonably well protected" (U.S. Department of Health, Education and Welfare, 1971).

The licensure process is a police power of the state. The state, through the legislative branch, determines what groups are to be licensed and the limitations of such licenses. Licensure laws may be either mandatory or permissive. A mandatory law requires any person who practices the profession or occupation to be licensed. A permissive law protects the use of the title granted in the law but does not prohibit persons practicing the profession or occupation if they do not use the title. All states now have a mandatory licensure law for the practice of nursing.

Just as the state has the power to issue a nursing license based upon established criteria, so does it retain the power to discipline a licensee for performing professional functions in a manner that is dangerous to patients or the general public. Discipline may include sanctions such as license suspension or revocation arising from unsafe, uninformed, or impaired practice by the nurse licensee.

Historically the nursing profession has demonstrated a commitment to the rehabilitation of nurses whose practice is below standard because of impairment by psychological dysfunction or substance abuse and misuse. In 1990, the ANA published suggested state legislation that included a Nursing Disciplinary Diversion Act (American Nurses Association, 1990). This publication recommended a diversion procedure, such as a peer assistance program to combat substance abuse, as a voluntary alternative to traditional disciplinary actions of suspension or revocation of a license. By 1995, at least 27 state boards of nursing had in place a disciplinary diversion process to assist impaired nurses to return to safe nursing practice.

In most states, state boards of nursing have the authority to enforce minimum criteria for nursing education programs. The practice act usually provides that an applicant for licensure must graduate from a state-approved nursing education program as a prerequisite for being admitted to the licensure examination.

State approval is different from national accreditation; many nursing education programs achieve accreditation by the nationally recognized accrediting agency, the National League for Nursing. Although many other professions and occupations require graduation from a nationally accredited educational program as a prerequisite for licensure, only state approval is required in nursing.

LICENSURE EXAMINATIONS

Since 1944, most state boards of nursing participated in a cooperative effort to develop an examination for licensure of RNs and LPNs that was adopted by each state and thus assisted in the interstate mobility of nurses. In describing this system, Schorr (1975, p. 1131) wrote:

> Ours (nursing) was the first health profession to have an examination that is used nationwide in judging a candidate's basic competence and right to be licensed. Because of this, the State Board Test Pool Examination (SBTPE) facilitates endorsement of a nurse's license by a state to which he or she is moving, providing the score on the SBTPE in the original state meets the required minimum score set by the board in the new state. Although the examination is used nationally and the questions on it are developed by nurses from all over the country, so that the tests really mirror practice nationwide, the principle of states' rights has also been worked into the system.

Because nurse licensure examinations are national examinations, they facilitate the system of **licensure by endorsement.** Endorsement means that RNs or LPNs/LVNs (licensed vocational nurses) can move from state to state without having to take another licensing examination. If they submit proof of licensure in another state and pay a licensure fee, they can receive licensure for the new state by endorsement. Licensure by endorsement is not available to all practice disciplines. Nursing's plan serves as a national model for other licensed professions and occupations.

Until 1978, the SBTPE was developed by the ANA's Council of State Boards of Nursing, and the National League for Nursing served as the testing service. In 1978, the National Council of State Boards of Nursing (NCSBN) was established and continued the activities of the ANA Council of State Boards. Through the NCSBN, each state still participates in the licensing process through test development and adoption of a minimum passing score.

The nurse licensure examinations are now called the National Council Licensure Examination for Registered Nurses (NCLEX-RN) and the National Council Licensure Examination for Practical Nurses (NCLEX-PN). The test was traditionally administered by paper and pencil; however the State Boards of

Nursing and the NCSBN began administering them by computerized adaptive testing (CAT) in 1994. The test plan for the NCLEX-RN licensure examination provides for the examination to measure critical thinking and nursing competence.

TRENDS IN LICENSURE

The climate for licensure of health professions became increasingly unstable in the mid to late 1990s, largely because of dramatic alterations in the financing and delivery of health services following the 1994 failure of health care reform. Federal and state governments indicated interest in examining all types of deregulation, and licensure of health professionals has no immunity to regulatory changes.

The Pew Charitable Trust funded extensive projects examining health care work force regulations, which may, over time, create a variety of regulatory schemes in different jurisdictions. The nursing community needs to be vigilant in the analysis of each proposal for regulatory change. Nursing has much to gain or lose in terms of its scope, authority, and accountability for practice should deregulation occur (Pew Health Professions Commission, 1995).

SPECIAL CONCERNS IN PROFESSIONAL NURSING PRACTICE

Nurses make decisions daily that affect the well-being of their patients. They often know personal information about patients and are in a position of great trust. Several areas of nursing practice are particularly fraught with legal risk. They include malpractice, delegation, assault and battery, informed consent, and confidentiality. Each of these areas is discussed.

Malpractice

Malpractice is the greatest legal concern of health care practitioners. To understand malpractice, it is necessary first to understand the legal concepts of torts and negligence. **Torts** are civil wrongs against a person and may be either intentional or unintentional. There must be harm resulting from the action, but the harm may be physical, emotional, or economic. An intentional tort refers to willful or intentional acts that violate another person's rights or property.

Negligence is the failure to act as a reasonably prudent person would have in specific circumstances. For example, if in burning yard debris on a windy day a man sets fire to his neighbor's garage, the neighbor may charge negligence. A reasonably prudent person would not have started a yard fire on a windy day, and an injury (the burned garage) can be shown to be a direct result of his failure to act prudently. The differences between negligence and intentional torts are summarized in Table 20–1.

Malpractice is negligence applied to the acts of a professional. In other words, malpractice occurs when a professional fails to act as a reasonably prudent professional would under specific circumstances. Malpractice is classified as an un-

TABLE 20–1
Differences Between Negligence and Intentional Torts

Negligence	Intentional Torts*
Intent	
May occur without any intent to act	Requires an intent to interfere with another's rights; a hostile motive not required
Proof of Damages	
Requires proof of a specific injury	Proof of actual injury not required
Duty or Standards of Care	
Relevant; Usually involves expert witnesses	Not needed
Consent	
Not necessarily a defense	Always may be a defense

*Examples of intentional torts include defamation (libel or slander), invasion of privacy, assault and battery, false imprisonment, and intentional infliction of emotional distress. Data from Aiken, T. (1994). *Legal, ethical, and political issues in nursing.* Philadelphia: F.A. Davis.

intentional tort. This means that it is not necessary to prove that the professional intended to be negligent. In malpractice, both *doing* things that should *not* be done (commissions) and *not doing* things that *should* be done (omissions) may be the basis of legal actions.

When a patient brings a malpractice claim against a nurse defendant, evidence is presented to the jury to determine if the elements of liability are present. At question is whether the nurse met the prevailing **standard of care.**

The nursing standard of care is what the reasonably prudent nurse, under similar circumstances, would have done. It is a peer standard of care that reflects not excellence but a minimum standard of "do no harm." The nursing standard of care is decided by the jury on a case-by-case basis and is developed through use of **expert witness** testimony; documents, including national **standards of nursing practice;** the patient record; and other pertinent evidence such as the direct testimony of the patient, the nurse, and others.

The prerequisite for a malpractice action is that the defendant (nurse) has specialized knowledge and skills and through the practice of that specialized knowledge caused the plaintiff's (patient's) injury. For a plaintiff patient to prove that the nurse defendant is liable for the injury, all elements of a cause of action for negligence must be proved. The elements are the same for any professional accused of malpractice. The elements necessary for a malpractice action are as follows:

1. The professional nurse has assumed the **duty of care** (responsibility for the patient's care).
2. The professional nurse breaches the duty of care by failing to meet the standard of care.
3. The failure of the professional nurse to meet the standard of care **proximately caused** the injury.

4. The injury is proved.

Setting forth all elements of a malpractice action requires a high degree of proof. Money damages are awarded when a patient plaintiff prevails. The money damages are based on proven economic losses, such as time missed from work or out-of-pocket health care costs, and remuneration for pain and suffering caused by the injury. In the case of a death, the next of kin can become the plaintiff on behalf of the deceased patient.

In the past, some malpractice lawsuits involved nurses but the physician or hospital defendants were traditionally called on to pay damages even when the substandard care was provided by nurses. In these instances, physicians were implicated through the **"captain of the ship" doctrine.** This doctrine implies that the physician is in charge of all patient care and thus should be responsible financially. Hospitals were implicated through the legal theory of **respondeat superior,** which attributes the acts of employees to their employer. As nurses increase their expertise, autonomy, credentials, and authority for nursing practice, however, liability for nursing care will correspondingly be increased. Nurses are expected to be defendants more often in the future (Sweeney, 1991).

A review of malpractice cases in which the liability of the nurse has been successfully litigated showed the categories of cases as follows:

1. The nurse failed to carry out the medical order (*Dobrzeniecki*, 1984).
2. The nurse carried out an order incorrectly (*Holbrooks*, 1983).
3. The nurse implemented a faulty medical order (*Doerr*, 1985).
4. The nurse failed to make an accurate assessment (*Harris*, 1985).
5. The nurse failed to act on an assessment (*Duren*, 1985).
6. The nurse failed to report inadequate patient care (*Utter*, 1977).
7. The nurse failed to secure adequate care for a patient (*Goff*, 1958).
8. The nurse abandoned a patient needing care (*Hiatt*, 1974).

Some examples of malpractice that included professional nurses were covered in the popular press. One such highly publicized case involved several nurses who, over a period of days, carried out a physician's faulty order and gave a cancer patient a 400 percent overdose of chemotherapy (*Doerr*, 1985). Another example is an operating room nurse who failed to follow well-established hospital policy for identifying and preparing patients for surgery. This breach of procedure resulted in the removal of one patient's only functioning kidney (*Holbrooks*, 1983). Although physicians and facilities are also involved in both of these cases, the nurse(s) are likely to be named as codefendants because they too fell below the standard of care and "but for" their actions, these serious injuries would not have occurred.

The lesson to be learned from such malpractice cases is that professional nurses must carefully consider the legal implications of practice and be willing and capable of conforming to professional standards and all legal expectations.

Delegation

Delegation, that is, "empowering one to act for another," is an issue gaining increasing importance in nursing practice. The ability to delegate has generally been reserved for professionals because they hold licenses that sanction the entire scope of practice for a particular profession. Professional nurses, for example, may delegate independent nursing activities and delegated medical functions to other nursing personnel. State nursing practice acts do not give delegatory authority to LPNs/LVNs.

Professional nurses retain accountability for acts delegated to another person and are responsible for determining that the delegatee is competent to perform the delegated act. Likewise, the delegatee is responsible for carrying out the delegated act safely. The professional nurse remains legally liable, however, for the nursing acts delegated to others unless the delegatee is a licensed professional whose scope includes the assigned act.

Delegatory acts must also be considered from the standpoint of their ethical implications. The *Code for Nurses* states, "The nurse exercises informed judgment and uses individual competence and qualifications as criteria in seeking consultation, accepting responsibilities, and delegating nursing activities to others" (American Nurses Association, 1985). An important point is that nurses are ethically bound to refuse to accept acts that are not within their area of expertise, even if a physician or hospital authority requests that they accept them.

Delegation is an important liability and one not fully appreciated by many practicing nurses. The professional nurse's primary legal and ethical consideration must be the patient's right to safe, effective nursing care.

Assault and Battery

Assault and battery is an intentional tort that is often the basis for legal action against a nurse defendant. **Assault** is a threat or an attempt to make bodily contact with another person without the person's consent. Assault precedes battery; it causes the person to fear that a battery is about to occur. **Battery** is the assault carried out, the unpermissible, unprivileged touching by one person of another. Actual harm may or may not occur as a result of assault and battery.

If, for example, a nurse threatens a patient with a vitamin injection if he does not eat his meals, the patient may charge assault. Actually giving the patient a vitamin injection against his will leaves the nurse open to charges of battery, even if there is a physician's order. It is important to remember that patients have the right to refuse treatment, even if the treatment would be in their best interest. Both by common law and by statute, **informed consent** is required in the health care context as a defense to battery (*United States Code*, 1990).

Informed Consent

All patients should be given an opportunity to grant informed consent before treatment unless there is an emergency that is life-threatening. Three major elements of informed consent include:

1. Consent must be given voluntarily.
2. Consent must be given by an individual with the capacity and competence to understand.

3. The patient must be given enough information to be the ultimate decision maker (Northrup and Kelly, 1987).

Informed consent is a full, knowing authorization by the patient for care, treatment, and procedures and must include information about the risks, benefits, side effects, costs, and alternatives. Consumers of health care need a great deal of information and should be told everything that they would consider significant in making a treatment decision (*Canterbury*, 1972).

For informed consent to be legally valid, elements of completeness, competency, and voluntariness are evaluated. Completeness refers to the quality of the information provided. **Competency** takes into account the capability of a particular patient to understand the information given and make a choice. Voluntariness refers to the freedom the patient has to accept or reject alternatives. When patients are minors, are under the effects of drugs or alcohol (including preoperative medications), or have other mental deficits, it is questionable that competency to consent exists.

The role of nurses in informed consent, unless they are themselves primary providers, is to collaborate with the primary provider, most often a physician. A nurse may witness a patient's signing of informed consent documents but is not responsible for explaining the proposed treatment (Fig. 20–2). The nurse is not responsible for evaluating whether the physician has truly explained the significant risks, benefits, and alternative treatments. Professional nurses *are* re-

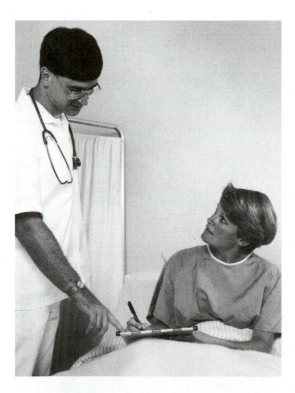

FIGURE 20–2
A nurse may be called upon to witness a patient's signing of informed consent documents. (Photo by Fielding Freed.)

sponsible for determining that the elements for valid consent are in place, providing feedback if the patient wishes to change consent, and communicating the patient's need for further information to the primary provider.

Confidentiality

Confidentiality is both a legal and an ethical concern in nursing practice. Confidentiality is the protection of private information gathered about a patient during the provision of health care services. The *Code for Nurses* states: "The nurse safeguards the client's right to privacy by judiciously protecting information of a confidential nature" (American Nurses Association, 1985).

The *Code* acknowledges exceptions to the obligation of confidentiality. The exceptions include discussing the care of patients with others involved in their direct care, quality assurance activities, and when the law demands disclosure (American Nurses Association, 1985). The *Code* also recognizes the need to disclose information without the patient's consent when the safety of innocent parties is in question (*Tarasoff*, 1976).

Although some professions have statutorily protected **privileged communication,** nurses are usually not included in such statutes. Thus, nurses may be ordered by a court to share information without the patient's consent. The principle of confidentiality is protected by state and federal statutes, but there are exceptions and limitations. It is essential for the professional nurse to understand these legal limitations.

In certain situations, through statute and common law, there has developed the antithesis of confidentiality—the **duty to report** or disclose. These laws require nurses and other health professionals to report child abuse, gunshot wounds, certain communicable diseases, and threats toward third parties. These laws vary by state and may be the responsibility of institutions providing health care services and not of an individual practitioner.

EVOLVING LEGAL ISSUES AND THE NURSE

Because of the dynamic nature of nursing and health care, legal issues affecting nursing practice are also evolving. Specific legal issues that illustrate the changing nature of nursing practice are related to role changes, supervision of assistive personnel, payment mechanisms, and a new law, the Patient Self-Determination Act (PSDA). Each of these issues is briefly discussed.

Role Changes in Health Care

Just as a nurse's knowledge base and the nurse's accountability for nursing practice have increased over time, so has the need to expand the **legal authority** for nursing practice. Even though the definitions and parameters of nursing outlined in nursing practice acts may seem to be an issue of concern only to nurses, this is not the case.

Nurses have found that as they worked through their state nurses associations to modify and update these acts, they met significant political resistance. This is due, in part, to the defensiveness of organized medicine, which often views an expansion of nurses' domain as a diminishment of physicians' roles or as a threat to physicians' economic base.

Professional nurses realize that it is important for a state nursing practice act to reflect nursing practice accurately and to keep up with changes in health care delivery as they occur. Otherwise, nurses have questionable legal basis for practice. Health care is becoming more specialized, so nursing specialties and subspecialties are increasing. Advanced practice nurses set the pace for evolving nursing practice, and the nursing practice act must support their ability to offer nursing services to consumers in various settings. Many functions defined as advanced practice have been absorbed into the statutory scope of professional nursing practice.

PRESCRIPTIVE AUTHORITY

An important role addition for advanced practice RNs is **prescriptive authority.** Prescriptive authority is defined as the legal acknowledgment of prescription writing as an appropriate act of nursing practice. The ANA supports prescriptive authority for advanced practice RNs, as distinguished from generalist RNs (American Nurses Association, 1990).

Several questions about prescriptive authority that nurses should consider include: Does the state recognize prescriptive authority for nurses? If so, is the state board of nursing the state regulatory authority for this practice? Does the law require physician collaboration or supervision or written protocols? What are the parameters for prescribing controlled substances, if any?

In late 1995, advanced practice RNs had some type of prescriptive authority in 48 states. This authority ranged from completely independent authority with no collaborative requirements in the District of Columbia to a pilot test in Louisiana granting limited prescriptive authority to nurses in underserved clinics. Most states require advanced practice status, the collaboration or supervision of a physician, and prescription writing protocols (American Nurses Association, 1995a).

In some states, nurses in advanced practice, such as nurse-midwives, nurse practitioners, and nurses in private practice, have not been supported by timely changes in the nursing practice act. For example, nurses in Missouri were sued for practicing medicine without a license in a women's health practice. After intense litigation, their practice was supported by the Missouri Supreme Court. The court found "legislative intent" in the nursing practice act not to limit nursing practice except to protect the public. The nurses in question were well credentialed and were practicing with the knowledge and support of the Missouri Board of Nursing and the Missouri Nurses Association, so the safety of the public was not in question (*Sermchief*, 1983). This is only one example of the legal exposure nurses face when their state's nursing practice act is not updated periodically to support explicitly an expanded scope of practice. Working within the state nurses association to expand the evolving scope of nursing practice appropriately ensures the growth of the profession and increases the number of primary care providers needed by the public.

Supervision of Unlicensed Assistive Personnel

Another evolving legal issue is the role expansion of unlicensed assistive personnel or limited licensed (LPN/LVN) personnel within health care institutions. Nurse aides (i.e., unlicensed assistive personnel) are increasingly being substituted for nurses, thus creating greater risks to patients and enlarging the liability of nurses, who supervise their work. Court decisions indicate that lack of professional nurse supervision poses a significant risk to patients, institutions, and nurses alike (Politis, 1983).

The substitution of unlicensed personnel for RNs is a strategy used by health care facilities to hold down costs. Such substitution is ill-advised because it jeopardizes quality of care and places the RN at increased risk for patient injury liability for acts performed by unlicensed assistive personnel. It is questionable whether, in the long-term, professional nursing care is actually more expensive than care provided by unlicensed personnel, who are less likely to do patient teaching and recognize complications.

In 1992, the ANA issued a *Position Statement on Registered Nurse Utilization of Unlicensed Assistive Personnel*. This statement indicated that the ANA recognizes that unlicensed assistive personnel provide support services to RNs that assist the RN in providing nursing care (American Nurses Association, 1992). The statement identified the need to clarify the activities that should be in the domain of the RN and those that can be safely delegated. Additional materials were developed by the ANA to provide RNs and health care facilities guidance on "best practice" use of unlicensed personnel (American Nurses Association, 1995c).

Historically, organized nursing has opposed the licensure or legal recognition of nurse aides and other nursing support personnel. This position needs further study, however, following congressional action mandating training and state registration of nurse aides in Medicaid-certified and Medicare-certified nursing facilities and Medicare-certified home health agencies. In January 1992, only 14 state boards of nursing regulated some aspect of the federally mandated requirements. Federal law allows the state Medicaid agency to contract with a state board of nursing to operate the required nurse aide registry; however, only the Medicaid agency can enter a finding of patient abuse, neglect, or misappropriation of patient property by individuals on the nurse aide registry.

Payment Mechanisms for Nurses

As discussed in Chapter 5, nurses are increasingly practicing in nontraditional roles and settings. Many professional nurses are both capable of and interested in offering nursing services as private practitioners, but current payment mechanisms may limit such activities. Nurses are concerned about offering services for which consumers are unable to obtain reimbursement from their insurance carriers, and third-party reimbursement has traditionally been limited to care provided by physicians.

Over the years, nurses have supported state and federal legislation to provide direct and indirect payments to nurses for nursing services rendered (American Nurses Association, 1991a). Changes in state insurance laws were enacted in many states to achieve direct payment for nursing services from private insurance companies. This means that consumers of health care may choose to receive services from physicians, nurses, or other qualified health professionals and receive insurance reimbursement for the chosen professional's fees. Nurses are concerned that these changes are often not implemented or nurses are paid less for similar services when provided by other health care professionals.

Laws are often passed that are not implemented. This occurs when the group affected by the law, for example, the insurance industry, is unwilling to implement the changes and no "watchdog" agency is created to ensure that changes occur. For example, federal legislation was enacted requiring state Medicaid agencies to pay certain nurses (nurse practitioners, nurse-midwives, and nurse anesthetists) directly for services provided to Medicaid recipients. As with the laws affecting private insurers, these requirements have not been implemented in every state. Nurses may need to seek legal remedies to require implementation of policies mandated by federal law (*Nurse Midwifery Associates*, 1990).

Following the failed 1994 efforts to overhaul the entire health care system, health care finance nevertheless underwent dramatic changes. One change, discussed in Chapter 16, was from fee-for-service provider reimbursement to capitation. Additionally, many individual and group insurance plans changed from indemnity plans to **managed care** plans, such as health maintenance organizations and preferred provider organizations. These shifts have posed new challenges for nurses because they are often not included on HMO and PPO provider panels. As a result of these new challenges, the ANA and state nurses associations are working to ensure that nurses are included on managed care panels, in "any willing provider" clauses, and in all federal insurance programs as appropriate providers of basic plan services.

Patient Self-Determination Act

As mentioned in Chapter 19, the federal **Patient Self-Determination Act** was effective December 1, 1991. The PSDA applies to acute care and long-term care facilities that receive Medicare and Medicaid funds. This act encourages patients to consider which life-prolonging treatment options they desire and to document their preferences in case they should later become incapable of participating in the decision-making process. Written instructions recognized by state law that describe an individual's preferences in regard to medical intervention should the individual become incapacitated is called an **advance directive.**

This act was passed partly in response to the U.S. Supreme Court's decision in *Cruzan v. Director* (1990), which was viewed as limiting an individual's ability to direct his or her health care when unable to do so. The PSDA requires the health care facility to document whether the patient has completed an advance directive.

The PSDA's basic assumption is that each person has legal and moral rights to informed consent about medical treatments with a focus on the person's right to choose (the ethical principle of autonomy). The act does not create any new rights, and no patient is required to execute an advance directive.

According to the PSDA, acute care (hospitals) and long-term care facilities must:

1. Provide written information to all adult patients about their rights under state law.
2. Ensure institutional compliance with state laws on advance directives.
3. Provide for education of staff and the community on advance directives.
4. Document in the medical record whether the patient has an advance directive.

There have been a number of widely publicized cases wherein families and providers disagreed about whether to terminate life support mechanisms (See News Note, Chapter 19). Widespread education of the public about advance directives should result in fewer such legal and ethical dilemmas in the future. Documentation of the existence of advance directives and use of them in planning care is an important patient advocacy role for nurses and is a legal requirement that needs careful implementation in clinical settings.

PREVENTING LEGAL PROBLEMS IN NURSING PRACTICE

Although the range of potential "hot spots" for health care litigation may seem enormous, there are a number of effective strategies that professional nurses can use to limit the possibility of legal action.

Practice in a Safe Setting

To be truly safe, facilities in which nurses work must be committed to safe patient care. The safest situation is one in which the agency:

1. Employs an appropriate number and skill mix of personnel to address the numbers and acuity of patients.
2. Has policies, procedures, and personnel practices that promote quality improvement.
3. Keeps equipment in good working order.
4. Provides orientation to new employees, supervises all levels of employees, and provides opportunities to learn new procedures consistent with the level of health care services provided by the agency.

In addition to an active quality improvement program, each health care institution should have a **risk management** program. Risk management seeks to identify and eliminate potential safety hazards, thereby reducing patient and staff injuries. Common institutional risks are medication errors, falls, assessment errors, and failure to communicate (Campazzi, 1980).

Communicate with Other Health Professionals

The professional nurse must have open and clear communication with nurses, physicians, and other health care professionals. Safe nurses trust their own assessments, inform physicians and others of changes in patients' conditions, and question unclear or inaccurate physicians' orders. A key aspect of communication essential in preventing legal problems is keeping good patient records. This written form of communication is called **documentation.** Current and descriptive documentation of patient care is essential, not only to quality care, but also to protecting the nurse. Assessments, plans, interventions, and evaluation of the patient's progress must be reflected in the patient's clinical record if malpractice is alleged.

The clinical record, particularly the nurse's notes, provides the core of evidence about each patient's nursing care (Kerr, 1975). No matter how good the nursing care, if the nurse fails to write it in the clinical record, in the eyes of the law the care did not take place.

Meet the Standard of Care

The most important protective strategy for the nurse is to be a knowledgeable and safe practitioner of nursing and to meet the standard of care with all patients. Meeting the standard of care involves being technically competent, keeping up-to-date with health care innovations, being aware of peer expectations, and participating as an equal on the health care team.

In addition to being current with the nursing literature, professional nurses must use national standards of practice as parameters for care giving, care planning, and care evaluation (American Nurses Association, 1991b). The ANA has promulgated generic and specialty standards of nursing practice. These national standards can be used by quality improvement programs in individual hospitals in establishing their own "local" standards of nursing care (Betts, 1978).

Carry Professional Liability Insurance

Despite the efforts of dedicated professionals, at times mistakes are made, and, unfortunately, patients are injured. It is essential for nurses to carry professional liability insurance to protect their assets and income, should they be required to pay monetary compensation to an injured patient. Nursing students should also carry insurance, and most nursing education programs require that they do so.

Professional liability insurance policies vary. Generally, they provide up to $1 million coverage for a single incident and up to $3 million total. The amount of coverage depends on the nurse's specialty. Nurse-midwives, for example, pay much higher liability insurance premiums than do psychiatric nurses because a nurse-midwife's potential for being sued is greater. Most policies also provide the defendant nurse with a defense attorney (American Association of Nurse Attorneys, 1984).

Professional liability insurance is available through most state nurses associations, nursing students' associations, and private insurers. Group policies, such as those available through professional associations, are usually less expensive than individual policies and are an important benefit of association membership. Box 20–1 displays information about the two main types of professional liability policies.

B O X   2 0 – 1

Basic Types of Professional Liability Insurance Policies

Occurrence Policies
Cover injuries that occur during the period covered by the policy

Claims-Made Policies
Cover injuries only if the injury occurs within the policy period *and* the claim

is reported to the insurance company during the policy period or during the "tail"*

*A "tail" is an uninterrupted extension of the policy period and is also known as the extending reporting endorsement.

National Practitioner Data Bank

The Health Care Quality Improvement Act (Public Law 100-177), was passed by Congress in 1986. It established a **National Practitioner Data Bank** (NPDB) to encourage identification and discipline of health care practitioners who engage in unprofessional behavior. An additional purpose was to restrict the ability of those practitioners to move from state to state without disclosing problems of damaging or incompetent practice. The Act requires that certain things be reported to a national data bank: any malpractice payments made to any licensed health practitioner, any licensure action taken by a licensing body, any clinical privilege suspension or revocation by a health care facility, and any clinical society censureship action.

The NPDB affects nurses in two major ways:

1. Malpractice payments made on behalf of a nurse are reported to the NPDB and copied to the state board of nursing.
2. An inquiry to the NPDB is required when nurses apply for hospital privileges and is required every two years for renewal of hospital privileges.

The NPDB reported in July 1995 that the number of malpractice payments was relatively constant, with the median amount of all malpractice payments being less than $60,000. It also reported that malpractice insurance premium costs in real dollars decreased by 20 percent between 1988 and 1991.

Malpractice payments in 1994 to various providers included the following ratios: one payment per 35 physicians; one payment per 52 dentists; one payment per 2500 RNs; one payment per 78 certified registered nurse anesthetists; one payment per 78 certified nurse-midwives; and one payment per 714 nurse practitioners (American Nurses Associations, 1995b).

Promote Positive Interpersonal Relationships

Even in the face of untoward outcomes from a health care provider, it is usually only the unhappy patient that sues. Therefore, the best strategy for the profes-

<table>
<tr><td colspan="2">

B O X 2 0 – 2
Guidelines for Preventing Legal Problems in Nursing Practice
</td></tr>
<tr><td>

- Practice in a safe setting.
- Communicate with other health professionals.
- Meet the standard of care.
</td><td>

- Carry professional liability insurance.
- Promote positive interpersonal relationships.
</td></tr>
</table>

sional nurse is prevention of legal actions through positive interpersonal relationships.

Prevention includes giving personalized, concerned care; including the patient and the family in planning and implementing care; and promoting positive, open interpersonal relationships that value the psychosocial aspects of care. The professional nurse who uses self as a therapeutic agent and acknowledges the holism of the patient is likely to prevent most legal problems. Box 20–2 summarizes the important steps nurses can take to avoid legal problems in professional practice.

SUMMARY

There are many legal issues for professional nurses. First, nurses must recognize that the law is a system of rules that governs conduct and attaches consequences to certain behavior. Such consequences include civil or criminal action or both. Nursing practice is limited by the definition of practice in the state nursing practice act and the qualifications for licensure to practice nursing in that state. Similar to nursing practice, the law is dynamic and must be responsive to society's needs. Advances in technology have increased the possibility for legal actions involving nurses. Technology has also increased concern about informed consent and patients' right to direct the care they choose to receive or refuse. Many nurses possess only a cursory knowledge of legal issues that affect nursing practice every day. These issues deserve increased attention by nurses in all areas of practice.

REVIEW AND DISCUSSION QUESTIONS

1. Using your state's nursing practice act, describe the scope of practice of the registered nurse. When was the last time the law was modified? Does it accurately reflect current nursing practice?
2. Read the section of the nursing practice act relating to advanced practice. What parameters, if any, do nurses have in the areas of practice and prescription writing in your state?
3. Go to the college library and browse through back issues of the *Regan Report on Nursing Law*. What kinds of legal issues do you find involving nurses?

4. Explain the Patient Self-Determination Act to your family and friends. What questions do they have about an advance directive? Find out what the laws regarding advance directives are in your state.
5. When interviewing for a position, what questions should you ask to determine if it is a legally safe setting in which to practice?

REFERENCES

Aiken, T. (1994). *Legal, ethical and political issues in nursing*. Philadelphia: F.A. Davis.

American Association of Nurse Attorneys. (1984). *Demonstrating financial responsibility for nursing practice*. Baltimore, MD: Author.

American Nurses Association (1996). *Model practice act*. Washington, DC: American Nurses Publishing.

American Nurses Association (1995a). *Analysis and comparison of advanced practice recognition with medical reimbursement and insurance reimbursement*. Washington, D.C.: American Nurses Publishing.

American Nurses Association (1995b). *Capital Update*, Vols. 13 and 14. Washington, D.C.: Author.

American Nurses Association (1995c). *Staff nurse guide to workplace restructuring*. Washington, D.C.: American Nurses Publishing.

American Nurses Association (1992). *Position statement on registered nurse utilization of unlicensed assistive personnel*. Washington, D.C.: Author.

American Nurses Association (1991a). *Pacesetter*, 18(2), Kansas City, MO: ANA Council of Psychiatric/Mental Health Nursing.

American Nurses Association (1991b). *Standards of clinical nursing practice*. Kansas City, MO: Author.

American Nurses Association (1990). *Suggested state legislation: Nursing practice act, nursing disciplinary diversion act, prescriptive authority act*. Kansas City, MO: Author.

American Nurses Association (1985). *Code for nurses*. Kansas City, MO: Author.

Betts, V. T. (1978). Using psychiatric audit as one aspect of a quality assurance program. *Current Perspectives in Psychiatric Nursing*, 2, 202–208.

Campazzi, M. (1980). Nurses, nursing, and malpractice litigation, 1967–1977. *Nursing Administration Quarterly*, 5(3), 1–8.

Canterbury v. Spense, 464 F^2 772 (1972).

Cruzan v. Director Missouri Department of Health, 110 Supreme Court 2841 (1990).

Dobrzeniecki v. University Hospital of Cleveland, 27 *ALTA Law Rpt.* 425 (1984).

Doerr v. Hurley, 28 *ALTA Law Rpt.* 42 (1985).

Duren v. Suburban Community Hospital. 28 *ALTA Law Rpt.* 168 (1985).

Goff v. Doctors General Hospital, 333 P^2 29 (1958).

Harris v. Skrocki, 28 *ALTA Law Rpt.* 420 (1985).

Hemelt, M., and Mackert, M. E. (1982). *Dynamics of law in nursing and health care*. Reston, VA: Reston Publishing.

Hiatt v. Groce, 523 P^2 320 (1974).

Holbrooks v. Duke Hospital, Inc., 305 SE^2 69 (1983).

Kerr, K. (1975). Nurses notes: That's where the goodies are. *Nursing*, 75(2), 34–41.

Northrup, C., and Kelly, M. (1987). *Legal issues in nursing*. St. Louis, MO: C.V. Mosby.

Nurse Midwifery Associates v. Hibbett, 918 Fed^2 605 (1990).

Pew Health Professions Commission. (1995). *Critical challenges: Revitalizing the health professions for the twenty first century*. San Francisco: Pew Health Trust.

Politis, E. (1983). Nurses' legal dilemma: When hospital staffing compromises professional standards. *University of San Francisco Law Review*, 3, 109–126.

Schorr, T. M. (1975). Securing licensure. *American Journal of Nursing*, 75(7), 1131.

Sermchief v. Gonzales, 660 SW^2 683 (1983).

Sweeney, S. (1991). Medical negligence: Proving nursing negligence. *Trial*, 91(5), 34–40.

Tarasoff v. Board of Regents of the University of California, 551 P^2 334 (1976).

42 *United States Code* 1395 cc. (1990).

U.S. Department of Health, Education and Welfare. (1971). *Report on licensure and related health personnel credentialing* (DHEW Publication No. [HSM] 72–11).

Washington, D.C.: Government Printing Office.

U.S. Department of Health, Education and Welfare. (1968). *Report of the National Advisory Commission on Health Manpower. II.* Washington, D.C.: Government Printing Office.

Utter v. United Hospital Center, Inc., 236 SE^2 213 (1977).

CHAPTER 21

Judith K. Leavitt
Virginia Trotter Betts
Cheryl Peterson

Nurses and Political Action

OBJECTIVES

- Differentiate between politics and policy.
- Explain the concept of personalizing the political process.
- Cite examples of sources of both personal and professional power.
- Describe how nurses can become involved in politics and policy development at the levels of citizen, activist, and politician.
- Explain how organized nursing is involved in political activities designed to strengthen professional nursing and influence health care policy.

VOCABULARY

adjudicate	nurse activist	politics
balance of power	nurse citizen	position power
electoral process	nurse politician	power grabbing
executive branch	pay equity	power sharing
general election	policy	powers of appointment
judicial branch	policy outcomes	primary election
knowledge-based power	political action	referendum
latent power	committees (PACs)	separation of powers
legislative branch		

Have you ever known a nurse member of Congress? Or a nurse mayor? Did you know that a nurse was responsible for developing the federal system for health care financing?

Nurses have served as head of the Social Security Administration, as head of Planned Parenthood of America, and as chief of staff for the Majority leader in the U.S. Senate. Nurses have held major leadership roles in government, professional and community organizations, and in the workplace. This chapter discusses the political process, describes how nurses can become politically active, and explains some of the ways nurse leaders have achieved positions of power and influence.

POLITICS: WHAT IT IS AND WHAT IT IS NOT

Politics is more than what is happening in Washington. It is part of our daily lives, both personal and professional. Ultimately, politics refers to the processes that influence the outcome of decisions among people. People often speak of politics with negative overtones. In reality, politics is neither good nor bad. It is the *outcome* of the political process that may be judged as positive or negative.

Politics is defined as the allocation of scarce resources. *Allocation* implies that decisions are made about how to use these scarce resources. Who distributes the resources, the amount of resources allocated, and who receives the allocated resources are all based on the application of politics to gain power.

Scarce connotes limits. There are never enough resources for everyone who wants or needs them. *Resources* usually indicates money. Resources, however, can also be people, time, status, power, and programs—any number of precious assets that are limited.

Policy is defined as the principles and values that govern actions directed toward given ends; policy statements set forth a plan, direction, or goal for action. Policies may be laws, regulations, or guidelines that govern behavior in government, workplaces, schools, organizations, and communities. Although different from politics, policy is *shaped* by politics (Mason, Talbott, and Leavitt, 1993).

Politics (*i.e.*, influencing the allocation of scarce resources) affects the development and implementation of policy. During the 1995–1996 balanced budget debate, congressional Republicans argued that the federal budget must be balanced within seven years (by the year 2002) through significant policy changes to slow the growth of domestic programs such as Medicare and Medicaid. The Clinton administration and many Democrats agreed that although there was a need for a balanced budget, the Republican-proposed Medicare and Medicaid changes would be overburdensome to the constituencies that these programs serve. This debate was not only about the allocation of scarce federal revenue, but also was an attempt to change the role of the federal government in health and human service programs.

Policy has significant impact on the practice of nursing. The ability of the individual nurse to provide care is affected by innumerable public policy decisions. As discussed in Chapter 20, state licensure as a registered nurse (RN) derives from legislation that defines the scope of nursing practice. The defined scope determines what a nurse legally can and cannot do. For example, giving intravenous medication, performing physical assessments, and taking blood pressures are now well accepted as falling within the scope of nursing practice. Twenty-five years ago, these activities were within the scope of the medical practice act rather than the nursing practice act, but as a result of nursing education and nursing's political influence on public policy, these changes were realized.

Regulations developed to implement legislation also affect practicing nurses and their work environments. For example, the protocols for administering and documenting the administration of narcotic drugs are promulgated by a regulatory agency of the federal government. The rules that define nurses' authority to order or administer narcotics depend on how regulations are written. If nurses do not actively participate in developing regulations, policy outcomes are likely to restrict rather than enhance nursing authority for regulated activities.

Broader issues affecting the nursing profession are also political in nature. Issues of **pay equity,** or equal pay for work of comparable value, are of concern to nurses because nurses have historically been underpaid for services. One of the first cases demonstrating the inequality of nursing salaries involved public health nurses in Colorado. They brought a case against the city of Denver, stating that they were paid considerably less than city tree trimmers and garbage collectors. The nurses demanded just compensation for their work by demonstrating that nursing requires more complex knowledge and is of greater value to society than tree trimming.

As a result of this suit, recognition of nursing's low pay was brought to public attention in such a way that public support was mobilized for increasing nursing salaries. This was an example of political action by nurses that resulted in both **policy outcomes** (regulations that expanded comparable pay issues to other jobs) and professional outcomes (salary increases for the individual nurse).

"THE PERSONAL IS POLITICAL"

Women involved in the feminist movement in the 1960s coined the phrase "The personal is political." The statement recognized that each individual—woman or man—could use personal experience to understand and become involved in broader social and political issues. It enabled individuals who did not consider themselves political to gain insight into what in society needed to be changed and how they could help bring about the change. It gave each individual power and resulted in people becoming involved in the political process—usually for the first time.

This premise of personalizing the political process has become a fundamental activity for organized nursing. Nurses at the grassroots become involved in advocating for legislation and supporting candidates for elective office because they understand the relationship between public policy and their professional and personal lives. The American Nurses Association (ANA) is actively involved in federal legislation, regulation, and electoral politics. The ANA and many of the state nurses associations, have government relations experts on their staffs, as do many other nursing and health organizations—such as the American Association of Colleges of Nursing, the American Hospital Association, and numerous specialty nursing organizations. They engage in lobbying to advocate for the professional concerns of their members (Fig. 21–1). Contemporary nursing leaders recognize that "being political," both through professional associations and as individuals, is essential to the practice and promotion of the profession and is a professional responsibility of all nurses.

POLITICS AND POWER

Politics connotes power. Without power, there cannot be influence. To be effective in influencing the outcome of decisions, an individual must ask: "Who has the power?" "How is it used?" "How can it be mobilized?"

There are numerous kinds of power. There is **position power,** such as that inherent in being a dean, vice-president for nursing, or chief executive of a com-

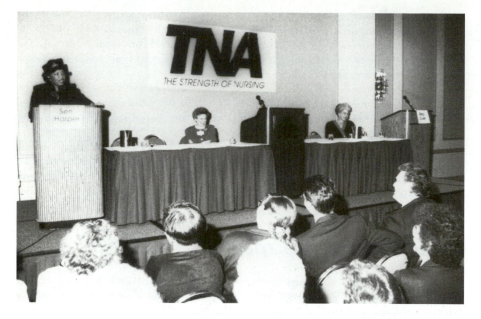

FIGURE 21–1
The members of a state nurses association exchange ideas and opinions with a state senator. (Courtesy of Tennessee Nurses Association. Photograph by Chip Powell.)

pany. There is **knowledge-based power,** such as the way information can be used by an expert to affect an outcome. There is power in numbers; a group is almost always more influential than an individual. There is power related to wealth. Wealth itself is a resource and provides access to other significant resources. There has always been power accorded to whomever belongs to the dominant race, gender, or class in a community or nation.

Latent power is untapped and underused. As the largest group of health providers, nurses have had latent power. Although there are more than 2 million nurses in the United States, nurses have only recently recognized the potential power that such numbers suggest. One in 44 women voters is a nurse. How powerful nursing's voice can be if that power is used wisely in the voting booth.

The power of nursing knowledge has also been underused. No other group of health care providers spends as much time in direct patient contact as do nurses. Nurses know what patients need and can use this knowledge to develop policies for meeting those needs both in the clinical setting and in the community at large. More nurses are using their expertise to participate in the development of health policy, share knowledge with legislators, and serve in community organizations to develop health services.

Power is neither good nor bad; it is how it is used that gives it value. If, for example, nurses use the power of persuasion to motivate patients to take prescribed medication, they are using the power of position and knowledge positively.

Power is not given; it must be taken. The taking of power converts latent power into action. Nurses are beginning to recognize that, to have power, they must want it and they must use it. Use of power is a hallmark of political activity.

There are differences in the way women and men have traditionally used power. The traditional male model of power has been described as **power grabbing.** It involves hoarding power and control, taking it from others, or wielding it over others. Women more often use **power sharing,** which is a process of equalizing resources, knowledge, or control. It is important to recognize that these two ways of using power are neither good nor bad. The most effective power brokers are those who can use both methods and know which is most effective in a given situation.

The nursing profession is beginning to use the media as a powerful political tool. It is the most effective way to get a message to the largest audience and thereby influence both the public and those who hold elective offices. Different media provide different ways to influence opinions. For example, talk radio has proven to be very influential. Talk radio hosts advocate certain opinions, often with little factual information. By controlling who gets to talk, they can control the kind of information and the level of feeling expressed and eliminate opposing viewpoints. Prior to the 1994 elections, when the Republican Party took control of both Houses of Congress, the majority of talk radio supported the Republican agenda. It is believed that their collective messages influenced the outcomes of the elections.

Television can be a forceful medium for visual influence, particularly advertisements. In 1993, the demise of President Clinton's national health care reform efforts was directly affected by television ads sponsored by the health insurance industry. Despite initial support for national health care reform from the Fortune 500 companies, health professional organizations, and major industry, the "Harry and Louise" advertisements were forceful enough to create a climate of fear and distrust about legislating health care. The power of those ads was partially credited with the defeat of federal health care legislation.

The print media are effective in disclosing detailed information supportive of a legislative issue. During the 1993–1994 health care reform debate, there were more than 300 articles in newspapers across the United States focused on nurses, especially nurses in advanced practice. Most were the result of news releases from the ANA's department of communications and other nursing organizations. Nursing's goal was to educate the public about the important role of nurses in delivering health care as well as to gain support for legislation that would enable these nurses to be directly reimbursed. The news articles were successful on both counts.

In 1995, during the flurry of hospital mergers and restructuring in the health care industry, nursing organizations used paid advertisements on television and in selected newspapers to counter hospital industry attempts to eliminate nursing positions. For example, the ANA's "Every patient deserves a nurse" campaign, raised public awareness of the need for adequate numbers of registered nurses for patient care. The strategy was to support legislative and regulatory measures that would ensure patient safety and job security for RNs.

The power of the media affects both legislators and the public at large. It is a tool that nurses will use even more widely in the future.

A LESSON IN CIVICS COMES ALIVE

No American student completes secondary school without one or more courses in civics or American government. Many students find these courses dull and not relevant to their lives. To many adults, however, American government is vibrant and fascinating. To impact the governmental process successfully, it is important that nursing and other health professions clearly understand how government works.

Three Branches of Government

The framers of the U.S. Constitution had a major objective—the **separation of powers**—to prevent the aggregation of power in any one person or branch of government. Thus, they set out a government with three branches—the legislative, executive, and judicial—and a mechanism of checks and balances for each. As intended by the founding fathers, U.S. history reveals a waxing and waning of the powers of each branch over time, depending on the personalities of incumbents, contemporary social problems, and world events.

Under the Constitution, each branch of the federal government has separate and distinct functions and powers. The function of the **legislative branch,** which includes the House of Representatives and the Senate, is to deliberate and enact laws. Example of legislative powers include setting and collecting taxes, overseeing commerce, declaring war, defining criminal offenses, coining money, and amending the Constitution. The legislative branch, particularly the House of Representatives, is assumed to be the government's closest link to the people and more susceptible to change through social pressure.

The chief function of the **executive branch** of government is to administer the laws of the land. At the federal level, power is vested with the president, who has a wide variety of governmental departments and employees (the bureaucracy) to carry out executive functions. The president has extensive **powers of appointment** (judges, ambassadors, agency heads) and is commander-in-chief of the armed forces. The president recommends legislation; gives the State of the Union report; and approves or vetoes the legislation of Congress, contributing to the balance of power.

The role of the **judicial branch** is to **adjudicate,** or decide "cases or controversies" on particular matters. The judicial branch is divided into the federal and state court systems. The greatest power of the courts is to provide judicial review over governmental activities to uphold the privileges of the Constitution. The Supreme Court is the ultimate legal authority of the land and reviews decisions from lower courts.

The **balance of power** among the three branches of government is illustrated in Figure 21–2. Notice that all three branches are involved in the legislative process.

Three Levels of Government

Government in the United States is organized at federal, state, and local levels. The Constitution established the relative powers of federal and state govern-

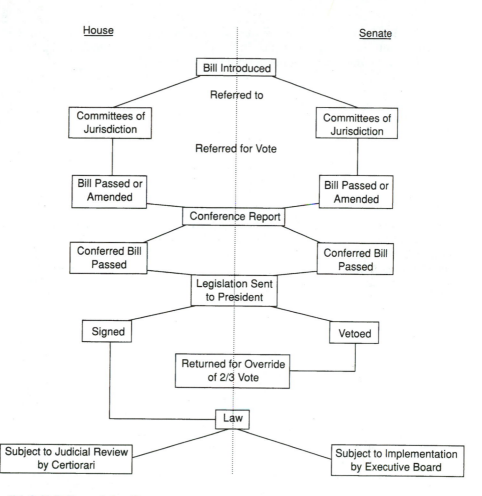

House   **Senate**

Bill Introduced

Referred to

Committees of Jurisdiction   Committees of Jurisdiction

Referred for Vote

Bill Passed or Amended   Bill Passed or Amended

Conference Report

Conferred Bill Passed   Conferred Bill Passed

Legislation Sent to President

Signed   Vetoed

Returned for Override of 2/3 Vote

Law

Subject to Judicial Review by Certiorari   Subject to Implementation by Executive Board

FIGURE   21–2
Legislation and the balance of power.

ments and the rights of the individual. The Constitution identified specific powers of the federal government as matters of national interest needing uniform policies and reserved all other powers for the states. States, in turn, have developed their own constitutions and delineated power relationships with local communities and between branches of state government.

Exclusive powers of the federal government include declaring war, making treaties, administering postal services, and developing relationships with foreign powers. State and local governments maintain internal order, regulate domestic relationships, and protect the people. Currently, both the federal and the state governments can tax and spend and promote health. In times of shrinking resources, programs that are considered to be costly, such as health services, may be shifted to state control, calling into question the federal government's role in ensuring uniform access to health services throughout the United States.

All levels of government are expected to maintain their activities within the parameters of the Constitution. The Bill of Rights serves to promote and protect the rights of the individual from governmental intrusion.

Electoral Process

The process of electing public officials to office is known as the **electoral process.** Governmental elections for the most part focus on selecting local, state, and federal legislators and executive branch leaders such as the president, governor, and mayor. Federal judges are appointed, although in some states judges are elected by the people.

In recent elections the American public appeared to be skeptical of politicians, the traditional political parties, and the entire electoral process. This was clearly evidenced in 1992 when Ross Perot of the United We Stand America Party (subsequently The Reform Party) received 19 percent of the votes cast for President. This was the highest percentage received by an independent or third-party candidate since the early 1900s (Congressional Quarterly, Inc., 1993). Many voters viewed the strong third-party showing as a message to long-term politicians and the traditional parties that they were not in touch with voters outside Washington, DC.

Voter discontent was again evident in the 1994 election cycle. Only 38 percent of eligible people voted. In addition, Congressional Democrats lost majority control of both the House of Representatives and the Senate. Democrats in the House of Representatives lost 52 seats, giving Republicans control of the House for the first time since 1954 (Healey, 1994). This shift from control by one party to the other was replicated in many state and local races. Clearly, voters were again sending a message, but its exact meaning remains unclear.

During the 1994 election, members of third parties, such as United We Stand America, not only impacted the outcome of the elections, but also shaped the issues that were discussed as part of a "change agenda." Heretofore the process of getting elected to office has occurred primarily through the two major parties—the Democratic and Republican parties. Third parties have become active in different regions at different times. Some of the more familiar third parties are the Reform Party (formerly United We Stand America), Right to Life, Conservative, Green, Socialist, Communist, and Rainbow Coalition parties. Other than Ross Perot's United We Stand America Party, none of the other third-party organizations has yet played a major role in national elections.

In most states, citizens declare party affiliation when registering to vote. There are three major types of elections: primary elections, general elections, and referendums.

Primary elections are those in which a party is choosing among several party-affiliated candidates for a particular office. The outcome of primary elections is that a party's candidate for a particular office is selected. In most states, voters may vote only in the primary of the party in which they are registered.

In **general elections,** all registered voters may vote. They need not vote a "straight party ticket"; that is, the voter can choose a candidate from any party on the ballot. Unless there is a tie or a challenge to the general election, the outcome is the selection of a governmental official such as a governor, senator, or president. Length of service as an elected official depends on the office. For example, U.S. senators serve six-year terms, and members of the House of Representatives serve two-year terms.

A **referendum** occurs when registered voters are asked to express directly their preferences on a policy issue. Usually these issues are referred to the public either by a legislative body or by civic activists who have gathered enough signatures to require a vote. For example, a county commission may seek a referendum on raising property taxes to support school reform. Activist groups may seek a state referendum on gay rights, assisted suicide, or other controversial issues.

Working on a campaign, raising money for a candidate, or running for office requires strict adherence to election laws. Rules vary from locality to locality and state to federal elections. Information about election regulations is available through local boards of election and from the National Election Commission.

HEALTH CARE LEGISLATION AND REGULATION

Many issues facing nursing professionals can best be addressed through public policy, which requires that nurses influence government. The key questions for nurses to ask when seeking governmental intervention to improve nursing practice and health care are: "Where can we play?" and "Where can we *win?*" The options to consider are the judicial, administrative, or legislative arenas.

There are local, state, and federal courts, all of which require standing (a *material* interest in the outcome of a case) to seek a judicial remedy. There are mayors, governors, presidents, their staffs, and department heads who make key decisions about how to implement (or not implement) health policy. Most often, nurses have sought legislative remedies for changes in health care policy. Historically, nurses have best learned to be effective with legislative branch relationships. Nursing has now broadened its focus to use the other two branches more effectively.

There have been three major eras in health policy development in the United States. As you learned in Chapter 16, the era extending from post–World War II through the 1960s served to increase health services dramatically and expand health delivery capacity. The 1970s and 1980s focused on enhanced research, technology development, and concerns about escalating costs in acute care. During the 1990s, several different issues predominate, including comprehensive health care reform addressing access, cost, and quality of health care. When attempts at comprehensive reform were unsuccessful, a dramatic restructuring of the health care payment and delivery systems to decrease aggregate health care costs followed.

Unfortunately the nursing profession was not well organized politically during the time of expanding health care capacity and access. Despite being the *only* health provider group in favor of the Medicare/Medicaid programs of the 1960s, nurses were not included as reimbursable providers. Times have changed, however. Nurses have increased their political savvy. Through the well-orchestrated efforts of the ANA, other professional organizations, state nurses associations, and their **political action committees** (PACs), nurses are now participating much more effectively in both governmental and electoral politics. Nursing PACs raise and distribute money to candidates who support the organization's stand on certain issues, and nurses' endorsements of candidates have become a valued political asset for many local, state, and federal candidates.

Influencing Public Policy

Nurses can make a difference in health policy outcomes. Through the political process, nurses influence the policy process by identifying health problems as policy problems, by formulating policy through drafting legislation with legislators and providing formal testimony, by lobbying governmental officials in the executive and legislative branches to make certain health policies a priority for action, and by filing suit as a party or as a friend of the court to implement health policy strategies on behalf of consumers.

Capitol Update, a newsletter published by the ANA, reports on the progress of nursing's influence with the President, members of Congress, their staffs, and the regulatory agencies that set policy for health programs. Such activity reflects the work of both ANA members and staff. The ANA's political activity in Washington, D.C., is mirrored throughout the United States by other nursing organizations and by state nurses associations conducting similar work with their state governments.

Two of nursing's major political activist programs are the Senator Coordinator and Congressional District Coordinator (SC-CDC) Networks and Nurses Strategic Action Teams (NSTAT). The SC-CDC Networks were developed by the ANA in 1985 and have been replicated on the state level by many state nurses associations. The purpose of the 535 member SC-CDC Network is to ensure that each member of Congress has a well-briefed professional nurse as an ongoing contact on matters of health and workplace legislation. This network seeks to enhance communication between nurses and members of Congress to educate legislators on matters of concern to the nursing profession. This one-on-one network has been a valuable instrument in helping the ANA achieve its legislative agenda.

During the health care reform debate of 1993–1994, the increasing ability of grassroots efforts to influence Congress became apparent. The ANA invested significant resources to develop NSTAT. In 1996, NSTAT consisted of approximately 40,000 state nurses association members who voluntarily mobilize using telephones, faxes, and mail to advocate for specific issues vital to nursing. NSTAT is effective because of the thousands of well-timed, well-targeted messages sent to members of Congress.

Organized activity in identifying, financially supporting, and working for candidates who are committed to nursing and "nurse-friendly" issues has dramatically increased in the last decade. Again, this electoral process is an essential function of the professional association. No better example for nursing, public policy, and political action exists than the 1992 Presidential election and its aftermath. In August 1992, the ANA-PAC endorsed the Clinton/Gore ticket at a nationally televised rally in California. Thousands of nurses were present along with patients and their families. The ANA became the first national health care organization to support Clinton's candidacy publicly, and nurses throughout the United States worked visibly and diligently during the campaign.

That early and visible political support meant that nursing enjoyed unprecedented access to the White House after President Clinton was elected. Nurses were involved significantly in the development of the President's Health Security Act of 1993, and nurses were included as qualified providers in that historic federal proposal. Despite the failure of the 103rd Congress to pass comprehensive health reform legislation in 1994, nursing achieved visibility, influence, and inclusion as a force in national health policy. As nursing united through the development of *Nursing's Agenda for Health Care Reform*, the latent power of nursing became evident to the public, to policymakers, and to nurses themselves.

Nurses working at the state level are also making their presence felt. In 1994, the Maine State Nurses Association endorsed Jill Goldthwait, an RN running as an Independent for election to the Maine State Assembly. After a successful race, State Senator Goldthwait entered the Maine Assembly and carried significant influence with Maine's newly elected Independent governor. Senator Goldthwait agreed to be the key sponsor of Maine State Nurses Association legislation to allow advanced practice nurses to have prescriptive authority and to enter into a collaborative practice with physicians.

This landmark legislation passed the State Senate and Assembly and was signed into law in June 1995. Thus, nursing political action through a state nurses association contributed to the election of a nurse politician, which, in turn, led directly to nursing's public policy ideal—independent practice and reimbursement for advanced practice nurses in Maine.

Individual nurses can make a difference in policy development, in elections, in speaking out for nursing, and by becoming policymakers. Either by election or by appointment, nurses need to be *making* health decisions, not just influencing them. Getting elected or appointed requires visibility, expertise, energy, risk taking, and a belief that policy and politics are critically important in achieving nursing's goals.

Getting Nurses Appointed

Becoming a policymaker involves either being elected or being appointed to office. Appointments are made by the chief executive of a city, county, state, or the nation. They are usually made in response to the expertise and visibility of the individual appointee, and to the power and influence of that appointee's membership in an organization that supported the elected official.

For example, after the 1992 elections, the ANA was asked to submit names of nurses for appointment to positions in the executive branch and to influential policymaking boards. The ANA began the Federal Appointments Project and worked with outstanding nurses throughout the United States to assemble a professional/political resume that would make them highly competitive for significant positions. Almost 500 nurses eagerly became part of the project, and many were successful. For example, Dr. Myra Synder, past executive director of the California Nurses Association, served on the Department of Health and Human Services Transition Team; Dr. Christine Gebbie was appointed National AIDS Policy Coordinator; Dr. Shirley Chater became Director of the Social Security Administration; and Pat Montoya and Pat Ford-Roegner became regional directors of the Department of Health and Human Services.

Virginia Trotter Betts, then ANA President, was appointed by the President as a Private Sector Delegate to the World Health Assembly in 1993 and 1996, a Private Sector Delegate to the United Nations Fourth World Conference on Women in Beijing, China, and to the Military Health Care Advisory Committee. Political activism has helped secure these and other key federal appointments of nurses.

The same process occurs at the state level. Many boards, commissions, and key government positions are made by the state executive, usually the governor. Thus, gubernatorial elections are of critical importance to state nurses associations. Qualified nurses who have supported the election of the governor and are known to their state nurses association are encouraged to seek appointments to regulatory bodies such as state boards of nursing. As previously discussed, state boards of nursing, through rules and regulations, make definitive health policy and are highly important to future nursing issues.

Working in a gubernatorial campaign, through the state nurses association, or through the candidate's party can be helpful in securing board of nursing appointments. Boards of health, health and human services commissions, and others all use similar processes of appointment and could benefit from nursing expertise.

GETTING INVOLVED

Although nurses are more active at all levels of the political process than ever before, there is still room for improvement. As can be seen in the accompanying Research Note, nurses tend to expect more in the way of political participation from fellow nurses than they themselves actually do. Three levels of political involvement in which nurses can participate are as nurse citizens, as nurse activists, and as nurse politicians. Each level is discussed briefly.

Nurse Citizens

A **nurse citizen** brings the perspective of health care to the voting booth, to public forums that advocate for health and human services, and to involvement in community activities. For example, budget cuts to a school district might involve elimination of school nurses. At a school board meeting, nurses can effectively speak about the vital role that school nurses provide to the health of children and the cost-effectiveness of maintaining the position.

Nurses tend to vote for candidates who advocate for improved health care. Here are some examples of how the nurse citizen can be politically active:

- Register to vote.
- Vote in every election.
- Keep informed about health care issues.
- Speak out when services or working conditions are inadequate.
- Participate in public forums.
- Know your local, state, and federal elected officials.
- Join politically active nursing organizations.

RESEARCH NOTE

A New York nurse, Margaret Leonard, wondered about the relationships among area of practice, educational level, and membership in professional organizations to political participation and political expectations of registered nurses (RNs). She hypothesized that nurse educators would have significantly higher levels of political participation and political expectation than clinical nurses, that nurses with master's or doctoral degrees would have higher levels of political participation and political expectation than nurses with baccalaureate or associate degrees or diplomas, and that nurses who were members of the New York State Nurses Association or the Nurses' Association of the Counties of Long Island would have significantly higher levels of political participation and political expectation than nurses who were not members of these professional organizations.

The data collection tool used in this study was the Political Expectations and Participation Questionnaire (PEPQ), which had been previously developed, validated, and established as reliable. It identifies nine politically active roles: voter, campaigner, player, monitor, networker, spokesperson, negotiator, leader, and lobbyist.

Using the PEPQ, Leonard surveyed 108 registered nurses who were attending a nursing association mini-convention. Subjects were 106 women and 2 men ranging in age from 27 to 70 years who had been RNs for 2 to 45 years. Most (77 percent) were members of a professional organization.

Leonard found that although there were no significant differences in political expectations between educators and clinical nurses, nurse educators scored significantly higher in political participation than did clinical nurses. Levels of political participation were significantly higher for master's or doctorally prepared nurses in all roles except that of spokesperson. Advanced degree nurses had significantly higher levels of political expectations in two areas—voter and monitor. In terms of organizational membership, subjects who were members of professional organizations had significantly higher levels of participation in campaigner, player, and leader roles. Overall findings confirmed that RNs have significantly higher levels of political expectations than they do levels of participation in all nine politically active roles.

As a result of this study, Leonard recommended that formal coursework in politics be added to nursing curricula to increase the political participation of all nurses and thereby increase nursing's political power. The desired result of increased political participation by nurses is improvement in the health care system to include universal access and reimbursement for RN-provided services.

(Adapted with permission of Leonard, M. [1994]. Levels of political participation and political expectations among nurses in New York State. *Journal of the New York State Nurses Association*, 25[1], 16–20.)

- Participate in community organizations that need health experts.
- Join a political party.

Once nurses make a decision to become involved politically, they need to learn how to get started. One of the best ways is to form a relationship with one or more policymakers. Box 21–1 contains several pointers for influencing policymakers.

BOX 21–1

Communication Is the Key to Influence

Cultivate a relationship with policymakers from your home district or state. Communicate by visits, telephone, letters. Letters need these elements:

- Use personal stationery.
- State who you are (a nursing student or registered nurse and a voter in a specific district).
- Identify the issue by a file number, if possible.
- Be clear on where you stand and why.
- Be positive when possible.
- Be concise.

- Ask for a commitment. State precisely what action you want the policymaker to take.
- Give your return address and phone number to urge a dialogue.
- Be persistent. Follow up with calls or letters.
- If you plan to visit your policymaker on a specific issue, be sure to make your appointment in advance in writing and indicate what issue you are interested in discussing.
- Be quick to thank and praise when policymakers do something you like.

Nurse Activists

The **nurse activist** takes a more active role than the nurse citizen and often does so because an issue arises that directly affects the nurse's professional life (Fig. 21–3). The need to respond moves the nurse to a more active level of participation. For example, a nurse in private practice who has difficulty getting private insurance companies or health maintenance organizations to honor patients' claims for reimbursement of nursing services may become active in lobbying state legislators for changes in insurance regulations.

Nurse activists can make changes by:

- Joining politically active nursing organizations.
- Contacting a public official through letters, telegrams, or phone calls.
- Registering people to vote.
- Contributing money to a political campaign.
- Working in a campaign.
- Lobbying decision makers by providing pertinent statistical and anecdotal information.
- Forming or joining coalitions that support an issue of concern.
- Writing letters to the editor of local papers.
- Inviting legislators to visit the workplace.
- Holding a media event to publicize an issue.
- Providing or giving testimony.

Box 21–2 includes some pointers on how to make a difference in health policy development.

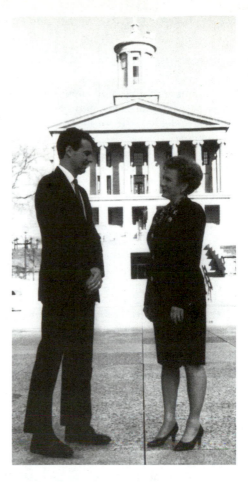

FIGURE 21-3

The nurse activist has a high level of
involvement in selected political issues.
(Courtesy of Tennessee Nurses
Association. Photograph by Chip
Powell.)

BOX 21-2

Key Questions for Nurses Who Want to Make a Difference in Health Policy

1. *Know the system.* Is it a federal, state, or local issue? Is it in the hands of the executive, legislative, or judicial branch of government?
2. *Know the issue.* What is wrong? What should happen? Why is it not happening? What is needed: leadership, a plan, pressure, data?
3. *Know the players.* Who is on your side and who is not? Who will make the decision? Who knows whom? Will a coalition be effective? Are you a member of the professional nursing organization?
4. *Know the process.* Is this a vote? Is this an appropriation? Is this a legislative procedure? Is this a committee or subcommittee report?
5. *Know what to do.* Should you write, call, go to lunch, organize a petition, show up at the hearing, give testimony, demonstrate, file a suit?

Nurse Politicians

Once a nurse realizes and experiences the empowerment that can come from political activism, he or she may choose to run for office. No longer satisfied to help others get elected, the **nurse politician** desires to develop the legislation, not just influence it.

In 1992, Congresswoman Eddie Bernice Johnson (D–TX) was the first nurse elected to the U.S. House of Representatives. Congresswoman Johnson successfully worked her way through the Texas state legislature to launch her career in national politics. In 1995, there were 69 nurse legislators in state government, numerous local mayors, city council members, and hundreds of nurses appointed to governmental regulatory agencies.

Nurse politicians use their knowledge about people, their expertise about health, their ability to communicate effectively, and their superb organizational skills in running for office. Because the public places a high value on nurses, nurse politicians are trusted. If nurses know how to run a campaign and can raise money, they stand a good chance of being elected.

Once nurses are elected, they can be available to sponsor legislation that reflects their professional experiences. Many of the laws that expand reimbursement for nursing services, funding for services to women and children, occupational safety and health issues, and research on women's health have been sponsored by nurse legislators and supported by nurses working as key legislative staff members.

Political life can be grueling, and the nurse politician must be ready to sacrifice a regular schedule and personal privacy. In addition, adequate financial resources are critical to a successful run for office. Fortunately, more nurses are willing to make this commitment because they believe in their own power and ability to enhance the well-being of the public. Individual nurses and nurse-specific PACs are increasingly willing and able to support nurse candidates financially at all levels of government.

The nurse politician can:

- Run for an elected office.
- Seek appointment to a regulatory agency.
- Be appointed to a governing board in the public or private sector.
- Use nursing expertise as a front-line policymaker who can enhance health care and the profession.

WE WERE ALL ONCE NOVICES

Nurses who have achieved success as leaders started with no knowledge of the political process and no expectation of the greatness they would achieve. Instead, they became involved because some issue, injustice, or abuse of power affected their lives. Instead of complaining or feeling helpless, they responded by taking an active role in bringing about change.

The mark of a leader is the ability to identify a problem, have a goal, and know how to join others in reaching that goal. A leader must know how to ask the right questions, analyze the positive and restraining forces toward meeting the goal, and know how to get and use power. A leader must know how to ask for help and how to give support to those who join the effort. These are the marks of nursing leaders who have been political experts.

A NURSE WHO KNEW HOW TO USE POLITICAL POWER

As discussed in Chapter 1, Florence Nightingale, the founder of modern nursing, was the consummate political woman. Her story exemplifies how she learned to use her skills and power to bring about revolutionary change in health care in the nineteenth century. She never anticipated that she would achieve greatness, especially as a nurse—a lifestyle Victorian society considered demeaning to a woman of her social standing.

Nightingale achieved incredible goals through her own intellect and determination and the utilization of the political influence of powerful friends in government. She was a strong-willed person with social and financial power. She had an excellent education and used theoretical knowledge as well as practical experience to learn about care of the sick. She developed and nurtured connections to powerful men (since there were few powerful women at the time other than Queen Victoria). She sought their support and, in turn, supported them when they needed her help.

Nightingale's goals changed as new problems arose because she recognized that being adaptable was a characteristic of leadership. In essence, she used her public support, her connections to people in powerful positions, and her intellectual skills to reach an unparalleled position of leadership. As a result, she was able to gain personal and professional power to move nursing and health care into the modern era. She was the first nurse politician.

NURSING AWAITS YOUR CONTRIBUTION

You can apply the skills discussed in this chapter. Look to teachers, family, friends, and community leaders whom you admire. What are the qualities they possess that you wish to have? Your role models can serve as inspiration for you to imitate.

You may also choose to form a relationship with a political mentor. A mentor is not only a role model, but also actively teaches, encourages, and critiques the process of growth and change in the learner. All nurses who have become political leaders have found mentors along the way to guide and support their growth. Your mentor could be a faculty member, such as the adviser to the nursing student organization or honor society, who can teach you leadership skills. Ask for help in running for a class office or student council president. If elected office does not appeal to you, use your political skills to develop a school or community project with other nursing students.

You may have a relative or friend involved in a political campaign who could help you learn about the political process. You might find a problem during a clinical experience that inhibits your ability to provide necessary care or the level of care that you wish. Seek a faculty member or nurse in the clinical facility who can guide you through the process of change.

Watch the communication skills of your role models or mentors. How does your own behavior compare with theirs? What enhances or impedes your progress? Get your friends and peers to join your activity. Seek their help and support. Always thank them and be ready to offer your help and support when they need it.

S U M M A R Y

Professional organizations and professional nurses have much to offer in formulating policy decisions at all levels and in each branch of government. Nursing—once called "the sleeping giant of the health care industry"—has awakened. Today, organized nursing is involved in politics at many levels in promoting:

1. *Nursing's Agenda for Health Care Reform*, discussed in Chapter 4.
2. Reimbursement for professional nurses at federal, state, and local levels.
3. Expanding the scope and authority of nursing practice in every jurisdiction.
4. Protection of the civil and privacy rights of clients, for example, in the areas of abortion rights, human immunodeficiency virus/acquired immunodeficiency syndrome (HIV/AIDS), and the terminally ill.
5. Prevention services and primary care services for women, children, and the elderly.

The list is almost limitless. The roles and opportunities for women and nurses in the field of policy development and politics are changing, and nursing can benefit from this "window of opportunity." Having more nurses involved in policy development and politics is good for nursing and for the United States.

Once you realize that becoming politically active is as easy as signing your name in support of an issue, registering to vote, organizing a project, or speaking out on an issue, you have started your political education. You will feel empowered. You will realize how important you can be—how *you* can make a difference. All of us, as nurses and as recipients of health care, will be better for your involvement.

R E V I E W   A N D   D I S C U S S I O N   Q U E S T I O N S

1. Conduct a class poll. Of those in the class who are eligible to vote, how many are registered? How many voted in the last local, state, or national election? Challenge those not registered to become registered before the end of the current school term.
2. List three types of power. How can nurses use these types of power on behalf of their profession and the health care system?
3. Because nurses have differing personal and political values, it has been a challenge to get them all united behind a single issue or candidate. If you were the president of the American Nurses Association, what techniques would you use to persuade the 2 million American nurses of the power of their numbers, their knowledge, and their commitment?

4. What types of political issues should nurses take a particular interest in? Do you see signs that nurses are actively involved in these issues in your community?
5. Find out whether the members of your state board of nursing are elected or appointed. What is the makeup of the board (how many registered nurses, licensed practical nurses, consumers, and so forth)? Do nurses hold most of the seats on the state board? Are these any other health professionals such as physicians on the board of nursing? If so, are there any nurses on the state board of medicine?

REFERENCES

Congressional Quarterly, Inc. (1993). *The 49th Annual CQ Almanac*. Washington, D.C.: Author.

Healey, J. (1994). Jubilant GOP strives to keep legislative feet on ground. *Congressional Quarterly Weekly Report*. 52(44), 3210–3215.

Leonard, M. (1994). Levels of political participation and political expectations among nurses in New York State. *Journal of the New York State Nurses Association*, 25(1), 16–20.

Mason, D., Talbott, S., and Leavitt, J. (Eds.) (1993). *Policy and politics for nurses: Action and change in the workplace, government, organizations, and community* (2nd ed.). Philadelphia: W. B. Saunders.

22

Kay K. Chitty

Nursing's Future Challenges

O B J E C T I V E S

- Review societal influences on the nursing profession anticipated during the next decade.
- Recognize the impact that changes in the health care system will have on the practice of nursing.
- Explain trends in nursing education needed to meet society's future nursing needs.

V O C A B U L A R Y

birthrate	euthanasia	mortality rate
centenarian	futurist	multiskilled worker
cultural diversity	heterogeneous	nursing informatics
demography	homogeneous	shared governance
differentiated practice	Human Genome Project	urbanization
disenfranchised	managed care	
epidemiologist	morbidity rate	

As you have seen throughout this textbook, the nursing profession is profoundly affected by changes in society and in the world. As we prepare to enter the twenty-first century, it is clear that nursing again faces many challenges, as it has in the past. The challenges nurses face relate to a variety of factors: changes in demographics, unhealthy lifestyles of many Americans, the continued deterioration of the environment, and rapid change in the health care system brought about by concern over increasing costs.

The World Health Organization (WHO) has set the goal of health for all by the year 2000. It is now clear that even in the United States, the wealthiest of the industrialized nations, we will fall far short of this goal. Millions of Americans have no health insurance, and many more have less than enough. Infant mortality rates remain unacceptably high. The fitness level of citizens, particularly young people, continues to decline. All these negative trends continue even though the United States spends more of its gross domestic product on health than any nation in the world. Many Americans believe that a complete overhaul of the health care system is required to begin to address these problems, and that process is underway.

Nursing enjoys high levels of respect and public confidence. It is a profession in heavy demand, and its practitioners enjoy more autonomy than ever. As the largest of the health care professions, nursing has enormous but largely untapped political power that would allow nurses to influence societal changes—rather than simply be influenced by them—if we would unify our efforts.

Everyone is excited about the dawning of a new millenium. The year 2000 will not be just another year but represents a milestone for humankind. Most of us know exactly how old we will be on New Year's Day in the year 2000 and know that it will be as memorable as where we were when President Kennedy was shot and astronauts first walked on the surface of the moon. This chapter explores some of nursing's challenges and opportunities as we enter the new millennium.

SOCIETAL CHALLENGES

At least five societal influences are expected to have major impact on the future of the nursing profession: demographic changes, environmental deterioration, unhealthy lifestyles and resulting illnesses, the need for cost controls, and the regulation of health care. Each of these influences is examined briefly.

Demographic Challenges

Demography is the science that studies vital statistics and social trends. Demographers examine vital statistics such as **birthrates** (births per thousand people), **morbidity rates** (illness), **mortality rates** (deaths), marriages, the ages of various populations, and migration patterns. From this wealth of information, **futurists,** people who predict what will occur, draw conclusions about what these trends mean for the future.

Four trends detected by demographers are particularly important to the future of nursing: rising numbers of elderly people, continuing increase in poverty in the United States, an increase in cultural diversity of the population, and a continuing trend toward urbanization. Each has implications for nursing.

RISING NUMBERS OF ELDERLY

Estimates vary, but demographers have predicted that the number of people between the ages of 65 and 74 in the United States by the year 2000 will exceed 18 million. The number of elderly people over age 75 is expected to exceed 16 million more, for a total of more than 35 million people aged 65 or older (U.S. Bureau of the Census, 1990). **Centenarians,** people over 100 years of age, represent one of the fastest-growing groups in the United States. The World Future Society predicts that by the end of the twenty-first century, the average life span will approach 100 years (Hendrick, 1995). Many elderly people are healthy, but the likelihood of illness becomes greater as people age. For example, indications are that by the age of 90, one of two people will develop Alzheimer's disease (Herbert et al, 1995). Clearly, nurses of the future must be prepared to work effectively with the rising numbers of elderly patients. Ethical issues such as **euthanasia** and assisted suicide will become increasingly important as technology enables people to sustain life far beyond the point of useful, meaningful existence. Society's views of assisted suicide and euthanasia are changing, as evidenced by the fact that juries have acquitted Dr. Jack Kevorkian of charges of murder in the assisted deaths of several terminally ill people.

CONTINUING POVERTY

Even though the United States is considered the world's wealthiest nation, the number of Americans living below the poverty line is increasing. This is particularly true of children and the elderly. The gap between the "haves" and the "have-nots" in the United States is ever widening, creating discontent and disillusionment. When basic needs for food, clothing, and shelter are unmet or uncertain, health care becomes a luxury. Children's immunizations, prenatal care for pregnant women, nutritious meals, and a variety of other health-maintaining factors are neglected. Poor people tend to put off seeking care until illness is advanced and thus harder to treat. Preventable conditions are often not prevented because of lack of education, lack of sanitation, crowded living conditions, improper shelter, homelessness, and a host of other poverty-related factors. Poverty will continue to create increasing numbers of **disenfranchised** people, that is, people who have no power in the political system, with limited access to health care. As their numbers grow, both federal and state governments will implement strategies that limit health care expenditures for these vulnerable populations. Nursing, as a profession, values providing nursing care to all people, regardless of social and economic factors. The increasing numbers of medically disenfranchised people and the increasing pressure to limit health care expenditures will collide to create a values conflict for nurses in the future.

INCREASING CULTURAL DIVERSITY

Cultural diversity refers to the array of people from different racial, ethnic, religious, social, and geographic backgrounds who make up a particular entity. Some countries, such as Japan, are **homogeneous** in culture. This means the citizens have similar cultural beliefs and practices. Others, such as the United States, have a **heterogeneous** cultural mix. This means that the cultural beliefs and practices of the citizens are quite different.

Immigration to the United States from Southeast Asia, Central America, Mexico, and the islands of the Caribbean has increased in recent years as a result of civil unrest, wars, and poor economic conditions (Fig. 22–1). This is the latest wave of newcomers to the United States, who join the European-Americans, African-Americans, and others whose ancestors came to this country earlier. Each group has its own nutritional practices, health beliefs, folk remedies, and conventional wisdom about health and sickness. Nurses need to take these beliefs into consideration when planning and implementing nursing care for indi-

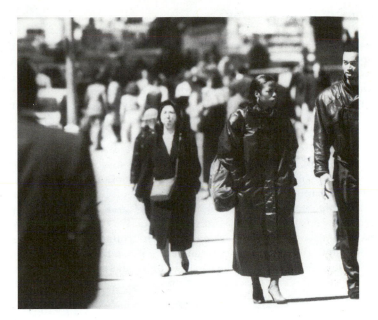

F I G U R E   2 2 – 1
Immigration to the United States from Southeast Asia, Central
America, Mexico, and islands of the Caribbean has increased in
recent years. (Courtesy of *Tennessee Nurse*. Photo by Thomas
Sconyers.)

viduals of diverse cultural backgrounds. Culturally sensitive care will be more
important in the future than ever before. Speaking a second language will be an
important skill for nurses in the future that will increase their marketability. The
nursing profession itself will become increasingly diverse as its membership reflects the diversity of the larger society.

CONTINUING URBANIZATION

Urbanization, that is, people moving from rural, farming areas to cities, has increased since the time of the industrial revolution. That trend continues today
and is expected to continue in the new century. As cities grow, suburbs flourish,
and most people who can afford to do so move away from the industrial centers
of cities. Decaying inner cities with large populations of poor people create major social problems such as homelessness, drugs, gangs, single-parent house-
holds, mental illness, violence, and crime. Despite the increase in public-private
partnerships designed to revitalize inner cities and programs designed to deal effectively with social problems, they continue to grow. These phenomena spill
over into the suburbs and rural areas, creating further social changes. Nurses of
the future will be increasingly confronted with health problems created by these
social phenomena.

Environmental Challenges

Every newspaper, news magazine, and television news program brings disturbing reports of the deterioration of our environment. Major environmental tragedies, such as the nuclear power plant accident at Chernobyl and 200 burning oil wells in Kuwait, overshadow the less dramatic but insidious gradual decline in the quality of the world's air, water, plant, and animal life. Acute and chronic respiratory diseases are increasing, as are debilitating allergic reactions to chemicals in the environment, and cancers of all types (Fig. 22–2). Reports of holes in the ozone layer, accidental lead and mercury poisonings, toxic shellfish beds, truckloads of pesticides spilling into streams and rivers, and the accidental release of radioactive steam from nuclear power plants occur with distressing regularity. **Epidemiologists,** who study the origins of diseases, believe that there is a relationship between environmental decline and increases in certain diseases, including epidemic diseases such as Hantavirus and Ebola virus.

Humans are responsible for destroying the environment, and the more human beings there are, the faster the environment will decline. Overpopulation contributes to the deterioration of the world's environment, yet, other than China, few countries are dealing effectively with issues of overpopulation. The United Nations has projected that the world's population will increase to 2.5 times its present size by the end of the twenty-first century (*Newsweek*, 1992). This rep-

FIGURE   22–2

This manufacturing plant, while providing jobs to scores of workers, has polluted the air and the ground around it and a nearby stream. (Photo by Kelly Whalin.)

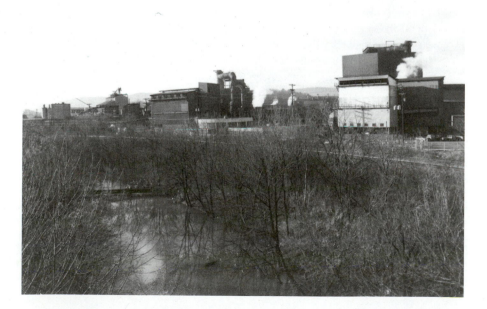

resents a total of 13 billion people, more than twice as many human beings than have ever lived. At the first Earth Summit Conference held in Rio de Janeiro in 1992, the analogy of the overloaded lifeboat was frequently used. The related problems of environmental deterioration and overpopulation are health care issues that future nurses will undoubtedly have to face, and there are no easy answers.

Lifestyle Challenges

Despite the focus on wellness in contemporary American society, unhealthy lifestyles still predominate; this trend shows no signs of changing. There are more obese Americans than ever before, even though obesity is known to predispose people to a number of illnesses. Futurists predict that Americans will eat more meals in restaurants in the future, but ordering a nutritious, well-balanced meal in a restaurant is a major challenge, even to people with a working knowledge of nutritional science. In acquiescence to the fast-food mentality of many families, nutritional consultants are now being hired by public school districts to teach cafeteria workers how to make nutritious school lunches look like fast foods. Apparently many modern children refuse to eat anything else.

As a result of pressure from health-conscious consumers, many of whom are now aging "baby boomers," some restaurant chains have introduced grilled foods and other "low-fat" items. Upon examination, however, the fat content of some of these foods is unacceptably high. The majority of the regular menu items are still loaded with animal fats, long known to cause cardiovascular disease, and sodium, known to aggravate a variety of health conditions. A taco salad, for example, can contain as many as 30 g of fat.

Yet another lifestyle issue is tobacco use. Smoking continues to increase among the young, especially young females and minorities, both of whom are targeted for increased marketing by tobacco companies. For years, smoking has been known to cause lung cancer, emphysema and other chronic lung diseases, low-birth-weight babies, and a host of other health problems. The incidence of lung cancer in older women has exceeded breast cancer, long the leading killer in this age group. The use of smokeless tobacco is rising, creating unhealthy oral mucous membranes and predisposing users to oral cancer. All these trends ensure that tobacco-related illnesses and deaths will rise in the future.

Lack of exercise is another lifestyle issue for Americans of the future, particularly the young. The ready availability of entertainment on television is at least partly to blame. Studies show the more television people of all ages watch, the more likely they are to be overweight. Snacking and television watching go hand in hand. Entire generations of Americans, raised watching several hours of television each day, are unlikely to give up the habit in the future, especially because more channels are added yearly. Other spend hours in front of computer screens or in other sedentary pursuits. These habits are expected to continue in the future.

Lack of exercise is not limited to the young, however. For every middle-aged jogger seen pounding the roadways, legions of sedentary adults remain unseen at home, gradually becoming less fit and more susceptible to disease. Browsing through mail-order catalogs aimed at the affluent middle-aged population reveals a plethora of labor-saving devices being developed and marketed to make Americans even less active in the future.

Advertising affects yet another lifestyle risk factor. With the emphasis on thinness in fashion advertising, many girls and young women resort to unhealthy habits such as starving or binging and purging. Rather than eating sensibly and engaging in exercise to maintain normal weights, they assume bizarre eating habits in the pursuit of the fashionable, if unnatural, degree of gauntness. Barring a dramatic change in the fashion industry, eating disorders and their resulting health hazards will continue to increase.

Another lifestyle issue is stress. The rapid pace of modern life creates stress, yet Americans continue to step up the pace with cellular telephones, fax machines, satellite communications, personal computers, paging devices, "call-waiting" options, and all the other fruits of modern technology. Although many Americans mourn the loss of leisure time, indications are that when given more leisure time, many people spend it working. This evidence indicates that stress-related diseases will increase in the next century.

The twin epidemics of acquired immunodeficiency syndrome (AIDS) and drug abuse are two lifestyle issues that will profoundly affect the future of nursing. When the AIDS epidemic began in the United States early in the 1980s, many of those affected were homosexual men. A few years later, infection rates among intravenous drug users began to rise. By the mid-1980s, AIDS moved into the general population of heterosexual adults, a trend already seen in other countries and now appearing in the United States. Another trend causing considerable concern is the spread to adolescents. Although optimists in the medical community continue to predict a vaccine against human immunodeficiency virus (HIV), millions of Americans are already infected, and no cure is on the horizon. Substance-abusing people suffer more accidents and illness than their nonabusing counterparts, thus requiring more medical and nursing care. They are also more likely to have unprotected sex, putting them at risk for acquiring HIV. Other health risks include hepatitis, noninfectious liver disorders, and kidney failure, among others. Nurses of the future will be called on to provide intensive nursing care to increasing numbers of substance abusers and people with AIDS.

Nurses' own lifestyle choices will come under scrutiny as the issue of HIV and hepatitis infections in physicians, dentists, nurses, and other health care workers will become a focus of public concern. Nurses will be involved in the development of sound public policies concerning these issues.

Given the predominance of unhealthy lifestyle factors, it is clear that nurses will play an increasingly important role in educating people about wellness and self-care in the years ahead. Nurses will also be instrumental in educating the public about how to be informed consumers of health care services. Nurses will continue to provide nursing care in acute care settings, such as hospitals, to those who choose not to listen.

Cost Control Challenges

During most of the 1970s, 1980s, and 1990s, governmental budget deficits reached all-time highs. At federal, state, and local levels, governments spent more money than was generated through taxes, and the pressure for health care for the elderly and poor created a significant part of those budgetary problems.

Society's poor, homeless, elderly, substance abusers, AIDS patients, and mentally ill are increasing in number and will increase into the new century. The question yet to be answered is: "How can we pay for health care for these vulnerable populations now and in the future when their numbers are expected to increase?"

Federal and state governments are seeking to answer that question. In many states, Medicaid is the largest and fastest-growing single state expense. If the U.S. economy continues to be flat and corporate down-sizing continues to put people out of work, more families will become eligible for Medicaid coverage. The aging of America will continue to create huge numbers of Social Security–eligible and Medicare-eligible citizens. The decrease in the ratio of these individuals to the number of those working and paying Social Security and income taxes will place an additional burden on the federal government's budget in the foreseeable future.

The next decade will see hospitals closing in record numbers, pressures continuing to mount from the business community forcing changes in financing health care, and significant health care reform. The nursing profession stands to benefit from these phenomena, because nursing has been shown to be a cost-conscious yet high-quality alternative to traditional medical care. In addition, nurses are well equipped to provide managed care. As a profession, nursing is expected to benefit from health care woes in the United States by expanding roles in prevention and community-based nursing.

One cost-effective method of providing basic health care to children is through school nurses. As the burden of providing care continues to shift from federal agencies to state and local agencies, local school boards will recognize the economies to be realized through school nursing. Health care reform will likely provoke a dramatic rise in state-mandated health services for schoolchildren. These services will be delivered largely by school nurses.

Regulation Challenges

Even if the cost of health care can be contained, health care expenses in the United States will continue to rise. This is due to the large number of aging Americans and the growing number of impoverished ones. This will force greater governmental regulation of health care in the future. Nurses will become increasingly active in developing health policies that improve access, quality, and value in the delivery of health services. Legislation mandating the direct reimbursement of nurses for their services will be a feature of most government-funded programs, despite the opposition of organized medicine and hospitals. Private **managed care** programs will also make increasing use of the services of advanced practice registered nurses (APRNs) as providers of primary care.

Nursing, through its professional associations, will continue to be a powerful player in health care politics in the United States. Nurses will form coalitions with consumer groups to influence consumer-friendly legislation at state and national levels. Individual nurses will become more politically active as voters, campaign workers, community health activists, and political candidates. As nursing's public profile becomes higher, public scrutiny of the profession will increase. Consumers of nursing services will exercise their political power to ensure that nurses and other primary care providers consistently offer first-class health care.

CHALLENGES IN NURSING PRACTICE

The societal changes just reviewed will necessarily create changes in nursing practice. Nurses in the next decade will face an ever-widening array of practice opportunities in hospital and community-based health care settings, each of which will bring its own set of challenges.

Challenges of Cost Containment

During the 1990s, cost-containment initiatives in hospitals eliminated layers of middle-management nurses. This represented a crisis for individual nurse managers but created an opportunity for a stronger voice for nurses involved in direct patient care. Future cost-containment measures will require nurses to demonstrate the cost-effectiveness of the care they provide. The "bottom line" will be an increasing focus of concern in all health care settings, and nurses will need resource management skills more than ever before.

Increasingly, nurses will work with unlicensed assistive personnel to deliver patient care. They will need communication skills, interpersonal skills, and delegation skills to make the new partnerships work. **Multiskilled workers** will take their place alongside nurses in all settings. Nurses will be challenged to expand their skills into areas formerly the domain of specialized workers, such as respiratory therapists and physical therapists. This will be essential if nurses are to cope with the periodic variations in supply and demand for traditional nursing positions.

Challenges of Autonomy and Accountability

Shared governance, that is, participation by nurses on strong policymaking hospital committees, is a trend already seen and mandated by accreditation bodies such as the Joint Commission on the Accreditation of Healthcare Organizations (JCAHO). Along with the empowerment of nurses, however, will come increased demand for accountability. Effective nursing care will be measured by patient outcomes. Continuous quality improvement of nursing care will be emphasized more than ever. Nurses must be able to show evidence that the care they provide makes a demonstrable difference in patient outcomes.

Challenges of Technology

Technology will continue to advance at a dizzying pace in the twenty-first century. **Nursing informatics,** the organization and use of nursing data, will change nursing practice dramatically. Computerized health information networks (CHINs) will allow immediate access to all patient data needed in refining the plan of care. The increased access to patient data will reinforce the need for patient confidentiality. Voice-activated bedside computers will allow nurses to record patient information literally "at the bedside," rather than making written notes and transferring them to the patient's chart at a later time.

Advances in telecommunications will improve access to medical services for rural and elderly Americans. Nurses and physicians will examine and treat patients who are hundreds of miles away using two-way television systems. They will evaluate and prescribe treatments via telephone. Telemedicine will become routine for those who live in remote areas or are homebound.

Genetic engineering will increase as the scientists participating in the **Human Genome Project** complete the mapping and sequencing of a composite set of human genes. This will make it possible to treat and prevent genetically transmitted and genetically predisposed diseases. It will also create ethical dilemmas of gigantic proportions as the ability to clone individuals and predetermine characteristics of human infants becomes a reality.

Nurses will continue to fight the dehumanizing tendency of technological advances such as patient monitoring devices. They will continue to value and provide a holistic, "high-touch" environment for patients. Nurses will realize that advanced technology and traditional nursing values are not mutually exclusive. Patients can have both if nurses stay patient centered rather than machine or monitor centered.

Advances in technology will bring new ethical dilemmas. Nurses will be more active in exploring ethical aspects of patient care, and their unique ethical perspective will be valued by other professionals. As a result, nurses will sit on ethics committees in increasing numbers.

Increasing numbers of Americans will turn away from mainstream medical care and seek alternative medical techniques as they take responsibility for their own health. Nontraditional care such as chiropractic, homeopathy, acupuncture, massage, therapeutic touch, and herbal remedies will become a focus of interest, study, research, and publication (McKenna, 1995).

Challenges of Practice in Expanded Settings

Community-based primary health care will continue to expand as cost-effectiveness remains a high priority. Nurse-managed clinics will increasingly serve inner-city and rural underserved populations. School nurses will be needed in large numbers, as will hospice nurses and those specializing in gerontology and chronic illnesses. For nurses who are willing to work outside traditional settings and their own "comfort zones," there will be no end to the available opportunities. Flexible scheduling and job sharing will increase in all professions and will become commonplace in nursing.

Nurse entrepreneurship will flourish in the future owing to changes in restrictive legislation, the resourcefulness and self-confidence of nurses, and the trust the public places in the nursing profession. Increasing numbers of nurses will own clinics and other health-related businesses, such as independent practice associations, free-standing wellness programs, dialysis care services, and worksite health programs.

Challenges of Differentiated Practice

In the past, there has been considerable resistance to differentiating levels of nursing practice, even though visionary nursing leaders have pointed out the need to do so. **Differentiated practice** means that nurses prepared in associate degree, baccalaureate degree, and higher degree programs should have different, well-defined roles. The competencies of nurses at each level should be clearly demonstrated. If differentiated practice became a reality, educational programs could be streamlined, employers could understand the differences, and patient care delivery systems could be reorganized to capitalize on the strengths of each level. Differentiated practice could help nurses be more cost-effective by determining who is best suited to perform certain nursing actions. Differentiated practice can become a reality in the twenty-first century only if practicing nurses are willing to give up the notion that "a nurse is a nurse is a nurse" and acknowledge that different educational programs do and should prepare different types of nursing practitioners.

CHALLENGES IN NURSING EDUCATION

As the profession of nursing matures, more nurses will recognize the value of bachelor's degrees for beginning professional practice and master's degrees for advanced practice. More nurses will pursue doctoral degrees to prepare for leadership roles in research and theory development. In response, colleges of nursing will expand flexible educational programs to improve access. They will also develop differentiated levels of nursing education that correspond to differentiated levels of practice.

Challenges of Outcome-Based Education

Just as nursing practice is being challenged to measure patient outcomes, nursing education is being challenged to develop student outcomes. In the future, the quality of educational programs will be judged by student competencies, that is, what students can actually do as a result of education. Nursing educational programs will monitor their graduates' activities and achievements as professional nurses. The emphasis on accountability of nursing education programs will increase as measures of competence in graduates are refined.

Accreditation of nursing education programs will become more difficult to achieve as national accrediting bodies come under increasing pressure to raise standards and to apply standards consistently. Substandard programs will be closed in increasing numbers.

Challenges of Diversity

In the twenty-first century, students in nursing education programs will reflect the demographics of the United States and become more diverse than ever before. More minorities, men, older students, and students with degrees in other fields will come into nursing because of the emotional rewards and professional image if offers. Access to education for nontraditional and traditional students will be an even greater issue. Schools will expand nontraditional curricula that enable adults to work and go to school simultaneously. Nursing courses delivered via telecommunications and satellite linkages will increase access for students living in remote areas. Fully articulated programs will become a requirement for state-supported schools.

Changes in demographics will affect the content of curricula as well as the methods by which content is delivered. As the population ages, the need for nurses prepared in gerontology, chronic disease management, and hospice care will give emphasis to educational programs at both undergraduate and graduate levels. Educational programs will develop and expand multicultural courses. Foreign languages will again become a graduation requirement in baccalaureate programs. International educational opportunities will increase as the global village concept takes hold.

Challenges of Technology and the Knowledge Explosion

Technological advances and the growth of nursing theories will create a knowledge explosion in nursing. Computer competence will not suffice for nurses of the future. They will need to master sophisticated information systems to use the wealth of available knowledge to improve patient care. Nursing faculty will be required to practice the profession actively to keep up with rapidly changing technologies.

Nurses of the future will need to be well versed in health care costs, budgeting, and financing of health care. Business education will be increasingly emphasized, particularly at the graduate level, as nurses pursue entrepreneurial and intrapreneurial roles.

It will be impossible for nursing education programs to include in their curricula everything nurses of the future need to know. Licensing examinations will change to reflect the expansion of nursing knowledge and the increase in community-based practice. Licensure at multiple levels will become a reality. Employers of new graduates will expect to provide internships designed to enable novices to make the transition from student to practicing nurse effectively.

Challenges of Collaboration

As nurses acquire more education, the resulting self-confidence will enable them to develop collaborative relationships on an equal footing with physicians and other highly educated health care professionals. This will enable nurses to be more assertive in patient advocacy and will improve patient care and strengthen the profession.

Nursing faculty, nurse managers, and practicing nurses will join forces to strengthen educational experiences for tomorrow's nurses and to mentor them. They will collaborate on clinical research that demonstrates the effectiveness of nursing care in terms of patient outcomes. They will collaborate with other nurses and consumer groups to remove regulatory restrictions that impede advanced clinical practice.

Nurse educators will recognize the need to treat students as professionals in training and will transform nursing education attitudes away from controlling students to collaborating with them. This will create a new generation of empowered nursing professionals.

Challenges of Health Care and Educational Reform

Many people believe that higher education will be the next "industry" to undergo public scrutiny and reform. It already suffers from serious underfunding. As governmental grants are reduced or eliminated to help balance the national budget, educational programs will experience even greater budgetary constraints. By the mid-1990s, several nursing education programs, including some well-regarded ones, had closed as a result of funding shortfalls. In many universities, autonomous schools and colleges of nursing were combined with health and human service programs into one administrative unit to save money. This often weakened the nursing program's voice on the campus. Budgets for operating expenses, equipment, and faculty salaries were under par in many locations even though the demand for nursing education remained high.

For a time, it appeared that hospitals could be a source of support for nursing education programs, but with their own significant budgetary constraints, it is unlikely that this will be a long-term solution. As long as they are able, however, hospitals will support nursing education with financial aid to students, subsidies of faculty salaries, joint appointments of faculty, and other forms of assistance.

Graduate education programs will change to produce practitioners who can meet consumer demands. Changes in hospital-based nursing practice will force a re-examination of the clinical nurse specialist and nurse practitioner roles (Williams and Valdivieso, 1994). The need for efficiency and cost-effectiveness will lead to a revision of advanced practice models, and educational programs will combine the two roles and emphasize community-based practice. Curricula at all levels will be standardized and streamlined to reduce cost and confusion and improve student mobility. The trend toward use of multiskilled workers will force nursing faculty to identify that which is uniquely nursing and to educate students for broader roles in the delivery of patient care (Blayney, 1994).

In the next decade, many longtime nursing faculty, educated at the master's level during the nurse-traineeship funding heyday of the 1960s, will retire. There will be no one to replace them because younger nurses are not entering teaching owing to the fact that nursing education salaries for faculty have not kept pace with those in practice settings. There will be a serious shortage of nursing faculty in the twenty-first century that will force a major curriculum reform in nursing education programs.

S U M M A R Y

Predicting the future is an occupation fraught with peril in a society and world that are changing rapidly. This chapter has highlighted some of the societal changes that seem likely to occur in the next decade as we enter the twenty-first century: changes in demographics, the deteriorating environment, risky lifestyles, economics of health care, and governmental regulation of health care. These changes will be accompanied by changes in both nursing practice and nursing education.

Nursing roles will be differentiated. Nursing practice will become more community-based. Nurses will be able to demonstrate that the care they provide makes a positive difference in patient outcomes, and they will continue to provide a warm, humanizing influence on patient care in potentially dehumanizing high-tech environments.

The major challenges for nursing education will be to respond to societal changes rapidly with appropriate curricular modifications; to produce a steady supply of well-prepared graduates in the face of an aging faculty, rapidly changing technology, and increasing cultural diversity of students and patients; and lack of human and budgetary resources in higher education.

A message for you, the users of this book, from a nurse who has practiced for more than 40 years is found in Box 22–1. In it, she addresses the need to embrace

---

BOX 22–1
Embrace the Change

Dear Students of Nursing,

The landscape in nursing changes constantly, but never quite so rapidly as it is changing now. How do we stay abreast of the changes? Even better yet, how do we look at the changes and create our own vision of how these changes will affect us, our colleagues, and our profession in the future? I can only tell you what has worked for me during these 40 plus years that I've been in nursing.

I believe it is imperative to develop inner strength to cope with change and the uncertainty of the future. This strength allows us to develop a personal and professional vision. Since I like to use acronyms, I will use the word *SAFE* to demonstrate this point because I believe that you have to feel safe before you can have inner strength.

S—Stop denial of abuse at home and at work. Denial is probably the number one addiction in our world today. As Claudia Black says, "Surround yourself with people who support you and treat you well." Relationships that you develop with supportive people provide a valuable network for safety.

A—Authentically be yourself. We put such stress on ourselves by being who we think others want us to be. Being honestly ourselves decreases stress and draws people of like mind toward us. Those of like mind are supportive, not abusive.

F—Find yourself in the moment, *live* in the moment, breathe, *be*. We can be-

come so busy and spend so much time in the past or in the future that we have no time to be or to develop relationships or vision.

E—Elicit unconditional love. Especially love yourself. This love includes staying in balance with your checkbook, your calendar, and your health. Your inner strength depends on it. It is impossible to create vision and embrace changes if you are broke, too busy, or sick.

Being SAFE strengthens us to embrace changes and visualize how these changes impact our lives and our futures. After we are SAFE, we can consider the best way to keep our knowledge current. Reading everything from *USA Today* to professional journals has always been a great resource to me. Just remember that what you read can be months old before it appears in professional journals. More current resources include the Internet, and tomorrow there will be other resources not yet known. We have to be willing to learn how to use the resources as soon as they are available if we want to keep ahead.

These ideas are just a start. Remember that there are no outcomes without risk. I will be sending you good vibes as you and the nursing profession meet the challenges of the future.

Sincerely,
Sylvia Rayfield

the changes that are sure to affect the health care system and the profession of nursing in the twenty-first century.

REVIEW AND DISCUSSION QUESTIONS

1. As the number of elderly Americans rises, the rate of chronic illness also rises. What challenges does this present for nurses of the future?
2. Take a position on the statement, "Nurses of the future will have an impact on the environment that exceeds that of the ordinary citizen." Be prepared to defend your position.
3. Describe economic issues that nurses of the future will be concerned about that today's nurses are not.
4. Initiate a classroom debate on the issue "HIV-positive nurses should not be limited in how they practice nursing."

REFERENCES

Blayney, K. D. (1994). The future of multi-skilling. Paper presented at the national conference Multiskilling and the Allied Health Workforce, co-sponsored by the Connelly Allied Health Education Center, Methodist Hospital, Indianapolis, IN, and the Health Resources and Services Administration, Bureau of Health Professions, Washington, D.C.

Hendrick, B. (1995). The coming millenium. *The Atlanta Journal/The Atlanta Constitution*. July 16, A-12.

Herbert, L. E., Scherr, P. A., Beckett, L. A., Chown, M. J., Funkstein, H. H., and

Evans, D. A. (1995). Alzheimer's disease. *JAMA*, 273(17), 1354–1359.

McKenna, M. A. J. (1995). Going mainstream. *The Atlanta Journal/The Atlanta Constitution*. May 17, C-8.

Newsweek. (1992). Why Rio will make history. June 15, 33.

U.S. Bureau of the Census. (1990). *Current population reports* (Series P. 25, No. 1018). Washington, D.C.: Author.

Williams, C. A. and Valdivieso, M. N. (1994). Advanced practice models: A comparison of clinical nurse specialist and nurse practitioner activities. *Clinical Nurse Specialist*, 8(6), 311–318.

Epilogue

You, our readers, are inheriting a rich legacy of achievement and progress in the nursing profession. Much remains to be done. You will be challenged to lead the way in your communities and regions in addressing the issues of health care costs and access to health care for the elderly, the poor, and others who are disenfranchised. You will be part of the solution.

It is the hope of all the nurses who have participated in writing this textbook that through this book you were stimulated to develop values, beliefs, knowledge, professionalism, and desire to be a nursing leader of the future and a positive force for change in the nursing profession.

Glossary

Acceptance See "nonjudgmental acceptance."

Accountability Responsibility for one's own behavior.

Accreditation A voluntary review process of educational programs or service agencies by professional organizations.

Action language A developmental phase in language development of older infants that consists of reaching for or crawling toward a desired object, or of closing the lips and turning the head when an undesired food is offered.

Active collaborator Engaged as a participant with another.

Active listening A method of communicating interest and attention using such signals as good eye contact, nodding, and encouraging the speaker.

Acuity Degree of illness.

Acute illness Sudden, steadily progressing symptoms that subside quickly with or without treatment, such as influenza.

Adaptation A change or response to stress of any kind.

Adaptation model A conceptual framework that focuses on the patient as an adaptive system; that is, one that strives to cope with both internal demands and the external demands of the environment.

Adjudicate To decide or sit in judgment, as in a legal case.

Administrative law Law created by a governmental agency to meet the intent of statutory law.

Advance directives Written instructions recognized by state law that describe individuals' preferences in regard to medical intervention should they become incapacitated.

Advanced degrees Degrees beyond the bachelor's degree; master's and doctoral degrees.

Advanced practice Nursing roles that require either a master's degree or specialized education in a specific area.

Aesthetics The study of the nature of beauty.

Affective goal Effort directed toward a change in a patient's values or belief system.

Alternative educational programs Programs other than basic nursing programs, such as baccalaureate programs for registered nurses and the New York Regents' External Degree Program.

Altruism   Unselfish concern for the welfare of others.

Ambulatory care   Health services provided to those who visit a clinic or hospital as outpatients and depart after treatment on the same day.

ANA Position Paper   A 1965 paper published by the American Nurses Association concluding that baccalaureate education should become the basic foundation for professional practice.

Analysis   The second step in the nursing process during which various pieces of patient data are analyzed. The outcome is one or more nursing diagnoses.

Ancillary workers   Nonprofessional auxiliary health care workers, such as nursing assistants.

Anxiety   A diffuse, vague feeling of apprehension and uncertainty.

Applied science   Use of scientific theory and laws in a practical way that has immediate application.

Appropriateness   A criterion for successful communication in which the reply fits the circumstances and matches the message, and the amount is neither too great nor too little.

Articulation   An educational mobility system providing for direct movement from a program at one level of nursing education to another without significant loss of credit.

Assault   A threat or an attempt to make bodily contact with another person without the person's consent.

Assessment   The first step in the nursing process involving the collection of information about the patient.

Associate degree program   The newest form of basic nursing education program leading to the associate degree (AD), consisting of three or fewer years, and usually offered in technical or community colleges.

Authority   Possessing both the responsibility for making decisions and the accountability for the outcome of those decisions.

Autonomy   Self-governing; freedom from the influence of others.

Baccalaureate degree program.   Basic nursing education offered in four-year colleges and universities leading to the bachelor's degree in nursing (BSN).

Balance of power   A distribution of forces among the branches of government so that no one is strong enough to dominate the others.

Ball, Mary Ann (1817–1901)   A Civil War woman who cared for the wounded and was known by them as "Mother Bickerdyke."

Barton, Clara (1821–1912)   A famous Civil War nurse and founder of the American Red Cross.

Basic program   Any nursing education program preparing beginning practitioners.

Battery   The unpermissible, unprivileged touching of one person by another.

Belief   The intellectual acceptance of something as true or correct.

Beneficence   The ethical principle of doing good.

Mother Bickerdyke   Affectionate nickname given by soldiers to Mary Ann Ball, a Civil War lay nurse.

Biculturalism   A term used to describe nurses who learn to balance the ideal nursing culture they learned about in school and the real one they experience in practice, using the best of both.

Bioethics   An area of ethical inquiry focusing on the dilemmas inherent in modern health care.

Biomedical technology   Complex machines or implantable devices used in patient care settings.

Birthrate   The number of births in a particular place during a specific time period, usually given as a quantity per 1000 people in a year.

Breckinridge, Mary   Founder of the Frontier Nursing Service in 1925.

BRN   Baccalaureate registered nurse, a term sometimes used to describe a registered nurse who has returned to school to earn a bachelor's degree.

Brown Report   A 1948 report recommending that basic schools of nursing be placed in universities and colleges and that efforts be made to recruit large numbers of men and minorities into nursing education programs.

Capitation   A cost management system wherein a certain amount of money is paid to a provider annually to take care of all of an individual's or group's health care needs.

"Captain of the ship" doctrine   A legal principle that implies that the physician is in charge of all patient care and, thus, should be financially responsible if damages are sought.

Caring   Watching over, attending to, and providing for the needs of others.

Case management nursing   A growing field within nursing in which nurses are responsible for coordinating services provided to patients in a cost-effective manner.

Case manager   An individual responsible for coordinating services provided to a group of patients.

Centenarian   A person who has reached the age of 100 or more years.

Certificate of need (CON)   A cost-containment measure requiring health care agencies to apply to a state agency for permission to construct or substantially add to an existing facility.

Certified nurse-midwife   A nationally certified nurse with advanced specialized education who assists women and couples during uncomplicated pregnancies, deliveries, and postdelivery periods.

Certified Registered Nurse Anesthetist (CRNA)   A nationally certified nurse with advanced education who specializes in the administration of anesthesia.

Certification   Validation of specific qualifications demonstrated by a registered nurse in a defined area of practice.

Change agent   An individual who recognizes the need for organizational change and facilitates that process.

Chief executive officer (CEO)   The senior administrator of an organization.

Chief nurse executive   The senior nursing administrator of an organization.

Chief of staff   A physician in a health care facility, generally elected by the medical staff for a limited term, who is responsible for overseeing the activities of the medical staff organization.

Chronic illness   Ongoing health problems of a generally incurable nature, such as diabetes.

Civil law   Law involving disputes between individuals.

Clarification   A therapeutic communication technique in which the nurse seeks to understand a patient's message more clearly.

Clinical coordinator   See "Clinical director."

Clinical director   Middle management nurse who has responsibility for multiple units in a health care agency.

Clinical ladder   Programs allowing nurses to progress while staying in direct patient care roles.

Clinical nurse specialist   A nurse with an advanced degree who serves as a resource person to other nurses and often provides direct care to patients or families with particularly difficult or complex problems.

Closed system   A system that does not interact with other systems or with the surrounding environment.

Coalition   A temporary alliance of distinct factions.

Code for Nurses   A statement of the nursing profession's code of ethics.

Code of ethics   A statement of professional standards used to guide behavior and as a framework for decision making.

Cognitive   Pertaining to intellectual activities requiring knowledge.

Cognitive goal   Effort directed toward a desired change in a patient's knowledge level.

Cognitive rebellion   A stage in the educational process wherein students begin to free themselves from external controls and to rely on their own judgment.

Collaboration   Working closely with another person in the spirit of cooperation.

Collective action   Activities undertaken by or on behalf of a group of people who have common interests.

Common law   Law that comes about as a result of decisions made by judges in legal cases.

Communication   The exchange of thoughts, ideas, or information; a dynamic process that is a primary instrument through which change is effected in nursing situations.

Competency   Refers to the capability of a particular patient to understand the information given and make an informed choice.

Concept   An abstract classification of data; for example, "temperature" is a concept.

Conceptual framework   A group of concepts that are broadly defined and systematically organized to provide a focus, a rationale, and a tool for the integration and interpretation of information.

Confidentiality   Assuring the privacy of individuals participating in research studies or being treated in health care settings.

Congruent   The form of communication that occurs when the verbal and nonverbal elements of a message match.

Consultation   The process of conferring with patients, families, or other health professionals.

Consumerism   A movement to protect consumers from unsafe or inferior products and services.

Contact hour   A measurement used to recognize participation in continuing education offerings, usually equivalent to 50 minutes.

Context   An essential element of communication consisting of the setting in which an interaction occurs, the mood, the relationship between sender and receiver, and other factors.

Continuing education (CE) Informal ways, such as workshops, conferences, and short courses, in which nurses maintain clinical expertise during their professional careers.

Continuous quality improvement (CQI) A management concept focusing on excellence and employee involvement at all levels of an organization.

Co-payment The portion of a provider's charges that an insured patient is responsible for paying.

Coping The methods a person uses to assess and manage demands.

Coping mechanisms Psychological devices used by individuals when a threat is perceived.

Cost containment An attempt to keep health care costs stable or increasing only slowly.

Criminal law Law involving public concerns against unlawful behavior that threatens society.

Cross-functional team People from all parts of an organization who contribute to a particular activity and outcome.

Cross-training Preparing a single worker for multiple tasks that formerly were performed by specialized workers.

Cultural care, theory of A nursing theory focusing on the importance of incorporating a patient's culturally determined health beliefs and practices into care.

Cultural diversity Social, ethnic, racial, and religious differences in a group.

Culture The attitudes, beliefs, and behaviors of social and ethnic groups that have been perpetuated through generations.

Culture of nursing The rites, rituals, and valued behaviors of the nursing profession.

Curtis, Namahyoke The first trained African-American nurse employed as a military hospital nurse during the Spanish-American War of 1898.

Data Information or facts collected for analysis.

Deaconess Institute A large hospital and planned training program for deaconesses established in 1836 by Pastor Theodor Fliedner at Kaiserswerth, Germany.

Decentralization An organizational structure in which decision-making authority is shared with employees most affected by the decisions rather than being retained by top executives.

Deductible The amount individuals must pay out-of-pocket before their health insurance begins to pay.

Deductive reasoning A process through which conclusions are drawn by logical inference from given premises; proceeds from the general case to the specific.

Defining characteristics Signs and symptoms of disease.

Delegate To refer a task to another.

Delegation The practice of assigning tasks or responsibilities to other persons.

Demographics The study of vital statistics and social trends.

Demography The science that studies vital statistics and social trends.

Deontology The ethical theory that the rightness or wrongness of an action depends on the inherent moral significance of the action.

Dependency   The degree to which individuals adopt passive attitudes and rely on others to take care of them.

Dependent intervention   Nursing actions on behalf of patients that require knowledge and skill on the part of the nurse but may not be done without explicit directions from another health professional, usually a physician.

Developmental theory   A theory in which growth is defined as an increase in physical size and shape to a point of optimal maturity.

Diagnosis   Identification of a disease or condition.

Diagnosis-related groups (DRGs)   A method of classifying illnesses according to similarities of diagnosis.

Dietitian   Bachelor's educated nutrition expert who specializes in therapeutic diet preparation and nutrition education.

Differentiated practice   Nursing practice at two levels, professional and technical, with differences in both educational preparation and clinical responsibilities.

Diploma program   The earliest form of formal nursing education in the United States, diploma programs are usually based in hospitals, require three years of study, and lead to a diploma in nursing.

Disease   A pathological alteration at the tissue or organ level.

Disenfranchised   The state of having no power or no voice in a political system.

Disseminate   Publish or widely distribute scientific information, such as the findings of a research study.

Dissonance   Lack of harmony.

Dix, Dorothea L.   A Boston schoolteacher, devoted to the care of the mentally ill, who served as the first superintendent of the Women Nurses of the Army during the Civil War.

Dock, Lavinia   A well-known early twentieth-century nurse who was actively involved in women's rights issues and the suffragette movement.

Documentation   Written communication about patient care, usually found in the patient record.

Dominant culture   Mainstream culture that contains one or more subcultures.

Duty of care   The responsibility of a nurse or other health professional for the care of a patient.

Duty to report   The requirement, according to state law, for health professionals to report certain illnesses, injuries, and actions of patients.

Economic and general welfare   Employment issues relating to salaries, benefits, and working conditions.

Educative instrument   A tool for increasing the knowledge and power of another.

Efficiency   A criterion for successful communication that consists of using simple, clear words timed at a pace suitable to participants.

Electoral process   The procedures that must be followed to select someone to fill an elected position.

Elliott, Francis Reed   The first African-American nurse accepted by the American Red Cross Nursing Service in 1918.

Empathy   Awareness of, sensitivity to, and identification with the feelings of another person.

Entrepreneur A person who sees a need for, organizes, manages, and assumes responsibility for a new enterprise or business.

Environment All the many factors, such as physical or psychological, that influence life and survival.

Epidemiologist A scientist who studies the origins and transmission of diseases.

Epistemology The branch of philosophy dealing with the theory of knowledge.

Ethical decision making The process of choosing between actions based on a system of beliefs and values.

Ethics The branch of philosophy that studies the propriety of certain courses of action.

Euthanasia The act of putting to death painlessly a person suffering from an incurable disease; mercy killing.

Evaluation Measuring the success or failure of the outputs and consequently the effectiveness of a system. It is the final step in the nursing process wherein the nurse examines the patient's progress to determine if a problem is solved, is in the process of being solved, or is unsolved. In communication theory, the analysis of information received.

Exacerbation Re-emergence or worsening of the symptoms of a chronic illness.

Executive branch The branch of government responsible for administering the laws of the land.

Experimental design Research designs that provide evidence of a cause-and-effect relationship between actions.

Expert witness An individual called upon to testify in court because of special skill or knowledge in a certain field, such as nursing.

Extended care Medical, nursing, or custodial care provided to an individual over a prolonged period of time.

Extended family A term used to describe nonnuclear family members such as grandparents, aunts, and uncles.

External degree program An alternative program in which learning is independent and is assessed through highly standardized and validated examinations.

External factors Impact on individuals of the values, beliefs, and behaviors of the significant people around them.

False reassurance A nontherapeutic form of communication.

Famous trio Three famous schools of nursing founded in 1873; the Bellevue Training School, the Connecticut Training School, and the Boston Training School.

Feedback The information given back into a system to determine whether or not the purpose of the system has been achieved. A major element in the communication process.

Feminism The study of gender inequalities; belief in the value and equality of women.

Flexibility A criterion for successful communication that occurs when messages are based on the immediate situation rather than preconceived expectations.

Flexible staffing A mechanism whereby nurses work at times other than the traditional hospital shifts.

Flexner Report   A 1910 study of medical education that provided the impetus for much-needed reform.

Formal socialization   The process by which individuals learn a new role through what others purposely teach them.

For-profit agency   A health care agency that is established to make a profit for the owners or stockholders.

Franklin, Martha   Founder, in 1908, of the National Association of Colored Graduate Nurses (NACGN).

Frontier Nursing Service   Founded in 1925, the Frontier Nursing Service provided the first organized midwifery service in the United States.

Functional nursing   A system of nursing care delivery in which each worker has a task, or function, to perform for all patients.

Futurist   An individual who studies trends and makes predictions about the future.

Galileo   An Italian physicist and astronomer who lived from 1564 to 1642.

Gatekeeper   An individual, generally a primary care physician, who controls patients' access to diagnostic procedures, medical specialists, and hospitalization.

General election   An election in which all registered voters may vote and may choose a candidate from any party on the ballot.

General systems theory   A theory promulgated by Ludwig von Bertalanffy in the late 1930s to explain the relationship of a whole to its parts.

Generalizable   Research findings that are transferable to other situations.

Generic master's degree   An accelerated master's degree in nursing for people with nonnursing bachelor's degrees.

Generic nursing doctorate   A doctoral degree program designed for individuals who are not already registered nurses and who possess baccalaureate degrees in other fields.

Goldmark Report   A major study of nursing education published in 1923 and named *The Study of Nursing and Nursing Education in the United States.*

Goodrich, Annie   Served as Assistant Professor of nursing at Teachers College, head of the Army School of Nursing (formed in 1918), president of the American Nurses Association, and first dean of the school of nursing at Yale University.

Governmental (public) agency   An agency primarily supported by taxes, administered by elected or appointed officials, and tailored to the needs of the communities served.

Growth   An increase in physical size and shape to a point of optimal maturity.

Hardiness   A personality characteristic that describes being able to manage the changes associated with illness and to have less physical illness resulting from stress.

Health   An individual's physical, mental, and social well-being; a continuum, not a constant state.

Health behaviors   Choices and habitual actions that promote or diminish health.

Health beliefs   Culturally determined beliefs about the nature of health and illness.

Health Care Financing Administration (HCFA)   The federal agency charged with the responsibility of overseeing the Medicare and Medicaid systems.

Health care network   A corporation with a consolidated set of facilities and services for comprehensive health care.

Health maintenance   Preventing illness and maintaining maximal function.

Health maintenance organization (HMO)   A network or group of providers who agree to provide certain basic health care services for a single predetermined yearly fee.

Health promotion   Encouraging a condition of maximum physical, mental, and social well-being.

Health promotion model   A theoretical nursing model that uses illness prevention and health promotion as a basic framework.

Helping professions   Professions such as social work, teaching, and nursing that emphasize meeting the needs of clients.

Henderson, Virginia   An influential twentieth-century nursing author and theorist who was widely known for her nursing textbooks, insightful definition of nursing, and identification of 14 basic patient needs.

Henry Street Settlement   A clinic for the poor founded by Lillian Wald and her colleague, Mary Brewster, on New York's Lower East Side.

Heterogeneous   Composed of parts of different kinds.

High-level wellness   Functioning at maximum potential in an integrated way within the environment.

High-tech nursing   Nursing care that involves the use of technical instruments such as monitors, pumps, and ventilators.

High-touch nursing   Nursing care that involves the use of interpersonal skills such as communication, listening, and empathy.

Hill-Burton Act   A 1946 federal law that called for and funded surveys of states' needs for hospitals, paid for planning hospitals and public health centers, and provided partial funding for constructing and equipping them.

Hippocrates (400 B.C.)   A Greek physician who believed that disease had natural, not magical, causes. Known as the father of medicine.

Holism   A school of health care thought that espouses treating the whole patient—body, mind, and spirit.

Home health agency   An organization that delivers various health services to patients in their homes.

Home health nursing   Rapidly growing field of nursing in which nursing care is provided to patients in their own homes.

Homeostasis   A relative constancy in the internal environment of the body.

Homogeneous   Composed of parts of the same or similar kinds.

Hospice   An agency that provides services to terminally ill patients and their families.

Human caring, theory of   Nursing theory emphasizing the nurturing aspects of professional nursing through which curative strategies are implemented.

Human Genome Project   A scientific project designed to map the genetic structure of composite human DNA.

Humanistic nursing care   Care the includes viewing professional relationships as human-to-human rather than nurse-to-patient.

Hypothesis   A statement predicting the relationship among various concepts or events.

Illness   An abnormal process in which an individual's physical, emotional, social, or intellectual functioning is impaired.

Illness prevention   All activities aimed at diminishing the likelihood that an individual's physical, emotional, social, and intellectual functions become impaired.

Implementation   A stage of the nursing process during which the plan of care is carried out.

Incongruent   Confusing form of communication that occurs when the verbal and nonverbal elements of a message do not match.

Independent intervention   Actions on behalf of patients for which the nurse requires no supervision or direction by physicians.

Inductive reasoning   The process of reasoning from the specific to the general. Repeated observations of an experiment or event enable the observer to draw general conclusions.

Inertia   Disinclination to change.

Informal socialization   The process through which individuals learn a new role by observing how others behave.

Information technology   Hardware and software used to manage and process information.

Informed consent   The process of asking individuals who are to undergo diagnostic procedures or surgery or who are asked to be research subjects to sign a consent form after describing the procedures and risks involved and assuring their privacy.

Infrastructure   Basic support mechanisms needed to ensure that an activity can be conducted.

Input   The information, energy, or matter that enter a system.

Institutional review board   A committee that ensures that research is well designed and ethical and does not violate the policies and procedures of the institution in which it is conducted.

Institutional structure   The way in which the workers within an agency are organized to carry out the functions of the agency.

Interdependent intervention   Actions on behalf of patients in which the nurse must collaborate or consult with another health professional before carrying out the action.

Interdisciplinary team   Group composed of individuals representing various disciplines who work together toward a common end.

Internal factors   Personal feelings and beliefs that influence an individual.

Internalize   The process of taking in knowledge, skills, attitudes, beliefs, norms, values, and ethical standards and making them a part of one's own self-image and behavior.

Internship   An apprenticeship under supervision.

Irrational belief   A fixed idea that is not affected by information to the contrary.

Issues management   Assisting a group to resolve a particular question to which there are significant differences of opinion.

Job hopping   Moving rapidly from job to job.

Judicial branch   The branch of government that decides cases or controversies on particular matters.

Justice   An ethical principle stating that equals should be treated the same and that unequals should be treated differently.

Knowledge-based power   Authority or control based upon the way information is used to effect an outcome.

Knowledge technology   The use of computer systems to transform information into knowledge and to generate new knowledge; expert systems.

Latent power   Untapped ability.

Law   All the rules of conduct established by a government and applicable to the people, whether in the form of legislation or custom.

Learned resourcefulness   An acquired ability to use available resources in one's behalf.

Legal authority   A group of people in whom power is vested by law, such as the powers vested in state boards of nursing by nursing practice acts.

Legislative branch   The branch of government consisting of elected officials who are responsible for enacting the laws of the land.

Leininger, Madeleine   Nurse theorist best known for her theory of cultural care.

Licensure   The process by which an agency of government grants permission to qualified persons to engage in a given profession or occupation.

Licensure by endorsement   A system whereby registered nurses or licensed practical/vocational nurses can, by submitting proof of licensure in another state and paying a licensure fee, receive licensure from the new state without sitting for a licensing examination.

Lobby   An attempt to influence the vote of legislators.

Logic   The study of correct and incorrect reasoning.

Long-term care   Care provided to individuals, such as people with Alzheimer's disease, who require lengthy assistance in the maintenance of activities of daily living.

Long-term goals   Major changes that may take months or even years to accomplish.

Lysaught Report   A 1970 report entitled *An Abstract for Action* that made recommendations concerning the supply and demand for nurses, nursing roles and functions, and nursing education.

Mahoney, Mary Eliza (1845–1926)   America's first African-American "trained nurse."

Malpractice   An unintentional tort that occurs when a professional fails to act as a reasonably prudent professional would under specific circumstances.

Managed care   A process in which an individual, often a nurse, is assigned to review patients' cases and coordinate services so that quality care can be achieved at the lowest cost.

Mandatory continuing education   The requirement that nurses complete a certain number of hours of continuing education as a prerequisite for relicensure.

Maslow, Abraham   An American humanistic psychologist who formulated a theory of human motivation in the 1940s.

Maximum health potential   The highest level of well-being that an individual is capable of attaining.

Medicaid   A jointly funded federal and state public health insurance that covers citizens below the poverty level and those with certain disabling conditions; established in 1965.

Medicare   A federally funded form of public health insurance for citizens 65 years of age and above; established in 1965.

Mentor   An experienced nurse who shares knowledge with less experienced nurses to help advance their careers.

Message   An essential element of communication consisting of the spoken word, plus accompanying nonverbal communication.

Metaphysics   The consideration of the ultimate nature of existence, reality, and experience.

Milieu   Surroundings or environment.

Model   A symbolic representation of reality.

Modeling   An informal type of socialization that occurs when an individual chooses an admired person to emulate.

Montag, Dr. Mildred   Originator, in 1952, of the concept of associate degree nursing education.

Moonlighting   The practice of working a second job after the regular one.

Moral development   The ways in which a person learns to deal with moral dilemmas from childhood through adulthood.

Morals   Established rules or standards that guide behavior in situations in which a decision about right and wrong must be made.

Morbidity rate   The incidence or occurrence of a certain illness in a particular population during a specific period of time, usually given as a quantity of 1000 people in a specific year.

Mortality rate   The number of deaths in a particular population during a specific period of time, usually given as a quantity of 1000 people in a specific year.

Multiskilled worker   Individual who has been cross-trained to perform a number of tasks formerly performed by a series of specialized workers.

Mutuality   Sharing jointly with others.

National Practitioner Data Bank   A national clearinghouse containing adverse information about physicians, nurses, and other health care providers that may be useful to potential employers or patients.

NCLEX-PN   National Council Licensing Examination for Practical Nurses, the examination graduates of practical nursing programs must take to become licensed to practice as licensed practical nurses (LPNs) or licensed vocational nurses (LVNs).

NCLEX-RN   National Council Licensing Examination for Registered Nurses, the examination graduates of basic nursing programs must take to become licensed to practice as registered nurses (RNs).

Negligence   The failure to act as a reasonably prudent person would have in specific circumstances.

Neuman, Betty   Nursing theorist who developed a systems model of nursing.

Newton, Isaac   English philosopher and mathematician who lived from 1642 to 1727.

Nightingale, Florence   Nineteenth-century English woman known as the founder of modern nursing and nursing education.

Nonexperimental design   Research design in which the research subjects are not influenced in any way.

Nonjudgmental   An attitude that conveys neither approval nor disapproval of patients' beliefs and respects each person's right to his or her beliefs.

Nonjudgmental acceptance   An attitude that conveys neither approval nor disapproval of patients, their personal beliefs, habits, expressions of feelings, or chosen lifestyles.

Nonmaleficence   To inflict no harm or evil.

Nonverbal communication   Communication without words; consists of grooming, clothing, gestures, posture, facial expressions, tone and loudness of voice, and actions, among other things.

North American Nursing Diagnosis Association (NANDA)   Group working since 1970 to establish a comprehensive list of nursing diagnoses.

Not-for-profit agency   An organization that does not attempt to make a profit for distribution to owners or stockholders. Money made by such organizations is used to operate and improve the organization itself.

Nuclear family   Term used to describe a mother, father, and their children.

Nurse activist   A nurse who works actively on behalf of a political candidate or certain legislation.

Nurse anesthetist   A nurse with specialized advanced education who administers anesthetic agents to patients undergoing operative procedures.

Nurse citizen   A nurse who exercises all the political rights accorded citizens, such as registering to vote and voting in all elections.

Nurse executive   The top nurse in the administrative structure of a health care organization.

Nurse manager   Also known as a head nurse, a nurse manager is in charge of all activities in a unit, including patient care, continuous quality improvement, personnel selection and evaluation, and resource (supplies and money) management.

Nurse-midwife   A nurse with advanced specialized education who assists women and couples during uncomplicated pregnancies, deliveries, and postdelivery periods.

Nurse-patient relationship   The mode of connection between a nurse and patient.

Nurse politician   A nurse who runs for political office.

Nurse practitioner   A nurse with advanced education who specializes in primary health care of a particular group, such as children, pregnant women, or the elderly.

Nursing   The provision of health care services, focusing on the maintenance, promotion, and restoration of health.

Nursing diagnosis   A process of describing a patient's response to health problems that either already exist or may occur in the future.

Nursing informatics   The branch of nursing that manages knowledge and data through technology with the goal of improving patient care.

Nursing information system   A software system that automates the nursing process.

Nursing orders   Actions designed to assist the patient in achieving a stated patient goal.

Nursing practice act   Law defining the scope of nursing practice in a given state.

Nursing process   A cognitive activity that requires both critical and creative thinking and serves as the basis for providing nursing care. A method used by nurses in dealing with patient problems in professional practice.

Nursing research The systematic investigation of events or circumstances related to improving nursing care.

Nutting, Adelaide An early twentieth-century nurse activist, first professor of nursing in the world, and a cofounder of the *American Journal of Nursing*.

Objective data Factual information obtained through observation and examination of the patient or through consultation with other health care providers.

Occupation A person's principal work or business.

Occupational health nurse A nurse specializing in the care of a specific group of workers in a given occupational setting.

Open-ended question An inquiry that causes the patient to answer fully, giving more than a "yes" or "no" answer.

Open posture Bodily position, squarely facing another person, with arms in a relaxed position.

Open system A system that promotes the exchange of matter, energy, and information with other systems and the environment.

Orem, Dorothea Nursing theorist known for her model focusing on patients' self-care needs and nursing actions designed to meet patients' needs.

Outcome criteria Patient goals.

Out-of-pocket payment Direct payment for health services from individuals' personal funds.

Output The end result or product of a system.

Paramedical Having to do with the field of medicine; generally used to describe ancillary workers such as emergency medical technicians.

Patient acuity Assessment of the degree of illness of a particular patient or group of patients, used to determine staffing needs.

Patient advocate One who promotes the interest of patients.

Patient classification system (PCS) Identification of patients' needs for nursing care in quantitative terms.

Patient-focused care A system that emphasizes coordinating patient care to maximize patient comfort, convenience, and security.

Patient interview A face-to-face interaction with the patient in which an interviewer elicits pertinent information.

Patient Self-Determination Act Effective December 1, 1991, this law encourages patients to consider which life-prolonging treatment options they desire and to document their preferences in case they should later become incapable of participating in the decision-making process.

Patients' rights Responsibilities that a hospital and its staff have toward patients and their families during hospitalization.

Pay equity Equal pay for work of comparable value.

Peer review process The process of submitting one's work for examination and comment by colleagues in the same profession.

Pender, Nola A nurse theorist best known for her health promotion model of professional nursing.

Perception The selection, organization, and interpretation of incoming signals into meaningful messages.

Person An individual—man, woman, or child.

Personal payment Direct payment for health services from individuals' personal funds.

Personal value system   The social principles, ideals, or standards held by an individual that form the basis for meaning, direction, and decision making in life.

Petry, Lucille   The first woman appointed to the position of Assistant Surgeon General of the United States Public Health Service in 1949.

Phenomenon   An occurrence or circumstance that is observable.

Philosophy   The study of the truths and principles of being, knowledge, or conduct.

Planning   The third step in the nursing process that begins with the identification of patient goals.

Point of care technology   Information system used for entering patient data directly from the bedside.

Point of service (POS)   A hybrid preferred provider organization in which the consumer selects a primary care physician gatekeeper.

Policy   The principles and values that govern actions directed toward given ends. Policy sets forth a plan, direction, or goal for action.

Policy development   The generation of principles and procedures that guide governmental or organizational action.

Policy outcome   The result of decisions made by governmental or organizational leaders who choose a certain course of action.

Political action committees (PACs)   Groups that raise and distribute money to candidates who support their organization's stand on certain issues.

Politics   The area of philosophy that deals with the regulation and control of people living in society; in government, the allocation of scarce resources.

Population   The entire group of people possessing a given characteristic, such as all brown-eyed people over the age of 65.

Position power   Authority and control accorded to an individual who holds an important role in an organization, profession, or government.

Power grabbing   Hoarding control, taking it from others, or wielding it over others.

Power sharing   A process of equalizing resources, knowledge, or control.

Powers of appointment   The authority to select the people who serve in positions such as judges, ambassadors, and cabinet officials.

Practical nurse program   A one-year educational program preparing individuals for direct patient care roles under the supervision of a physician or registered nurse.

Preceptor   A teacher; in nursing, usually an experienced nurse who assumes responsibility for teaching a novice.

Preferred provider organization (PPO)   A group of physicians or institutions to which insurance companies direct their policyholders for care.

Premium   The amount paid for an insurance policy, usually in installments.

Primary care   Basic health care including promotion of health, early diagnosis of disease, and prevention of disease.

Primary election   An election in which voters who are declared members of a political party choose among several candidates of that same party for a particular office.

Primary nursing   A system of nursing care delivery in which one nurse has responsibility for the planning, implementation, and evaluation of the care of one or more clients 24 hours a day for the duration of the hospital stay.

Primary source   The patient is considered a primary source of data about himself or herself.

Private insurance   Insurance obtained from a privately owned company, as opposed to public or governmental insurance.

Private practice   Nursing practice, engaged in by nurses with advanced education, that takes place outside of a health care delivery setting and is usually provided on a fee-for-service basis, similar to medical practice.

Privileged communications   The principle that information given to certain professionals is so confidential in nature as not even to be disclosed in court.

Problem solving   A method of finding solutions to difficulties specific to a given situation and designed for immediate action.

Profession   Work requiring advanced training and usually involving mental rather than manual effort.

Professional   A person who engages in one of the professions, such as law or medicine.

Professional accountabilities   A basic set of responsibilities of all professional nurses regardless of practice setting.

Professional association   An organization consisting of people belonging to the same profession and thereby having many common interests.

Professional boundary   The dividing line between the activities of two professions.

Professional governance   The concept that health care professionals have a right and a responsibility to govern their own work and time within a financially secure, patient-centered system.

Professionalism   Professional behavior, appearance, and conduct.

Professional review organization (PRO)   Organizations that review Medicare hospital admissions and Medicare patients' lengths of stay.

Professional socialization   The process of developing an occupational identity.

Proposition   A statement about how two or more concepts are related.

Prospective payment system (PPS)   A cost-containment mechanism wherein providers, such as physicians and hospitals, receive payment on a per case basis, regardless of the cost of delivering the services.

Protocol   A written plan specifying the procedure to be followed.

Provider   An deliverer of health care services, hospital, clinic, nurse, or physician.

Proximate cause   Action occurring immediately before an injury occurred, thereby assumed to be the reason for the injury.

Psychomotor goal   Effort directed toward a change in motor skills or actions by a patient.

Pure science   Summarizes and explains the universe without regard for whether the information is immediately useful; also known as "basic science."

Qualitative research   Answers questions that cannot be answered by quantitative designs and that must be addressed by more subjective methods.

Quality management   See "total quality management."

Quantitative research   Research that is objective and uses data gathering techniques that can be repeated by others and verified. Data collected are quantifiable; that is, they can be counted, measured with standardized instruments, or observed with a high degree of agreement among observers.

Receiver   An essential element of communication consisting of the person receiving the message.

Re-engineering Radical redesign of business processes and thinking to improve performance.

Referendum An election resulting from the registered voters being asked to express a preference on a policy issue by a legislative body.

Reflection A communication technique that consists of encouraging patients to think through problems for themselves by directing patient questions back to the patient.

Registered nurse (RN) An individual who has completed a basic program for registered nurses and successfully completed the licensing examination.

Rehabilitation services Those activities designed to restore an individual or a body part to normal or near-normal function following a disease or an accident.

Reliable Yielding the same values dependably each time an instrument is used to measure the same thing.

Reality shock The feelings of powerlessness and ineffectiveness often experienced by new nursing graduates.

Remission A period of chronic illness during which symptoms subside.

Replication Repeating a research study as closely as possible.

Research process Prescribed steps that must be taken to plan and conduct meaningful research properly.

Research question A statement, question, or hypothesis that a research study is designed to answer.

Resocialization A transitional process of giving up part or all of one set of professional values and learning new ones.

Respondeat superior Legal theory that attributes the acts of employees to their employer.

Retrospective reimbursement Insurance payment made after services are delivered.

Richards, Linda In 1873, she became the first "trained nurse" in the United States.

Risk management A program that seeks to identify and eliminate potential safety hazards, thereby reducing patient injuries.

RN-to-BSN education Programs for registered nurses who hold associate degrees or diplomas in nursing enabling them to acquire baccalaureate degrees in nursing.

Robb, Isabel Hampton An outstanding turn-of-the-century American nurse who was instrumental in forming the forerunners of the National League for Nursing and the American Nurses Association as well as co-founding the *American Journal of Nursing*.

Role A goal-directed pattern of behavior learned within a cultural setting.

Role model An individual who serves as a model of desirable behavior for another.

Role strain Stress created by difficulty experienced in adjusting to a life or occupational role.

Rogers, Martha Nursing theorist who developed a model known as the "science of unitary human beings."

Roy, Sister Callista Nursing theorist who developed an adaptation model based on general systems theory.

Salary compression A phenomenon in which pay increases are limited during an individual's career, so that the salary of a veteran nurse may be little higher than a recently hired nurse's salary as a novice.

Sample   A subset of an entire population that reflects the characteristics of the population.

Sanger, Margaret   Founder of the first birth control clinic in the United States in 1916 and an ardent proponent of women's rights to use contraception.

Scales, Jessie Sleet   Became the first African-American public health nurse in 1900.

School nurse   Nurse specializing in the care of school-age children or adolescents and who practices in school settings.

Scientific discipline   A branch of instruction or field of learning based on the study of a body of facts about the physical or material world.

Scientific method   A systematic, orderly approach to the gathering of data and the solving of problems.

Secondary care   An intermediate level of health care performed in a hospital having specialized equipment and laboratory facilities.

Secondary source   Sources of data such as the nurse's own observations or perceptions of family and friends of the patient.

Self-actualization   A process of realizing one's maximum potential and using one's capabilities to the fullest extent possible.

Self-awareness   Understanding of one's own needs, biases, and impact on others.

Self-insurance   An individual or business who pays for care directly rather than purchasing insurance.

Self-care model   Nursing theoretical model based on the concept of ability to care for self.

Self-directed work team   A method of decentralizing decision making using cross-functional groups united around common goals.

Self-efficacy   A belief in self as possessing the ability to perform an activity, such as administering daily insulin.

Sender   An essential element of communication consisting of the person sending a message.

Separation of powers   Under the Constitution, each branch of the federal government has separate and distinct functions and powers.

Set   A group of circumstances or situations joined and treated as a whole.

Sex-role stereotyping   The practice of automatically and routinely linking positive or negative characteristics to either males or females.

Shared goverance   See "professional goverance."

Short-term goals   Specific, small steps leading to the achievement of broader, long-term goals.

Sign   Outward evidence of illness visible to others, such as a rash.

Skill mix   The ratio of registered nurses to licensed practical nurses and nursing assistants in each hospital unit.

Socialization   The process whereby values and expectations are transmitted from generation to generation.

Social services   Services designed to assist individuals and families in obtaining basic needs, such as housing, food, and medical care.

Somatic language   Language used by infants to signal their needs to caretakers, such as crying; reddening of the skin; fast, shallow breathing; facial expressions; and jerking of the limbs.

Spellman Seminary   Site of the first nursing program for African-Americans, founded in Atlanta, Georgia, in 1886.

Staff nurse   The bedside nurse who cares for a group of patients but has no management responsibilities for the nursing unit.

Stage theory   A theory that views human development as a series of identifiable stages through which individuals and families pass.

Standard of care   What the reasonably prudent nurse, under similar circumstances, would have done.

Standard of nursing practice   Those nursing actions that are generally agreed upon, by nurses, as constituting safe, effective patient care.

Statutory law   Law established through formal legislative processes.

Stereotypes   Prejudiced attitudes developed through interactions with family, friends, and others in an individual's social and cultural system.

Stress   Any emotional, physical, social, economic, or other factor that requires a response or change.

Stressors   Stimuli that tend to disturb equilibrium.

Subacute care   A level of care between hospital-based acute care and long-term residential care.

Subjective data   Information obtained from patients as they describe their needs, feelings, and strengths, and their perceptions of the problem.

Subjects   The individuals who are studied in a research project.

Subsystems   The parts that make up a system.

Supervision   The initial direction and periodic inspection of the actual accomplishment of a task.

Suprasystem   The larger environment outside a system.

Symptom   An indication of illness felt by the individual but not observable to others, such as pain.

System   A set of interrelated parts that come together to form a whole.

Systems theory   See "general systems theory."

Taylor, Susie (1848–1912)   A young, African-American Civil War nurse who knew and was influenced by Clara Barton.

Team nursing   A system of nursing care delivery in which a group of nurses and ancillary workers are responsible for the care of a group of patients during a specified time period, usually 8 to 12 hours.

Tertiary care   Specialized, highly technical level of health care provided in sophisticated research and teaching hospitals.

Tertiary source   Sources of data including the medical records and health care providers, such as physical therapists, physicians, or dietitians.

Theory   A general explanation scholars use to explain, predict, control, and understand commonly occurring events.

Theory of human motivation   Abraham Maslow's theory of human needs and their relationship to the stimulation of purposeful behavior.

Therapist   Any of several health care workers with differing educational backgrounds who work with patients with specific deficits; examples include physical therapists and occupational therapists.

Third-party payment   Payment for health services by an entity other than the patient or the provider of services.

Tort   A civil wrong against a person; may be intentional or unintentional.

Total quality management (TQM)   Management philosophy and activities directed toward achieving excellence and employee participation in all aspects of that goal.

Transcultural nursing Nursing care that is based on the patient's culturally determined health values, beliefs, and practices.

Transmission The expression of information verbally or nonverbally.

Truth, Sojourner (1797–1881) A famous African-American nurse and former slave who was an abolitionist and underground railroad agent during the Civil War.

Tubman, Harriet Ross (1820–1913) An African-American Civil War nurse who helped more than 300 slaves to freedom on the underground railroad.

Unitary human beings, science of A nursing theory developed by Martha Rogers.

Universal care Provision of health care to all people.

Unlicensed assistive personnel Individuals who are not extensively educated or licensed but provide direct patient care under the supervision of licensed personnel.

Urbanization The process of population migration to cities.

Utilitarianism An ethical theory asserting that it is right to maximize the greatest good for the happiness or pleasure of the greatest number of people.

Valid Measuring what it is intended to measure, as in a valid test question or research instrument.

Values The social principles, ideals, or standards held by an individual, class, or group that give meaning and direction to life.

Ventilation The verbal "letting off steam" that occurs when people talk about concerns or frustrations.

Veracity Telling the truth.

Verbal communication All language whether written or spoken; represents only a small part of communication.

Voluntary (private) agency An agency supported entirely through voluntary contributions of time and/or money.

Wald, Lillian Founder of the Henry Street Settlement and public health nursing in the United States. She later formed the National Organization of Public Health Nurses (1912), marking the beginning of specialization in nursing.

Watson, Jean Nursing theorist who emphasizes human caring as a focus of nursing.

Whole system shared governance Involving people at all levels of an organization in decision making within the organization.

Worker's compensation A federally mandated insurance system covering workers injured on the job.

Work ethic A belief in the importance of work; an appreciation for the characteristics employers desire in employees and a commitment to providing it.

Yale School of Nursing The first school of nursing in the world to be established as a separate university department with an independent budget and its own dean, Annie W. Goodrich.

Index